From Algorithms to Ailments

Madhu Chetty • Jennifer Hallinan
Editors

From Algorithms to Ailments

AI in Innovative and Translational Healthcare

Springer

Editors
Madhu Chetty
Federation University Australia
Churchill, VIC, Australia

Jennifer Hallinan
BioThink Pty Ltd
Redcliffe, QLD, Australia

ISBN 978-3-032-11022-0 ISBN 978-3-032-11023-7 (eBook)
https://doi.org/10.1007/978-3-032-11023-7

This Springer imprint is published by the registered company Springer Nature Switzerland AG
The registered company address is: Gewerbestrasse 11, 6330 Cham, Switzerland

Preface

Artificial Intelligence (AI) is revolutionizing the world of health and healthcare, offering groundbreaking possibilities to redefine the way in which we predict, prevent, diagnose, and treat illnesses. The aim of this book is to bridge the gap between two rapidly evolving domains—technology and health—by exploring the diverse ways in which AI is transforming healthcare practices and systems. From early disease prediction to personalized therapies, AI holds the promise of enhancing patient outcomes and addressing challenges that were previously insurmountable. This book aspires to provide readers with an insightful overview of the innovations, applications, and implications of AI in healthcare.

The eight chapters in this book traverse a wide range of topics, with the opening chapter tracing the historical evolution of AI in healthcare and shedding light on milestones that have paved the way for its current capabilities. Following the foundational concepts of AI in Chap. 1 and molecular biology in Chap. 2, subsequent chapters dive into specific areas such as AI application in genetics, cancer, eye care, mental health, and more. Through case studies, real-world examples, and in-depth analysis, we highlight the way in which AI-driven methods are being implemented in research, clinical settings, and public health initiatives.

We live in an era of increasing application of artificial intelligence to medicine. Beginning with *Chapter 1: From Data Science to Artificial Intelligence*, we introduce the foundational principles of AI and data science that underpin the innovations presented in this book. While recent advances have focused on deep learning, these and other bio-inspired methods of computational intelligence have their own long history. The interplay and evolution of hardware and software has led to an explosion of new directions and tools, some of which are described in other chapters in this book. This chapter reviews the history of computational intelligence and provides a survey of methods and approaches that introduce the reader to concepts and briefly touches on future directions. Thus, this chapter, aimed mainly at biologists, focuses on introducing the background and essentials of data science and artificial intelligence.

While there is a tendency for bioinformatics and biomedical researchers to focus their attention mainly on AI algorithms and their application to health, it is equally important to have a clear understanding of the biological basis of the problems that are being dealt with. Hence, the narrative then transitions to the fascinating world of molecular biology in *Chapter 2: From Genomes to Proteins: Molecular Biology Lite*, offering a concise yet rich introduction to the biological processes that AI is beginning to decode. This chapter covers the basics of molecular biology from genomes to proteins, including those areas in which AI has been applied, and those which were investigated before the development of AI algorithms. While a lot of basics of molecular biology were developed before the advent of computers, AI has been applied to the data thus generated with valuable results. This chapter, aimed mainly at computer scientists, provides a concise introduction to biology, available bioinformatics tools, and some useful bioinformatics datasets.

The advent of advanced natural language processing (NLP) finds its place in *Chapter 3: Natural Language Understanding, Large Language Models, and their Applications to Genetic Diseases and Healthcare*. This chapter sheds light on how NLP is revolutionizing healthcare and genetic research by enabling machines to comprehend and analyze English text generated from diverse sources. Recent advancements in large language models (LLMs), such as BioGPT and BioBERT, have significantly enhanced the ability to extract, interpret, and synthesize information from vast biomedical datasets. These models excel at tasks such as named entity recognition, information retrieval, relationship extraction, and summarization, making them invaluable to applications in healthcare and genetic diseases. The chapter elaborates on the basic principles of NLP and its relevance in processing and analyzing unstructured text in healthcare and genetics, the application of NLP in biology and healthcare, and state-of-the-art NLP techniques in the context of genetic and clinical research.

In *Chapter 4: Modeling Genetic Networks*, we delve into the complex interplay of genes and the potential of AI to model and understand these relationships, via accurate reconstruction of gene regulatory networks (GRNs). Mathematical modeling in computational systems biology has become essential for comprehending intricate biological processes; specifically, the regulatory mechanisms that govern these biological systems. Among the various computational paradigms, GRN inference plays a vital role in unraveling gene-gene interactions and elucidating the regulatory architecture of living organisms and provides valuable insights into the key biological interactions among various genes, including those involved in disease progression. In this chapter, we review some of the key computational methodologies employed in GRN inference and describe how these different methods can be combined to address the challenges faced in GRN inference. The GRAMP approach, proposed by the authors is shown to pave the way for advances in predictive models of cellular behavior, facilitating personalized medicine, and drug discovery.

There is considerable interest in the development of novel proteins for two main reasons. First, and perhaps most importantly, is that the ability to design new proteins on-order allows the production of enzymes which are more efficient than existing proteins; those which perform entirely novel functions, unknown in nature, or any other application. The second reason is that novel proteins, even those which perform the same functions as existing proteins, can be patented by industrial companies, potentially generating considerable revenue. *Chapter 5: Genomics and Synthetic Biology* takes a step further, showcasing AI's ability to drive innovation in genome editing and the engineering of biological systems. While Chap. 2 looked at the mechanism of protein production, with the unspoken assumption that we are dealing with naturally evolved proteins, this chapter emphasizes the role of AI methods in the design and synthesis of novel proteins. In this chapter, we review some major aspects of the use of AI in the design of novel proteins.

Cancer poses a significant threat to human life. Early detection and treatment is very important for enhancing survival rates. *Chapter 6: AI-Driven Innovations in Cancer Care and Research* focuses on the way in which machine learning is transforming oncology, from early detection and personalized treatment plans to cutting-edge cancer research. The research typically requires multi-omic data consisting of genomics, epigenomics, transcriptomics, proteomics, and more. These omics technologies give a deeper understanding about cancer cells at different molecular layers, but each type generates a complex high-dimensional data, making manual analysis impractical. This chapter deals with the utilization of multi-omics big data and Artificial Intelligence (AI), machine learning which has fueled the progress of cancer research.

In the last two decades, ophthalmology has seen rapid technological developments, in particular in medical imaging and the use of AI for image interpretation. *Chapter 7: Artificial Intelligence for the Eye* highlights AI's pivotal role in diagnosing and managing ophthalmic conditions, showcasing the blend of precision and care that defines modern medicine. The chapter discusses some of the innovations in imaging, for example, optical coherence tomography, and computer vision techniques such as convolutional neural networks, that have led to revolutionary advances in the detection of two vision-threatening conditions: diabetic retinopathy and glaucoma. Throughout medical history the eye has been seen and used as a "window" into the body's internal state. Hippocrates, the father of Western medicine, identified a variety of eye characteristics associated with systemic conditions like hepatitis, which causes yellowing of the sclera. In modern medicine, the eye continues to play a role in the management of systemic, cardiovascular, and neurological conditions. We therefore also include recent advances in the analysis of retinal vasculature and optic nerve tissues, and the insights these approaches provide.

The journey continues with *Chapter 8: AI and Mental Health Research*: a deep dive into the way in which AI is being used to understand and address the growing challenges of mental health, especially Alzheimer's disease Artificial intelligence (AI) has a significant role in the development of computer-assisted mental health research. The chapter starts by elaborating why early diagnosis is crucial in reducing the societal and economic burden of Alzheimer's disease. The chapter provides an overview of the clinical features of Alzheimer's related language impairments based upon theories such as the Wernicke-Geschwind model and connectionist views. We also outline the publicly available datasets like the Pitt and ADReSS corpora, used as benchmarks for the development of AI models. This coverage is followed by a discussion on building an Alzheimer's dementia recognition pipeline and various types of features used, such as acoustic, textual, and disfluency-based elements.

Finally, the Epilogue reflects on the transformative potential of AI and considers the ethical, social, and future-oriented questions that this technological revolution brings. We address some of the promise of these approaches to the understanding and maintenance of human health and indicate the issues which should be addressed. AI has the potential to make a significant positive impact upon healthcare but, as with any technological advance, its limitations must be understood and taken into account. We therefore discuss the most important of the limitations of this technology, as it currently stands.

This book is intended for a diverse audience—healthcare professionals, researchers, technologists, and curious readers—who are eager to understand the intersection of AI and health. This book is a journey through the diverse and transformative applications of AI in health and healthcare, framed by the exploration of its impact across genetics, disease prediction, and clinical care. As we navigate the opportunities and challenges that AI brings to healthcare, our hope is to inspire thoughtful dialogue and foster a shared vision for a future where technology and human expertise work in harmony to improve human lives. We invite you to join us on this journey as we explore the transformative potential of AI in shaping a healthier tomorrow.

Churchill, VIC, Australia — Madhu Chetty
Redcliffe, QLD, Australia — Jennifer Hallinan

Contents

Chapter 1
From Data Science to Artificial Intelligence

Gary B. Fogel

Abstract We live in a new era of increasing application of artificial intelligence in medicine. While recent advances have focused on deep learning, these and other bio-inspired methods of computational intelligence have their own long history. The interplay and evolution of hardware and software methods has led to an explosion of new directions and tools, some of which will be described in other chapters in this book. This chapter reviews the history of computational intelligence and provides a survey of methods and approaches that introduces the reader to concepts and briefly touches on future directions.

Introduction

In the midst of this dynamic time for informatics and healthcare, it's hard to remember how challenging bioinformatics and its application to medicine was at the time of the initial working draft of the human genome a short 25 years ago. Society tends to view Moore's Law[1] from the present looking to the future in an ever-increasing race for faster processing speeds, but occasionally there is value in remembering where we've been. Roughly 25 years ago, in 2001, a state-of-the-art Apple Powerbook G4 offered a 400 MHz processor with 128 MB of RAM. Just 3 years later a 2004 Sony Vaio Pentium 4 offered a 2.6 GHz processor with 512 MB of RAM. While amazing in their day, these devices pale in comparison to modern gaming desktop computers with their 64 GB of RAM and Nvidia GeForce graphics cards. Today we even find chips designed specifically for AI applications, such as

[1] Moore's Law, named after Gordon Moore, co-founder of Intel and Fairchild Semiconductor, was formulated in 1965, and states that the number of transistors in a microchip doubles roughly every 2 years.

G. B. Fogel (✉)
Natural Selection, Inc., San Diego, CA, USA
e-mail: gfogel@natural-selection.com

M. Chetty, J. Hallinan (eds.), *From Algorithms to Ailments*,
https://doi.org/10.1007/978-3-032-11023-7_1

the wafer-scale engine (WSE-3) offered by Cerebras with its whopping 900,000 independently programmable cores suited to function as a single processor and specifically designed for deep learning. In the hope that Moore's Law continues unabated, it is somehow inconceivable to think that 25 years from now these same chips could feel like the Apple Powerbooks of 2001. But despite the hardware restrictions in 2001, plenty of excellent work in bioinformatics was ongoing, including the Human Genome Project. As this book focuses on the use of artificial intelligence (AI) for healthcare, it is useful to be reminded of the software development that existed in parallel to these hardware achievements and led to the progress in AI that we observe today.

Background

The software approaches considered central to the current wave of AI trace their ancestry to well before the 2000s and in many cases even to the time of Bardeen, Brattain, and Shockley's invention of the modern transistor in 1947. It is interesting to realize that for nearly as long as we've had sufficiently large computers at our disposal, researchers have been interested in mimicking biological systems for learning or engineering purposes. Biomimicry itself is central to engineering, and it is especially pleasing and circular to apply those bio-inspired methods of computing to help understand the very biological systems that were considered their inspiration.

Artificial neural networks (ANNs) were first developed by Frank Rosenblatt in 1958 at Cornell. His "perceptron" networks were implemented on an IBM 704 at Cornell Aeronautical Laboratory [1]. These efforts in biomimicry were the first demonstrations of a computer learning new skills through a model of how a brain works, led by the seminal effort of Warren McCulloch and Walter Pitts to describe the electrical circuits of brains in 1943 and the realization that networks of such neurons could be used to represent any finite logical expression [2]. Donald Hebb's approaches to update the weights associated with McCulloch-Pitts networks published in 1949 showed how such networks could learn given new information [3]. While Rosenblatt's invention applied these concepts successfully within a computer for the first time, it wasn't until the 1960s when a larger computing community began to offer additional significant advances such as Bernard Widow and Marcian (Ted) Hoff's efforts to automatically adjust neural network weights given the error of the output from the model. These approaches set forth methods to optimize neural network models in the light of training data [4, 5]. A complete listing of the history of neural networks is well beyond the scope of this chapter, but must include Paul Werbos' contribution to develop backpropagation as a method of neural network optimization in 1974, as this finally represented a method to update the weights associated with a neural network with training data [6]. John Hopfield's effort to consider the optimization of neural networks as equivalent to the minimization of an energy function was also seminal [7]. Again, entire books have been written on this history, but it is important to note that these efforts were now more than 40 years ago. And while neural networks suffered through the first AI winter of 1974–1980[2] and a second AI winter of 1987–2000, their importance to bioinformatics and healthcare grew in the 1990s and 2000s leading to significant recent advances. A survey of these recent uses is supplied later in this chapter.

Other bioinspired approaches were also developed earlier than many realize. For instance, in 1953, Nils Barricelli at Vanderbilt University investigated simulated evolution using an environment of numbers in a grid competing for survival [8] In the mid to late 1950s, independent efforts were made by George Friedman at UC Los Angeles, Alex Fraser in Australia, George Box in England, and Richard Friedberg at IBM to either understand natural evolutionary or genetic processes using simulation or for engineering, for improved production or to evolve computer programs themselves [9–13]. These approaches ran contrary to the prevailing computational approaches of the day that used "expert systems" for reasoning. With expert systems, human experts were polled on how they would respond to a problem, this approach was then coded in a computer program, and when the computer faced the same problem, the computer would answer in a manner similar to that of a human expert. This approach is not what we would consider today to be intelligence coming directly from a computer on its own accord. But in the 1950s and 1960s it was believed that methods of random variation and selection inherent to evolution would be incapable of finding useful solutions in a computer in any real time. Despite these issues, in the 1960s researchers continued to explore the use of evolutionary computation for improved understanding of biological systems or engineering. Such efforts included work by Hans Bremmerman at UC Berkeley in 1962 to examine neural systems as models of an environment that could be learned over time [14]. While at the National Science Foundation in 1960, Lawrence Fogel wondered if simulated evolution would be able to generate artificial intelligence on their own, for engineering applications, this in direct contrast to expert systems. This approach was shown to be successful soon thereafter at General Dynamics (Convair) in San Diego by the team of Fogel, Alvin Owens, and Michael Walsh, leading to a method termed "evolutionary programming" [15, 16]. Independently in Germany, engineers Ingo Rechenberg and Hans-Paul Schwefel reasoned that it would be possible to optimize airfoil shapes in wind tunnels to minimize drag. This was first done by hand but then later through their method of "evolution strategies" and applied not only to airfoil optimization but other problems as well [17, 18]. John Holland at the University of Michigan also focused on the modeling of adaptive systems in 1967 through 1975 with an approach that emphasized genetic optimization called "genetic algorithms" [19]. All three of these approaches were deployed across many problem domains in the 1960s–2000s, despite the relatively lower performance of computers. Similarly to neural networks, these approaches have been used by bioinformaticians to improve a wide range of healthcare efforts over time.

[2] The history of AI is a pendulum, moving from "these algorithms are going to solve everything!" to "these algorithms are fundamentally flawed". The term "AI winter refers to those periods when this research fell out of favour, and funding and publications were hard to obtain.

While neural networks can be useful for pattern recognition, not all problems, especially those in healthcare, conveniently fall into well-defined classes. Biology itself tends to be continuous and dynamic rather than discrete and static, even though it is easy for us to comprehend complex systems through discrete units such as genes. The dynamics of gene expression may lack complete precision, yet in the majority of cases biology can go on just fine. In the mid-1960s, Lotfi Zadeh at UC Berkeley described methods for decision making where the decision classes were ill-defined [20]. Through his approaches for what were termed "fuzzy logic," each class or category to be predicted was defined by a membership function that could range from 0 to 1. In this manner the color orange, for instance, could be described as having a membership of 0.5 in red and 0.5 in yellow, and differing shades of orange could be described by different degrees of membership. Such membership functions allow for a mathematical representation of continuous classification and the opportunity to compute using the vagaries that are common to human language. These approaches were at first eschewed by the AI community, especially during the first AI winter. However, their direct utility in engineering applications in Japan and in the United Kingdom led to further interest [21–23]. The use of fuzzy logic as fuzzy systems is now worldwide in common appliances such as rice cookers, washing machines, air conditioners, and even for the docking of spacecraft. Their use in healthcare is equally impressive, as shown in the examples provided below.

These three main lines of computational biomimicry (neural networks, evolutionary computation, and fuzzy logic) form the basis of what is now called "computational intelligence." Practitioners feel that nothing is "artificial" about the learning that is being generated through these methods. At the time of their development, all three approaches ran contrary to the standard belief in the community that "intelligence" in computers should be pre-programmed through heuristics; rules that represented the best in human thinking as humans were clearly smarter than machines. An unfortunate byproduct of the timing was resistance between the key leaders in the rule-based "expert systems" approach and these new directions. It did not help matters that the hardware was in its infancy and that truly showing the societal impact of a neural network on any meaningful task was daunting. It also did not help that despite efforts in areas such as natural language processing, and its promise even in the 1940s, predictions of future success failed to show immediate returns, and by the late 1960s funding for such research became difficult to obtain. The same was true for neural networks, and by the 1970s it was hard to find any funding for anything other than a theoretical understanding of how neural networks worked. Through the 1970s and into the 1980s expert systems still represented the main opportunity for AI. It is no wonder, then, that the community currently practicing computational intelligence would seek to call itself something other than AI, as the pioneers in the field were largely eschewed by the AI community at the time. It is interesting to reflect on the conditions that impeded software development, as today we no longer doubt their considerable utility. However, in the late 1990s and through to today, AI and the opportunity to extract knowledge from data through broad methods of data science witnessed a resurgence, mainly and lately led by methods that trace their roots back to these earlier pioneering approaches. The rate and scale of their utility is tied closely to the continued growth in hardware and processing capability, which today allow for computation that no mainframe computer or collection of mainframes in the 1970s could have achieved.

Modern Approaches

Deep learning methods (artificial neural networks typically with many processing layers and large numbers of inputs) have fundamentally reshaped analytics in healthcare, particularly convolutional neural networks (CNNs) and transformer models. For instance, these approaches can take features directly from raw images, yielding a decision as output as to whether the image is representative of a medical decision such as its relation to cancer. Following the promise of deep learning for image analysis shown by Krizhevsky et al. [24] and others on images, these methods were adopted quickly for the analysis and classification of medical images. Popular tools quickly emerged such as ResNet [25] and U-Net [26] to segment images, classify images into categories or detect specific anomalies in images. These approaches could be used across many different types of images.

Transformer models such as those developed by Vaswani et al. [27] extended deep learning to convert text into numerical representations called tokens. These approaches led to the development of large language models (LLMs) and have revolutionized natural language processing (NLP). The "bidirectional encoder representations from transformers" (BERT) language model developed at Google [28] used supervised learning to represent text as a sequence of vectors, becoming a new standard for NLP. These models excelled at capturing contextual nuances [27] especially those in unstructured biological and medical data. For example, ClinicalBERT, developed by Huang et al. [29] successfully fine-tuned clinical narratives from electronic health records, enhancing the extraction of clinically relevant information and predictive analytics for hospital readmissions. SciBERT [30], was developed as a pre-trained language model for scientific papers. This program has been applied successfully for document classification and information retrieval within the scientific literature. BlueBERT [31], was pre-trained on both PubMed abstracts and clinical notes, yielding robust performance in both research and medical settings. BioBERT [32], was among the first adaptations specifically pre-trained on large amounts of biomedical text including abstracts and full articles from PubMed and focused on informatics in healthcare. PubMedBERT refined this approach further, establishing new state-of-the-art benchmarks on various biomedical NLP tasks [33].

In addition to these text-based models, the BERT architecture has been useful for genomics. For example, the now very popular DNABERT [34], tokenized DNAsequences as *k*-mers to help identify and interpret genetic variants and improve genome annotation. RNABERT [35] adapted the BERT architecture for sequence alignment, the prediction of RNA secondary and tertiary structures. CodonBERT used codons as inputs to enable the selection of mRNAs with improved expression or stability. This model was trained on more than ten million mRNAs across a diverse set of organisms [36]. Still other transformer-based approaches have been developed for genome annotation. For instance, Enformer leverages the information in long-range genomic contexts to predict gene expression and regulatory elements in genomes more accurately than previous approaches [37]. LLMs tailored for healthcare, such as MedLM [38] and LLaVA-Med [39] have recently emerged to support clinical decision-making and medical education. The tremendous explosion of different BERT-derived tools has been amazing and has far-reaching implications for bioinformatics and healthcare.

Protein Folding

One of the long-standing "Holy Grail" problems central to molecular biology has been the protein structure prediction problem: To be able to take a one-dimensional protein sequence and automatically calculate its native folding in three dimensions *de novo*. Traditional methods of x-ray crystallography and NMR spectroscopy are time-consuming and costly. Despite many attempts, this problem went unsolved for decades other than for the smallest proteins. There were some in the community (including myself), who wondered if this quest would ever be achieved. Then in 2021, a team from Google DeepMind released AlphaFold, a tool that combined deep learning and information about protein evolution resulting in near perfect accuracy to known crystal structures in the popular CASP competitions [40]. In this one tool, the entire field took a giant leap forward. Since its inception, AlphaFold has been applied to a very wide range of proteins from viruses to bacteria to humans, helping to revolutionize our understanding of viral-host interactions and enabling improved rational design of novel anti-viral drugs. It has been extended through additional versions—AlphaFold2 [41] and AlphaFold3 [42]—leading to improved understanding of molecular interactions between proteins, new strategies for drug development, new enzymes, and biomaterials. In less than 5 years the field has progressed with amazing speed in this direction, a wonderful example of the power of novel AI approaches and growth in processing speed. Chapter 5 of this book provides examples of the use of CNNs and other methods for protein design.

Drug Design

In parallel, a similar revolution has taken place in cheminformatics, with advantages to medicine as AI rapidly transforms the pharmaceutical pipeline by accelerating the drug discovery process and reducing the traditionally high failure rates of clinical trials. AI platforms are now capable of reducing drug discovery timelines from the typical 10–15 years to as little as 5–7 years in some cases [43, 44]. These systems optimize target identification and minimize experimental failures, leading to an estimated reduction in R&D costs by 30–50%. Enhanced predictive modeling and virtual screening methods have improved the probability of clinical trial success by approximately 20–30%, thereby increasing the overall efficiency of the drug development pipeline. New AI models emerging in 2025 have provided mechanistic insights into cancer cell signaling pathways, offering novel therapeutic targets and approaches. As a result, these advances are expected to bring life-saving medicines to market more rapidly, improving the quality of life for many. The understanding of genetic regulatory networks for cellular biology helps to define opportunities to design drugs that can affect more than one protein on the same pathway, or drugs targeting proteins that are at the hub of many pathways. Chapter 3 provides insight into these approaches including methods of nonlinear analysis and fuzzy logic.

Medical Imaging

The image analysis tools developed as a part of the deep learning revolution have been tailored over time to be used in the field of medical imaging, enabling precise and efficient diagnostic workflows. CheXNet [45] employed a 121-layer CNN to analyze chest X-rays for pneumonia detection. Trained on over 100,000 x-ray images, its performance was comparable to that of experienced radiologists. The approach can be integrated into hospital picture archiving and communication systems (PACS) to offer analysis alongside x-rays to decision makers. Such tools can help reduce diagnostic errors in multiple ways [46, 47]. Beyond pneumonia detection, CNNs for image segmentation such as U-Net [26] have been used for accurate segmentation of anatomical structures in MRI, CT, and ultrasound images, while ResNet [25] facilitated the detection and classification of lesions and tumors. Generative adversarial networks (GANs) [48] are a coupling of two neural networks, one a generator, the other a discriminator. Applied to the context of imaging, a generator network generates images that look like those that might be representative of cancer, while the discriminator network attempts to determine if that image is real or fake. Over time the coupling of these two networks generates a latent space that can be used to understand more about what cancer means in this context, and a well-trained generator can be used to generate additional synthetic images that could be used for the training of other models. These approaches continue to be refined, especially for medical imaging [49, 50]. The synthetic images are now so realistic that it is difficult for a trained human to distinguish between real or fake images. Chapter 4 provides an overview of many modern methods used to address cancer from CNNs to GANs to LLMs.

Electronic Health Records

Studies have revealed that physicians spend ~37% of their workday on electronic health record (EHR)-related tasks [51]. AI-based tools, such as ClinicalBERT and scalable deep learning models described by Rajkomar et al. [52], have demonstrated that it is possible to reduce the time required for EHR documentation considerably, allowing clinicians to devote more time to direct patient care, and ultimately improving healthcare outcomes. The popular large language model ChatGPT offered by OpenAI and its many derivatives can also be used in medicine, for instance in medical writing or documentation and discharge summaries, remote patient monitoring and a host of other activities that center on writing. Moreover, tools like Deep Patient [53] were developed on hundreds of thousands of EHR records and can be used to make clinical predictions for a wide variety of diseases, advancing patient management and ensuring timely intervention. Some of these models perform so well that it is now possible to find associations that were previously not realized in medicine, or to diagnose someone as having a high risk of Alzheimer's from a retinal scan. We live in a new age where the mix of AI and medicine promises new diagnostics, new interventions, even new ways of thinking about how to use AI for medicine itself. For example, Moor et al. [54] recently proposed "generalist medical AI" (GMAI). Such models trained on large datasets of across multiple formats (text, images, genomics, graphs) could produce human-interpretable text explanations or even spoken recommendations with advanced medical reasoning. Natural language processing approaches and their opportunity in healthcare are highlighted in Chapter 6.

Computational Intelligence

However, as noted earlier, the field of computational intelligence has three pillars (neural networks, evolutionary computation, and fuzzy logic). The vast majority of the applications I've mentioned so far have been associated solely with neural networks, and while the field is definitely focused in that direction, important advances in the application of evolutionary computation and fuzzy logic to medicine should not be ignored.

For example, Alderdice et al. [55] used an evolutionary algorithm to mine The Cancer Genome Atlas for clinically relevant associations and identified a new factor, IL2RB, associated with immune checkpoints in colorectal cancer. Their work included both a bioinformatics analysis and experimental validation of IL2RB in this role. Within the field of evolutionary computation, one must define an objective function that represents the worth of alternative solutions so that they can be ranked as a judgement of fitness. Typically, such an objective function has one term, but it is possible to define objective functions that have many terms that are all to be optimized simultaneously. In some cases these terms can conflict, leading to solutions that are suboptimal in any one dimension but optimal over all terms combined. Such strategies are known as multi-objective evolutionary algorithms (MOEAs) or multi-objective optimization. Zhao et al. [56] used MOEAs to cluster single-cell transcriptomes from single-cell RNA sequencing (scRNA-seq) and spatial imaging. This approach outperformed other methods for clustering and holds promise for the discovery of novel disease biomarkers in light of the more properly clustered single-cell transcriptomics. It is also possible to use evolutionary algorithms for feature selection or optimizing neural network or other model architectures for pattern recognition considering the data. Such approaches can be used in virology to identify signatures associated with coreceptor usage [57], tissue localization [58], or immunoregulation [59]. For additional information the reader is referred to other recent surveys [60].

The field of medical decision-making has inherent uncertainty and ambiguity handled well by fuzzy logic. Korkmaz et al. [61] used fuzzy logic for risk assessment of metabolic syndrome and cardiovascular diseases, achieving over 92% accuracy. Ali et al. [62] provides an excellent review of fuzzy approaches to cardiovascular disease, showing how similar approaches can be applied to other medical needs. Fuzzy cognitive maps (FCMs) have been used to relate biological factors to diagnosis, prognosis, and treatment for more than 20 years [63]. It is even possible to use fuzzy approaches to evaluate the use and appropriateness of large language models in medical settings [64].

Looking Ahead

In this brief introductory chapter, I hope it has become clear that AI is having an amazingly transformative and positive impact on medicine and healthcare worldwide. Sahini et al. [65] estimate that the adoption of AI can lead to a 5–10% savings in US healthcare costs ($200B–$360B annually). A recent Forbes analysis noted that private payers could see savings of $80B–$110B annually over the next 5 years, while physicians could save 3–8% of their costs ($20B–$60B) [66]. Such savings will only increase as AI improves over time.

However, we must realize that these same AI tools are used to influence life-or-death decisions. Issues of ethics and patient confidentiality must remain forefront, so that the approaches remain trusted. Regulation has developed specifically around the use of AI in medicine, such as the European Union's General Data Protection Regulation (GDPR) and the U.S. Health Insurance Portability and Accountability Act (HIPAA). The GDPR explicitly mandates stringent rules on data processing and patient consent to ensure that AI applications do not compromise personal privacy. Similarly, HIPAA sets rigorous standards for protecting health information in the United States. Global guidelines issued by organizations such as the OECD and UNESCO further emphasize that AI systems used for critical decision-making should be transparent, interpretable, and ethically sound. The reader is directed to other surveys for more information in this area [67–69] Many in the AI community remain equally concerned about these issues and monitor applications as they come online [70]. Within the U.S., the Center for Drug Evaluation and Research (CDER) at the U.S. Food and Drug Administration has recently published draft guidance towards the use of AI in regulatory decision-making to approve drug and biological products, as it is clear that AI will be accelerating the advancement of new medical entities (https://www.regulations.gov/docket/FDA-2024-D-4689).

Over the last decade, as the field focuses on varieties of deep learning methods, larger datasets are required for model development, larger models with hundreds of thousands of features, each with hundreds of processing layers become common, and so forth, all at high expense to develop in terms of computational resources, time, and energy. While this approach has led to amazing progress, the resulting energy demands are so high that companies such as Microsoft, Amazon, and Google are now investing in nuclear power generation. But is bigger and faster truly always better? Perhaps we should be focused on doing more with less. One can use evolutionary computation to help optimize models, reduce their size, and reduce the number of features used, while still retaining reasonable performance. One can use fuzzy logic to abstract decision-making in ways that may avoid use of a large model. One can hybridize methods of neural networks, evolutionary computation, and fuzzy logic to improve efficiency while not sacrificing performance and perhaps even improving human interpretability. Not every problem is difficult, and we shouldn't be forced into thinking that all problems should be solved with complex tools. It is critical that AI researchers apply the right methods to the right problems, keeping efficiency in mind.

As a researcher who has been interested in this area for more than 30 years, it is impressive to realize that the number of papers in PubMed has continued to increase dramatically. It is estimated that in 2000 there were roughly 1600 papers about the application of AI to medicine. By 2022, this number had increased to 58,000, an increase of 36-fold [71]. The rate of publication shows no sign of slowing; in fact, it is accelerating. This results in considerable difficulty for any researcher to remain current with the expanding literature. Books such as this one are instrumental in doing so. However, despite all the interest, success, and publications, in many ways we still lack a granular level understanding of the mechanics of biology. Perhaps in the near future we will have models that can help determine the fate of cells and rationalize why cellular development went one direction versus another through intricate dynamics of gene regulation and help us choose certain cell fates over others. Perhaps AI will allow us to monitor the dynamics of cell biology in real time in ways that we do not yet comprehend. Perhaps we can fully understand the relationships between genetics and environment that can result in disease development, with AI helping to provide us with the tools and medicines necessary to intervene in advance of disease progression. Many such significant challenges remain in biology. However, in just a short 25 years we've come a long way and have leveraged many computational intelligence methods for some truly exceptionally impressive gains. The next 25 years promise to be even more exciting than the last, and I hope that the chapters of this book serve as a foundation for interdisciplinary thought and growth towards a similarly impressive future.

References

1. F. Rosenblatt, "The perceptron: a probabilistic model for information storage and organization in the brain," *Psych. Rev.*, vol. 65, pp. 386–408, 1958. https://doi.org/10.1037/h0042519
2. W. McCulloch and W. Pitts, "A logical calculus of the ideas immanent in nervous activity," *Bull. Math. Phys.*, vol. 7, pp. 115–133, 1943. https://doi.org/10.1007/BF02478259
3. D. Hebb, *The Organization of Behavior*, Wiley, 1949.
4. B. Widrow, "Generalization and information storage in networks of adaline neurons," in *Self-Organizing Systems*, M. C. Yovits, G. T. Jacobi, and G. D. Goldstein, Eds., Washington D.C.: Spartan Books, 1962.
5. B. Widrow and M. Hoff, "Adaptive switching circuits," Western Electronic Show and Convention, Vol. 4, pp. 96–104. *Institute of Radio Engineers.*, 1960.
6. P. Werbos, *Beyond Regression: New Tools for Prediction and Analysis in the Behavioral Sciences*. Doctoral dissertation, Harvard University, Cambridge, MA, 1974.
7. J.J. Hopfield, "Neural networks and physical systems with emergent collective computational abilities," *Proc. Natl. Acad. Sci., U.S.A.*, Vol. 79, pp. 2554–2558, 1982. https://doi.org/10.1073/pnas.79.8.2554
8. N. A. Barricelli, "Esempi numerici di processi di evoluzione," *Methodos*, pp. 45–68, 1954.
9. G.E.P. Box, "Evolutionary operation: A method for increasing industrial productivity," *Appl. Statistics*, Vol. 6, pp. 81-101, 1957. https://doi.org/10.2307/2985505
10. A.S. Fraser, "Simulation of genetic systems by automatic digital computers," *Australian Jour. Biol. Sci.*, Vol. 10, pp. 484-491, 1957. https://doi.org/10.1071/BI9570484
11. R.M. Friedberg, "A learning machine: Part I," *IBM J. Res. Dev.*, Vol. 2, pp. 2-13, 1958. https://doi.org/10.1147/rd.21.0002
12. R.M. Friedberg, "A learning machine: Part II," *IBM J. Res. Dev.*, Vol. 3, pp. 282-287, 1959. https://doi.org/10.1147/rd.33.0282
13. G. J. Friedman, *Selective Feedback Computers for Engineering Synthesis and Nervous System Analogy*, Masters thesis, UC Los Angeles, 1956.
14. H.J. Bremmerman, M. Rogson, and S. Salaff, "Global properties of evolution processes," In *Natural Automata and Useful Simulations*, H.H. Pattee, E.A. Edlsack, L. Fein, and A.B. Callahan (Eds.), Washington, D.C.: Spartan Books, pp. 3–41, 1966.
15. L.J. Fogel, *On the Organization of Intellect*, Ph.D. dissertation, UCLA, 1964.
16. L.J. Fogel., A.J. Owens, and M.J. Walsh, *Artificial Intelligence Through Simulated Evolution*, John Wiley, New York, 1966.
17. I. Rechenberg, "Cybernetic solution path of an experimental problem," *Royal Aircraft Establishment*, Library translation, 1122, 1965.
18. H.-P. Schwefel, Numerische Optimierung von Computer-Modellen mittels der Evolutionsstrategie. Birkhäuser, Basle, *Interdisciplinary Systems Research* 26, 1977.
19. J.H. Holland, "Genetic algorithms and the optimal allocation of trials," *SIAM J. Comput.* Vol. 2, pp. 88-105, 1973. https://doi.org/10.1137/0202009
20. L. Zadeh, "Fuzzy sets," *Inf. Control.*, Vol. 8, pp. 338-353, 1965. https://doi.org/10.1016/S0019-9958(65)90241-X
21. E.H. Mamdani and N. Baaklini, "Prescriptive method for deriving a control policy in a fuzzy logic controller," *Electronics Letters*, Vol 11, p. 625, 1975.
22. M. Sugeno, *Theory of Fuzzy Integrals and its Applications*, Doctoral dissertation, Tokyo Institute of Technology, 1974.
23. T. Terano, K. Asai, M. Sugeno, *Fuzzy Systems Theory and its Applications*, San Diego, CA: Academic Press Professional, Inc., 1992.
24. Krizhevsky, A., Sutskever, I. and Hinton, G.E. (2012) ImageNet Classification with Deep Convolutional Neural Networks. Advances in Neural Information Processing Systems, 25, 1097–1105.

25. He, K., Zhang, X., Ren, S. and Sun, J. (2016) Deep Residual Learning for Image Recognition. Proceedings of the IEEE Conference on Computer Vision and Pattern Recognition, Las Vegas, 27–30 June 2016, 770–778.
26. Ronneberger, O., Fischer, P. and Brox, T. (2015) U-Net: Convolutional Networks for Biomedical Image Segmentation. In: Navab, N., Hornegger, J., Wells, W., Frangi A., Eds., International Conference on Medical Image Computing and Computer-Assisted Intervention, Springer, Cham, 234–241.
27. Vaswani, A., Shazeer, N., Parmar, N., Uszkoreit, J., Jones, L., Gomez, A.N., Polosukhin, I., et al. (2017) Attention Is All You Need. 31st Conference on Neural Information Processing Systems (NIPS 2017), Long Beach, CA, 5998–6008.
28. Devlin, J., Chang, M.W., Lee, K., Toutanova, K.: Bert: Pre-training of deep bidirectional transformers for language understanding. NAACL pp. 4171–4186 (2019)
29. Huang, K., Altosaar, J. and Ranganath, R. (2019) ClinicalBERT: Modeling Clinical Notes and Predicting Hospital Readmission. arXiv:1904.05342.
30. I. Beltagy, K. Lo, A. Cohan, SciBERT: A Pretrained Language Model for Scientific Text. EMNLP/IJCNLP (1) 2019: 3613–3618.
31. Peng, Y., Yan, S., & Lu, Z. (2019) BLUE: A Pre-trained Language Model for Biomedical Text. arXiv preprint arXiv:1909.04164.
32. J. Lee, W. Yoon, S. Kim, D. Kim, S. Kim, C. H. So, and J. Kang, "BioBERT: a pre-trained biomedical language representation model for biomedical text mining," Bioinformatics, vol. 36, no. 4, pp. 1234–1240, 2020. https://doi.org/10.1093/bioinformatics/btz682
33. Y. Gu, R. Tinn, H. Cheng, M. Lucas, N. Usuyama, X. Liu, T. Naumann, J. Gao, and H. Poon, "Domain-specific language model pretraining for biomedical natural language processing," 2020. https://doi.org/10.48550/arXiv.2007.15779
34. Ji Y., Zhou Z., Liu H., Davuluri R.V. "DNABERT: pre-trained bidirectional encoder representations from transformers model for DNA-language in genome. Bioinformatics, 37 (15) (2021), pp. 2112–2120. https://doi.org/10.1093/bioinformatics/btab083
35. Manato Akiyama, Yasubumi Sakakibara, Informative RNA base embedding for RNA structural alignment and clustering by deep representation learning, *NAR Genomics and Bioinformatics*, Volume 4, Issue 1, March 2022, lqac012, https://doi.org/10.1093/nargab/lqac012
36. Sizhen Li, Saeed Moayedpour, Ruijiang Li, Michael Bailey, Saleh Riahi, Lorenzo Kogler-Anele, Milad Miladi, Jacob Miner, Dinghai Zheng, Jun Wang, Akshay Balsubramani, Khang Tran, Minnie Zacharia, Monica Wu, Xiaobo Gu, Ryan Clinton, Carla Asquith, Joseph Skaleski, Lianne Boeglin, Sudha Chivukula, Anusha Dias, Fernando Ulloa Montoya, Vikram Agarwal, Ziv Bar-Joseph, Sven Jager, (2024) "CodonBERT: Large Language Models for mRNA design and optimization." Genome Research https://doi.org/10.1101/gr.278870.123
37. Avsec Ž, Agarwal V, Visentin D, Ledsam JR, Grabska-Barwinska A, Taylor KR, Assael Y, Jumper J, Kohli P, Kelley DR. Effective gene expression prediction from sequence by integrating long-range interactions. Nat Methods. 2021 Oct;18(10):1196–1203. https://doi.org/10.1038/s41592-021-01252-x
38. Yagnik, N., Jhaveri, J., Sharma, V., Pila, G., Ben, A. and Shang, J., 2024. MedLM: Exploring Language Models for Medical Question Answering Systems. *arXiv preprint arXiv:2401.11389*.
39. Chunyuan Li, Cliff Wong, Sheng Zhang, Naoto Usuyama, Haotian Liu, Jianwei Yang, Tristan Naumann, Hoifung Poon, and Jianfeng Gao. 2023. LLaVA-med: training a large language-and-vision assistant for biomedicine in one day. In Proceedings of the 37th International Conference on Neural Information Processing Systems (NIPS '23). Curran Associates Inc., Red Hook, NY, USA, Article 1240, 28541–28564.
40. Jumper, J., Evans, R., Pritzel, A. *et al.* Highly accurate protein structure prediction with AlphaFold. *Nature* 596, 583–589 (2021). https://doi.org/10.1038/s41586-021-03819-2
41. Yang, Z., Zeng, X., Zhao, Y. *et al.* AlphaFold2 and its applications in the fields of biology and medicine. *Sig Transduct Target Ther* **8**, 115 (2023). https://doi.org/10.1038/s41392-023

42. Abramson, J., Adler, J., Dunger, J. *et al.* Accurate structure prediction of biomolecular interactions with AlphaFold 3. *Nature* **630**, 493–500 (2024). https://doi.org/10.1038/s41586-024-07487-w
43. Mak KK, Pichika MR. Artificial intelligence in drug development: present status and future prospects. Drug Discov Today. 2019 Mar;24(3):773–780. https://doi.org/10.1016/j.drudis.2018.11.014
44. Topol, E.J. High-performance medicine: the convergence of human and artificial intelligence. *Nat Med* 25, 44–56 (2019). https://doi.org/10.1038/s41591-018-0300-7
45. Rajpurkar, P., Irvin, J., Zhu, K., Yang, B. Mehta, H., Duan, T., Ding, D. Bagul, A., Langlotz, C., Shpanskaya, K., Lungren, M.P., Ng, A.Y. "CheXNet: Radiologist-Level Pneumonia Detection on Chest X-Rays with Deep Learning." *ArXiv abs/1711* 5225 (2017).
46. Burti, S., Zotti, A., Banzato, T. "Role of AI in diagnostic imaging error reduction," Front. Vet. Sci. 2024 https://doi.org/10.3389/fvets.2024.1437284
47. Katal, S., York, B., Gholamrezanezhad, A. (2024) "AI in radiology: From promise to practice—A guide to effective integration," European Journal of Radiology, Vol. 181. https://doi.org/10.1016/j.ejrad.2024.111798
48. I. Goodfellow, J. Pouget-Abadie, M. Mirza, B. Xu, D. Warde-Farley, S. Ozair, A. Courville, and Y. Bengio. "Generative adversarial nets" Advances in neural information processing systems, pp. 2672–2680. (2014) https://doi.org/10.1145/3422622
49. Ahmad, W., Ali, H., Shah, Z. *et al.* A new generative adversarial network for medical images super resolution. *Sci Rep* **12**, 9533 (2022). https://doi.org/10.1038/s41598-022-13658-4
50. Skandarani Y, Jodoin PM, Lalande A. GANs for Medical Image Synthesis: An Empirical Study. J Imaging. 2023 Mar 16;9(3):69. https://doi.org/10.3390/jimaging9030069
51. Sinsky C, Colligan L, Li L, Prgomet M, Reynolds S, Goeders L, Westbrook J, Tutty M, Blike G. Allocation of Physician Time in Ambulatory Practice: A Time and Motion Study in 4 Specialties. Ann Intern Med. 2016 Dec 6;165(11):753–760. https://doi.org/10.7326/M16-0961
52. Rajkomar A, Oren E, Chen K, Dai AM, Hajaj N, Hardt M, Liu PJ, Liu X, Marcus J, Sun M, Sundberg P, Yee H, Zhang K, Zhang Y, Flores G, Duggan GE, Irvine J, Le Q, Litsch K, Mossin A, Tansuwan J, Wang D, Wexler J, Wilson J, Ludwig D, Volchenboum SL, Chou K, Pearson M, Madabushi S, Shah NH, Butte AJ, Howell MD, Cui C, Corrado GS, Dean J. Scalable and accurate deep learning with electronic health records. NPJ Digit Med. 2018 May 8;1:18. https://doi.org/10.1038/s41746-018-0029-1
53. Miotto, R., Li, L., Kidd, B. *et al.* Deep Patient: An Unsupervised Representation to Predict the Future of Patients from the Electronic Health Records. *Sci Rep* **6**, 26094 (2016). https://doi.org/10.1038/srep26094
54. Moor, M., Banerjee, O., Abad, Z.S.H. *et al.* Foundation models for generalist medical artificial intelligence. *Nature* **616**, 259–265 (2023). https://doi.org/10.1038/s41586-023-05881-4
55. Alderdice M, Craig SG, Humphries MP, Gilmore A, Johnston N, Bingham V, Coyle V, Senevirathne S, Longley DB, Loughrey MB, McQuaid S, James JA, Salto-Tellez M, Lawler M, McArt DG. Evolutionary genetic algorithm identifies *IL2RB* as a potential predictive biomarker for immune-checkpoint therapy in colorectal cancer. NAR Genom Bioinform. 2021 Apr 20;3(2):lqab016. https://doi.org/10.1093/nargab/lqab016
56. Zhao K, Grayson JM, Khuri N. Multi-Objective Genetic Algorithm for Cluster Analysis of Single-Cell Transcriptomes. J Pers Med. 2023 Jan 20;13(2):183. https://doi.org/10.3390/jpm13020183
57. Fogel GB, Lamers SL, Liu ES, Salemi M, McGrath MS. Identification of dual-tropic HIV-1 using evolved neural networks. Biosystems. 2015 Nov;137:12–19. https://doi.org/10.1016/j.biosystems.2015.09.007
58. Lamers SL, Fogel GB, Liu ES, Barbier AE, Rodriguez CW, Singer EJ, Nolan DJ, Rose R, McGrath MS. Brain-specific HIV Nef identified in multiple patients with neurological disease. J Neurovirol. 2018 Feb;24(1):1–15. https://doi.org/10.1007/s13365-017-0586-0

59. S.L. Lamers, G. B. Fogel, E. S. Liu, D.J. Nolan, R. Rose, M.S. McGrath "HIV-1 subtypes maintain distinctive physicochemical signatures in Nef domains associated with immunoregulation," Infection, Genetics, and Evolution Vol 115, https://doi.org/10.1016/j.meegid.2023.105514
60. Holmes JH. Methods and applications of evolutionary computation in biomedicine. J Biomed Inform. 2014 Jun;49:11–15. https://doi.org/10.1016/j.jbi.2014.05.008
61. Korkmaz H, Canayaz E, Birtane Akar S, Altikardes ZA. Fuzzy logic based risk assessment system giving individualized advice for metabolic syndrome and fatal cardiovascular diseases. Technol Health Care. 2019;27(S1):59–66. https://doi.org/10.3233/THC-199007. Erratum in: Technol Health Care. 2019;27(6):681. https://doi.org/10.3233/THC-199041
62. Ali ML, Sadi MS, Goni MO (2024) Diagnosis of heart diseases: A fuzzy-logic-based approach. PLoS ONE 19(2): e0293112. https://doi.org/10.1371/journal.pone.0293112
63. Apostolopoulos ID, Papandrianos NI, Papathanasiou ND, Papageorgiou EI. Fuzzy Cognitive Map Applications in Medicine over the Last Two Decades: A Review Study. Bioengineering (Basel). 2024 Jan 30;11(2):139. https://doi.org/10.3390/bioengineering11020139
64. Alamoodi AH, Zughoul O, David D, Garfan S, Pamucar D, Albahri OS, Albahri AS, Yussof S, Sharaf IM. A Novel Evaluation Framework for Medical LLMs: Combining Fuzzy Logic and MCDM for Medical Relation and Clinical Concept Extraction. J Med Syst. 2024 Aug 31;48(1):81. https://doi.org/10.1007/s10916-024-02090-y
65. Sahini, N.R., G. Stein, R. Zemmel, D. Cutler, "The potential impact of artificial intelligence on health care spending," in *The Economics of Artificial Intelligence: Health Care Challenges*, National Bureau of Economic Research, 2024. ISBN 978-0-226-83311-8.
66. Kazyanau, A. (2024) "Balancing the cost of AI in healthcare: Future savings vs. current spending," https://www.forbes.com/councils/forbestechcouncil/2024/04/17/balancing-the-cost-of-ai-in-healthcare-future-savings-vs-current-spending/
67. Reddy S "Navigating the AI Revolution: The Case for Precise Regulation in Health Care," J Med Internet Res 2023;25:e49989 doi: https://doi.org/10.2196/49989
68. Trotsyuk AA, Federico CA, Cho MK, Altman RB, Magnus D. Stronger regulation of AI in biomedicine. Sci Transl Med. 2023 Sep 13;15(713):eadi0336. https://doi.org/10.1126/scitranslmed.adi0336
69. Palaniappan K, Lin EYT, Vogel S. Global Regulatory Frameworks for the Use of Artificial Intelligence (AI) in the Healthcare Services Sector. Healthcare (Basel). 2024 Feb 28;12(5):562. https://doi.org/10.3390/healthcare12050562
70. Haltaufderheide, J., Ranisch, R. The ethics of ChatGPT in medicine and healthcare: a systematic review on Large Language Models (LLMs). *npj Digit. Med.* **7**, 183 (2024). https://doi.org/10.1038/s41746-024-01157-x
71. Shi J, Bendig D, Vollmar HC, Rasche P. Mapping the Bibliometrics Landscape of AI in Medicine: Methodological Study. J Med Internet Res. 2023 Dec 8;25:e45815. https://doi.org/10.2196/45815

Chapter 2
Molecular Biology Light

Jennifer Hallinan

Abstract In this book we provide an overview of some of the important applications of AI to medicine. In order to fully understand the implications of this work, it is important to understand the molecular basis of the biology of human cells. In this chapter we briefly cover the basics of molecular biology, from the discovery of the structure of DNA to our current knowledge of the field. Some of these discoveries were made with the aid of AI, but many preceded the advent of the algorithms and computing power of which current AI is composed. Many of the readers will already be familiar with this material, in which case feel free to skip this chapter. For other readers this chapter provides information essential to the application of AI in a medical setting.

Introduction

The advent of AI has produced major changes in our understanding of the link between genomes and proteins, which bodes well to change our entire view of the genetic basis of medicine. In this chapter, we examine the genome sequence and the relationships between the genome and the proteome, laying the basis for some of the work reported in more detail in later chapters of the book.

Estimates of the number of species of organisms currently living on Earth vary widely, from two million [1] to three trillion [2]. However, the most widely accepted estimate appears to be about 8.75 million [3], of which about 1.5 million have been named [4]. Despite the enormous diversity of size, shape and behavior apparent amongst these organisms, there is little doubt that all organisms alive today share a common heredity. The basic biochemistry and genetics of all organisms are identical; all organisms known to science use deoxyribose nucleic acid (DNA) or the closely related ribose nucleic acid (RNA) as the fundamental information-carrying

J. Hallinan (✉)
BioThink, Brisbane, QLD, Australia

M. Chetty, J. Hallinan (eds.), *From Algorithms to Ailments*,
https://doi.org/10.1007/978-3-032-11023-7_2

molecule in the cell, and they all process that information using practically identical cellular machinery. It is highly unlikely that these similarities are the result of coincidence. Life on earth appears to have a single, common, ancestor. This ancestor even has a name: LUCA, the Last Universal Common Ancestor, and lived about 3.8 billion years ago [5].

From this single root the tree of life has developed over time, giving rise to ever more branches. Many of the branches terminate in extinction; some persist relatively unchanged for long periods, occasionally giving rise to an offshoot; and some diverge rapidly into a mass of related but different forms. The biosphere that we observe today is a slice in time across the branches of the tree.

Co-existing organisms can therefore be organized into more-or-less closely related groups. The result is a hierarchical taxonomy, the top level of which contains five major Kingdoms: the Prokaryotae (bacteria); the Protoctista (algae and protozoans); the Fungi (mushrooms, molds and lichens); the Animalia (animals); and the Plantae (plants) [6]. The Kingdoms are divided into Orders, which in turn are split into Phyla, then Families, Genera and Species. Sub or super taxa or both may also be defined for some organisms.

Individual organisms are commonly referred to using the genus and species names, a convention known as *binomial nomenclature*. This convention was devised by Carl von Linné, aka Linnaeus,[1] in his *Systemae Naturae* in 1735. In text, the entire name is italicised or underlined, the genus name is capitalized and the species name starts with a lower case letter the genus name is frequently shortened to a single letter when there is no chance of confusion. The domestic dog, for example, is a member of the genus *Canis* and species *familiaris*; it is therefore referred to as *Canis familiaris* (or *C. familiaris*). The closely related wolf is *Canis lupus*: same genus but different species. Figure 2.1 shows the full phylogenetic tree of *C. familiaris* and *C. lupus*.

Perhaps the most fundamental distinction between organisms is that between the *prokaryotes* and the *eukaryotes*. Prokaryotes are single-celled organisms which carry their DNA as a circular chromosome floating free in the cell. There are two main groups within the prokaryotes, the "true bacteria" or *eubacteria*, which include familiar bacteria such as human skin colonists and human pathogens, and the *archaebacteria*, which were only discovered in the 1970s, and tend to live in extreme environments [7].

Prokaryotes do not necessarily restrict themselves to a single chromosome; some have several. Many prokaryotes also carry a range of *plasmids*, small extrachromosomal circles of DNA, carrying a few genes. Plasmids are readily swapped between cells, resulting in *lateral gene transfer* between bacteria. Lateral gene transfer is an important mechanism by which antibiotic resistance spreads.

Prokaryotes living in extreme conditions are particularly prone to having multiple chromosomes. *Deinococcus radiodurans*, for example, has an amazing ability to withstand radiation, being able to withstand, without loss of viability, a level of

[1] Biologists in the eighteenth century commonly used a latinized version of their names, a hangover from the Middle Ages, when Greece and Rome were regarded as the fonts of all knowledge.

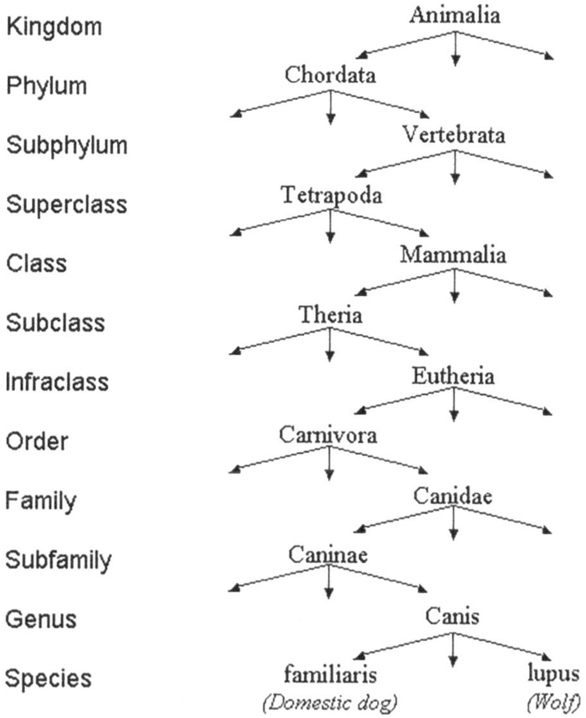

Fig. 2.1 Phylogenetic tree for the domestic dog, *Canis familiaris* and wolf, *Canis lupus*

radiation 3000 times greater than that which would kill a human. It has a complex genome, consisting of two chromosomes, a small plasmid and a megaplasmid [8]. It carries four to ten copies of the genome, and it is this redundancy, together with efficient DNA repair mechanisms, which enables it to survive intense radiation by rapidly repairing radiation-induced breaks in the chromosomes.

Eukaryotes are distinguished from prokaryotes by having compartmentalized cells. Their DNA is isolated from the main body of the cell inside a *nucleus*, which is surrounded by a nuclear membrane. The remainder of the cell, the *cytoplasm*, contains cellular organelles specialized for functions such as the production of energy (mitochondria), the manufacture of proteins (ribosomes) and the transport of molecules (endoplasmic reticulum and others). All of the multicellular organisms, the macroscopic plants and animals making up the visible world around us, are eukaryotes. Not all eukaryotes are multicellular, however; there are a number of single-celled eukaryotes.

Eukaryotic DNA is organized into linear segments called *chromosomes*. Different species have different numbers of chromosomes,[2] but in general organisms have two

[2] An irresistible statistic: the Adder's Tongue Fern, *Ophioglossum reticulatum* has been estimated to have up to 1020 chromosomes!

copies of each chromosome, one of which comes from the mother and one from the father. This is known as a *diploid* chromosome number.[3] Most eukaryotes are diploid, although organisms which reproduce asexually may be haploid, and some plants may duplicate their entire set of chromosomes several times (*polyploidy*).

DNA and RNA are fundamental to life. What makes these molecules so special?

The Molecules of Life

In this post-genomic era, we tend to be blasé about the amazing machinery that gives rise to life. Biologists routinely sequence entire genomes and can map many of the genes in these genomes to their physical location on the chromosomes. DNA, RNAs, and their associated molecules tend to be seen simply as raw materials to be "engineered" into whatever products society may desire: transgenic pigs for infection-free organ transplantation, pesticide-resistant crops, and so forth. This is a common attitude in the popular press, engendered by the enormous growth in our knowledge of molecular biology over the last 50 years, but it belies the fact that a cell is an incredibly complex system, about which we currently know only a fraction of what there is to be known. A relatively large amount is known, however, about the structure and function of the fundamental molecules of life: DNA and RNA.

Deoxyribose Nucleic Acid (DNA)

The cell is an information processing system, and protein is the primary physical manifestation of that information. Proteins are used for building bodies, transporting molecules around the cell, catalysing reactions, and many other functions. Estimates of the number of proteins in the human body range from 100,000 or so, up to over a million. The basic recipe for these proteins is encoded in the DNA of the cells of most organisms, although some viruses use the closely related ribose nucleic acid (RNA) instead. The DNA inside each of the cells of a human, if stretched to full length, would be approximately two meters long.

Human DNA is divided into 46 chromosomes: 22 pairs of *somatic* (or body) chromosomes, possessed by both males and females, and one pair of *sex chromosomes*. The sex chromosomes comprise two X chromosomes in females, and one X and one Y in males. Other organisms have different numbers of chromosomes. One chromosome of each pair, somatic or sex, is inherited from the mother, and one from the father. There are many variations of this genetic structure. Individuals may have multiple X or Y chromosomes, and different combinations have different

[3] Cells with a single copy of each chromosome are said to have a *haploid* chromosome number.

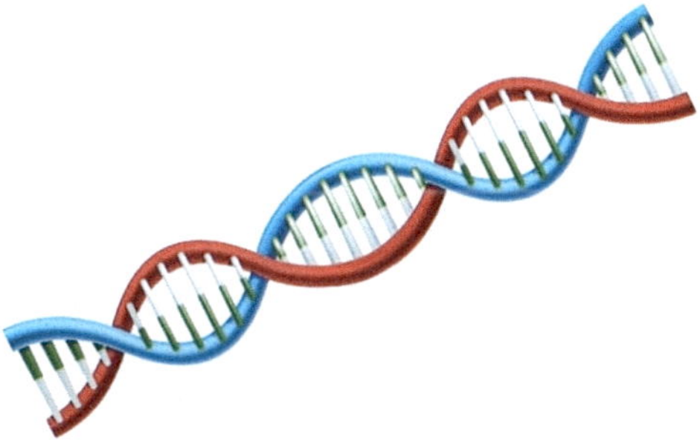

Fig. 2.2 Deoxyribose nucleic acid. (Image courtesy of https://www.freepik.com/free-photos-vectors/dna-structure)

physical effects on the body. Biological sex is a complex issue, but most humans are either XX or XY.

Each of the strands of a DNA molecule consists of a chain of alternating sugars (deoxyribose) and phosphate groups. The carbon atoms in the deoxyribose molecules are, by convention, numbered from 1′ (pronounced "one prime") to 5′. This numbering allows a directionality to be defined for the DNA molecule, with a 5′ carbon exposed at one end and a 3′ carbon at the other. DNA runs from the 5′ to the 3′ end. Since DNA is a double stranded molecule, the strand complementary to that running 5′–3′ runs 3′–5′.

Attached to each deoxyribose is one of four *bases*. The four bases are *adenine* (generally designated A), *guanine* (G), *cytosine* (C) and *thymine* (T). The bases bind to each other—A with T and C with G—to form the "rungs" of the DNA "ladder" (Fig. 2.2). This ladder twists lengthwise to form the familiar DNA double helix.

The DNA sequence can be modified by various types of mutation: changes to a single base, known as *point mutations* and insertions or deletions of DNA from other sources. These mutated sequences are passed on to an individual's descendants. However, DNA can be modified in other ways, which do not alter the sequence itself. This phenomenon is known as *epigenetics*, and includes modifications such as the methylation of bases and modifications to the histone proteins around which the DNA is wrapped in the chromosomes [9]. These modifications, particularly methylation, have been associated with a number of disease conditions, including cancer [10], Alzheimer disease [11], obesity [12], asthma [13], and ageing [14].

Epigenetic changes may increase over time; identical twins generally tend to have similar methylomes at birth, but due to environmental and chance factors, the methylomes may diverge over the course of their lives [15]. The changes are also hereditary. Natural "experiments", such as the Dutch Hunger Winter, a famine caused by a German blockade of the Western Netherlands lasting from late 1944 to Spring 1945 have facilitated large-scale studies of these effects. Children conceived during the famine were undernourished *in utero* and grew up to be thin adults with faster aging than well-nourished individuals. This trend, which appears to be due to epigenetic changes, was evident in their children, and even grandchildren. One study found accelerated ageing after six generations [16].

DNA has a threefold role: to carry the information required to build the cell; to participate in cell functioning by producing the proteins and RNA required on a minute-to-minute basis; and to transport this information from generation to generation. The latter role, as the fundamental molecule of inheritance, carrying information from parent to child, is most often discussed in the context of evolution. Evolutionary biologists tend to take a long-range view of the processes of life. However, it is important to realize that inside each of the cells of a living organism DNA is a dynamic molecule, constantly being unpackaged and repackaged in order to expose genes to the transcriptional machinery of the cell. Every cell in an organism contains the same DNA, but different genes are active at different times and in different tissues. Different subsets of proteins are thus constantly being produced and metabolised in response to events both internal and external to the cell.

DNA to RNA: The Genetic Code and Transcription

For the information encoded in the DNA to be useful, it must ultimately be translated into physical form. The intermediary between DNA and protein is RNA deoxyribose, and the base uracil (U) replaces DNA's thymine (T).

DNA is *transcribed* into a form of RNA known as messenger RNA (mRNA) in the nucleus. The mRNA is then transported from the nucleus, where it is produced, into the cytoplasm. Before the mRNA can be *translated* into protein it undergoes post-transcriptional processing. In prokaryotes genes occur as a single stretch of DNA delimited by a start codon and a stop codon. In most eukaryotes, however, the gene is divided into variable-length stretches of protein-coding DNA, known as *exons*, and segments of non-protein-coding DNA, known as *introns*. Before translation the introns are spliced out of the mRNA, a nucleotide cap is added to the 5′ end, and a string of alanine molecules, known as a *poly A tail* is added to the 3′ end. Different exons may be spliced out of identical RNA sequences under different circumstances, leading to the production of different proteins from the same gene.

Further processing may also occur, in the form of *RNA editing*. Two main types of RNA editing have been identified: the insertion or deletion of individual bases, mediated by RNA guide molecules; and the substitution of one base for another, catalysed by proteins. RNA editing can also lead to the production of different proteins from the same gene. Indeed, many different proteins may be produced, and they may bear little or no resemblance to each other. A gene called *cacophony* in the vinegar fly *Drosophila melanogaster* can generate more than 1000 different proteins via RNA editing alone.[4] In conjunction with differential splicing of introns, RNA editing means that the *proteome* (the set of all proteins present at any time in an organism) is generally much more diverse than the genome.

Following any required splicing and editing, the mRNA is translated into a string of amino acids which subsequently folds into a three-dimensional structure: a protein.

[4] https://www.ncbi.nlm.nih.gov/gene?Db=gene&Cmd=DetailsSearch&Term=32158

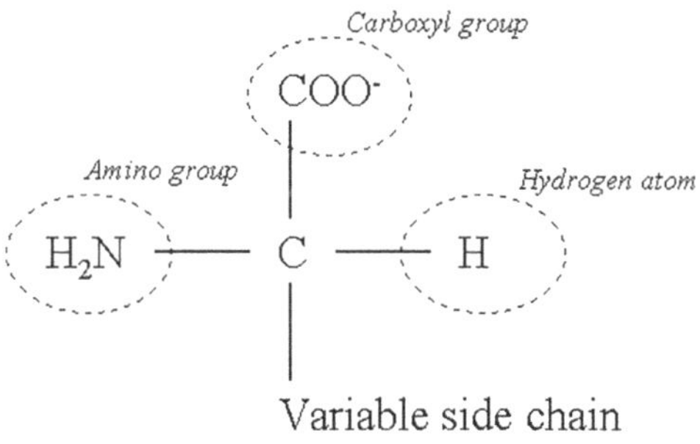

Fig. 2.3 Generic structure of an amino acid

Table 2.1 Amino acid nomenclature

Name	Three-letter code	One-letter code
Alanine	Ala	A
Cysteine	Cys	C
Aspartate	Asp	D
Glutamate	Glu	E
Phenylalanine	Phe	F
Glycine	Gly	G
Histidine	His	H
Isoleucine	Ile	I
Lysine	Lys	K
Leucine	Leu	L
Methionine	Met	M
Asparagine	Asn	N
Proline	Pro	P
Glutamine	Gln	Q
Arginine	Arg	R
Serine	Ser	S
Threonine	Thr	T
Valine	Val	V
Tryptophane	Trp	W
Tyrosine	Tyr	Y

Amino acids are molecules consisting of a central carbon atom attached to four chemical groups; an *amino group* (-NH_2); a *carboxyl group* (-COO^-); a hydrogen atom; and a variable side chain (Fig. 2.3). The variable side chain determines the physical, chemical and electrical characteristics of the amino acid.

Each amino acid has both a three-letter and a one-letter designation and a name (Table 2.1).

mRNA is read by the cellular machinery in groups of three bases, referred to as *codons*. Each codon codes for a single amino acid. Since there are 64 ways to combine four letters into groups of three, but far fewer amino acids, there is considerable redundancy in the genetic code, with many amino acids being coded for by more than one codon (Table 2.2). In addition to the codons representing amino acids, there is one start codon, which signals the cellular machinery to commence transcription

Table 2.2 The genetic code, organized by middle letter, then first letter, then third letter

T	C	G	A
Phe: TTT	Ser: TCT	Cys: TGT	Tyr: TAT
Phe: TTC	Ser: TCC	Cys: TGC	Tyr: TAC
Leu: TTG	Ser: TCG	Trp: TGG	Stop: TAG
Leu: TTA	Ser: TCA	Stop: TGA	Stop: TAA
Leu: CTT	Pro: CCT	Arg: CGT	His: CAT
Leu: CTC	Pro: CCC	Arg: CGC	His: CAC
Leu: CTG	Pro: CCG	Arg: CGG	Gln: CAG
Leu: CTA	Pro: CCA	Arg: CGA	Gln: CAA
Val: GTT	Ala: GCT	Gly: GGT	Asp: GAT
Val: GTC	Ala: GCC	Gly: GGC	Asp: GAC
Val: GTG	Ala: GCG	Gly: GGG	Glu: GAG
Val: GTA	Ala: GCA	Gly: GGA	Glu: GAA
Ile: ATT	Thr: ACT	Ser: AGT	Asn: AAT
Ile: ATC	Thr: ACC	Ser: AGC	Asn: AAC
Met: ATG	Thr: ACG	Arg: AGG	Lys: AAG
Ile: ATA	Thr: ACA	Arg: AGA	Lys: AAA

of a gene, and three stop codons (in general; recent research has indicated that this is not always true in a small number of cases). Premature termination codons (PTCs) cause ~10–20% of inherited diseases, and are involved in cancer [17].

When the genetic code was first cracked in the 1960s it appeared that the genome coded for 20 amino acids. More than these 20 do occur in proteins, but some "non-standard" amino acids are formed from the genomically encoded ones by chemical modifications following translation. There is order in the way in which codons are used (Table 2.2); it is clear that in the course of evolution codons have not been associated with amino acids at random.

Table 2.2 is laid out in such a way as to make these regularities more apparent. Each column of the table contains codons whose middle position is identical. Within a column, the rows are ordered by first position, then by second position. The third base in a triplet is sometimes known as the "wobble base" because mutation in this position is least likely to affect the amino acid coded for. As can be seen in the table, codons coding for the same amino acid tend to cluster together.

The regularities go further than that, though. The first column of the table contains amino acids with hydrophobic (water repelling) residues in the variable side chain; the second column lists amino acids with small side chain residues; the third group have residues which are mutated comparatively rarely, and the right-hand column contains amino acids with hydrophilic (water loving) residues. The code is highly error tolerant, both because it is redundant and because similar codons code for amino acids with similar chemical properties, meaning that many mutations have minimal effect on the chemical properties on the resulting protein.

It might be expected that the alternative codons coding for a single amino acid are selectively neutral; that is, that one codon has no selective advantage over its alternatives. In this case all codons for a single amino acid should be more-or-less equally represented in the genome. This does not appear to be the case. In some genomes some codons are favored over others which code for the same amino acid, a situation known as *codon usage bias*.

The most striking patterns of codon usage bias occur in unicellular organisms, probably because their very large population sizes allow very weak selection pressures to be effective. There tends to be preferential usage of codons which bind more efficiently to the transfer tRNA, or which are recognized by a more abundant tRNA, particularly in highly expressed genes. These codons probably have slightly higher translational efficiency than their alternatives and therefore have a small selective advantage.

The "universal" genetic code depicted in Table 2.2 has been modified slightly by a few organisms. For example, in some species of starfish, the codons UGA and AGR specify Trp and Ser, respectively, when they occur in mitochondrial mRNA, but the same codons specify Stop and Arg in nuclear mRNA. In a few organisms with small genomes, rarely used codons are permanently reassigned. This variation in the code appears to have arisen in the course of evolution from an ancestor using the "default" code. There is no evidence that this differential codon usage reflects a different evolutionary origin for the organisms involved.

RNA to Protein: Translation

One of the major challenges of computational biology has long been "how do we determine protein structure from a DNA sequence?" Protein structure has traditionally been determined using X-ray crystallography, a process in which proteins are crystallized and thensubjected to a beam of X-rays. The resulting diffraction pattern is then analyzed to determine the structure of the crystal. This process has several problems. The process of creating protein crystals is time consuming, expensive, and requires considerable skills and specialized equipment. Not all proteins can be coaxed into forming crystals. Protein structure, particularly that of protein complexes, can be complex and hard to determine. And finally, many proteins are dynamic, folding, unfolding, and refolding repeatedly, with different conformations potentially performing different tasks within the cell.

RNA is translated into protein on ribosomes in the cytoplasm. The RNA is read linearly, commencing with a start codon. Each codon is read in turn, and the corresponding amino acid added to the end of the growing amino acid chain, until a stop codon is encountered.

At the stop codon the amino acid string detaches from the ribosome. It then folds and refolds into a complex three-dimensional protein whose structure is determined by short-range and long-range physical and chemical interactions between the amino acids themselves, and between the protein and the cellular environment. An overview of the entire process of producing a protein from information contained in the DNA is illustrated in Fig. 2.4.

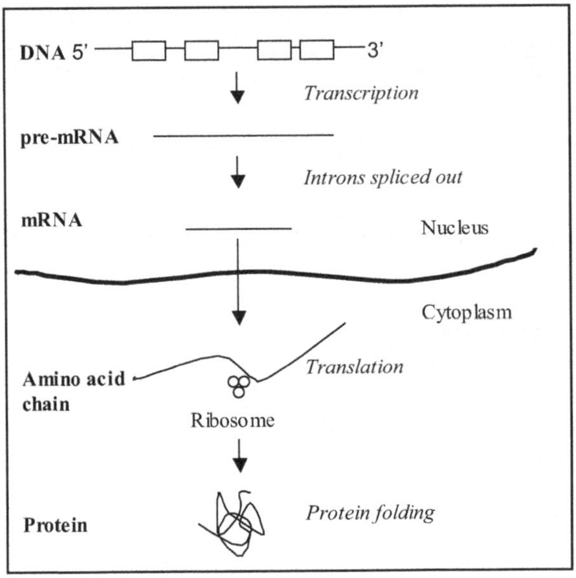

Fig. 2.4 The path from gene to protein

Twist and Shout: The Problem of Protein Folding

The activity of most proteins is critically dependent upon their final shape, as well as their amino acid composition. For a protein to interact with other proteins, DNA, or other molecules, it must possess the correct three-dimensional shape, with the appropriate amino acids positioned at the right place on the protein surface. Protein folding occurs in stages. The initial amino acid chain initially folds into structures such as helices and sheets, forming the *two-dimensional structure*. The two-dimensional structure then folds into the final *tertiary structure* of the protein.

Protein folding occurs spontaneously within the cell. The process is known to involve long-distance as well as local interactions between amino acids, and sometimes the assistance of helper or *chaperone* proteins, but is far from understood in detail. Much work has gone into the development of computer algorithms for the prediction of protein 3D structure from the amino acid sequence information. For many years, the prediction of the 3D structure of a protein from its DNA sequence was considered to be a major challenge in bioinformatics. In 2020, however, DeepMind announced the development of an AI algorithm called AlphaFold, which could carry out structure prediction with considerable success. By mid 2021, AlphaFold had been used to predict the structure of 95.8% of human proteins, and by 2022 it had been used to predict the structures of nearly all the proteins stored in the UniProt database; more than 200 million proteins. This use of AI has the potential to significantly affect the field of bioinformatics, particularly in drug discovery and design. Since AlphaFold was developed, several other successful protein structure algorithms have been developed; some of these are covered in more detail in Chap. 5.

Although the majority of proteins fold spontaneously and correctly within the cell, the process does occasionally go awry. Protein misfolding can cause disease, and many such diseases have devastating results. The most notorious disease caused by protein misfolding is undoubtedly Bovine Spongiform Encephalopathy (BSE, or Mad Cow Disease) and its human form, Creutzfeld-Jacob Disease (CJD). Related diseases also occur naturally in sheep, deer and mink, and can be transmitted experimentally to rodents, pigs and primates.

CJD appears to be caused by the abnormal folding of a protein called the prion protein (PrP) which is part of the usual protein complement of an organism. In familial forms of the disease the patient has inherited a mutation in PrP which predisposes it to abnormal folding. The so-called variant CJD (vCJD) appears to be induced by the consumption of the abnormal form of the protein. It appears that eating meat from cattle affected with BSE can lead to vCJD in humans with a normal PrP gene. Abnormally folded PrP is not broken down by most cooking procedures or by the digestive process. It is absorbed into the bloodstream and transported to cells in the central nervous system. There the abnormally folded PrP binds to the normal protein and induces it to fold the "wrong" way. The presence of misfolded PrP leads to a cascade of protein refolding and the formation of *amyloid plaques* in the brain, leading to behavioral changes, dementia and eventually death. There is currently no treatment for CJD.

CJD is remarkable because it is the first disease believed to be caused by an infectious agent which is not based on DNA or RNA. The very idea of an infectious protein was extremely controversial when it was first proposed. The further suggestion that the protein in question was causing infections via the food chain, through the consumption of cattle infected with BSE provoked intense debate. The term "prion", together with the theory that these degenerative brain diseases were caused by misfolded proteins, were put forward by Stanley B. Prusiner, of the University of California, San Francisco School of Medicine, in 1982, and was initially roundly rejected. In 1997 Prusiner won the Nobel Prize in Physiology or Medicine for his discovery.

The Gene Genie

A stretch of DNA delimited by a start codon and a stop codon is an *open reading frame* (ORF) or *gene*. Not all DNA gives rise to proteins. In eukaryotes there are long stretches of non-protein-coding DNA between genes. Recent work suggests that much of the non-coding DNA is transcribed into mRNA but not translated into protein. There are several types of non-protein-coding RNA, which play a range of roles within the cell. Mutations and other forms of modification of these RNA systems can lead to a range of diseases, including cancer [18].

The concept of a "gene" is becoming less clear cut as we learn more about the way in which the cell operates. It was originally believed that a gene was a stretch of DNA coding for a single protein, which had a clear-cut role in the functioning of the cell: as a transport molecule, perhaps, or as a structural protein. Information flow was perceived as strictly one-way, from DNA through RNA to protein. For a long

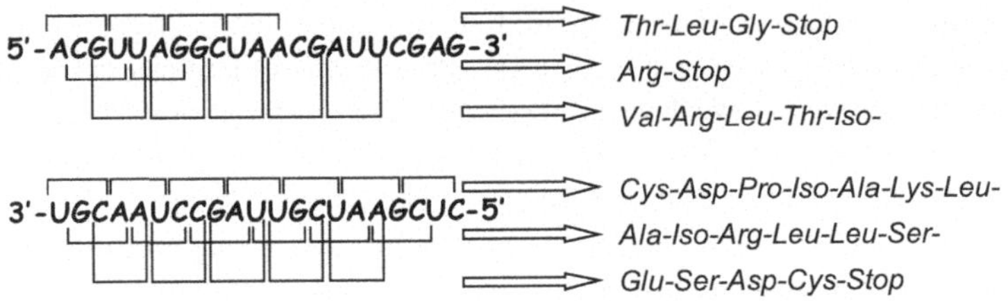

Fig. 2.5 Six possible alternative reading frames for RNA generated by a double-stranded DNA molecule Eukaryotes, however, appear to be much more profligate with their DNA

time, this was the Central Dogma of genetics and could be summarized as "one gene: one protein".

More recently, it has become apparent that the process of protein production is not so straightforward. This finding should come as no surprise; the various genome sequencing projects have demonstrated that most organisms examined have many fewer genes in the genome than there are proteins in the proteome. It is now clear that a single "gene" may give rise to dozens or even hundreds of proteins, many of which may bear no chemical or structural relationship to each other. There are several mechanisms leading to the production of multiple proteins from a single gene.

Prokaryotes, with their small circular chromosomes, generally pack genes in closely, and can even increase the effective number of genes in the genome by using a different reading frame on the same sequence to generate different proteins. Since the code for a single amino acid consists of three bases, a stretch of double stranded DNA may be read in any of six *reading frames*, three on one strand and three on the other (Fig. 2.5).

In addition to differential splicing, mRNA may undergo *RNA editing*, in which the RNA sequence is altered by the deletion, addition or substitution of bases. Overall, the basics of DNA transcription and translation, and the production of proteins, appears to be relatively straightforward. However, many of the details of molecular biology are complex and context dependent. AI has the potential to assist with the process of understanding these details in ways which have not been possible to date.

Summary

Most of the molecular details described above were elucidated without the aid of computation, and certainly without the use of AI (Table 2.3).

It is clear from Table 2.3 that most of the major advances in the development of AI occurred after the basics of molecular biology were understood. These basics were elucidated by a process of experimentation on so-called *model organisms* and required considerable time and skill. There used to be, in my working life, a saying: "one gene, one PhD" reflecting the fact that understanding the structure and

Table 2.3 A timeline of developments in molecular biology

Date	Achievement	Role of computation	Notes	Reference
1953	Structure of DNA	X-ray crystallography		[19]
1958	Central dogma	None	Now discredited	[20]
1958	Role of RNA	None		[20]
1958	Transcription	None	Beautiful comment at the end of Watson and Crick's paper	[19]
1958	Translation	None		[21]
1958	*First artificial neural networks*			[22]
1960s	*Evolutionary computation developed*		*Earlier work was done, but this is a classic reference*	[23]
1961	Genetic code	None	Link between codons and amino acids	[24]
1965	Role of non-coding RNA	None	First non-coding RNA described	[25]
1970	*Backpropagation algorithm for ANNs*		*Enabled ANNs to learn to solve nonlinear problems*	[26]
1971	*PCs developed*		*John Blankenbaker's Kenbak-1*	*https://www.computerhistory.org/revolution/personal-computers/17/297*
1973	Protein folding	None	However, AI currently widely used for this application	[27]
1977	Introns/exons	None	And other challenges to the "gene" concept	[28]
1996	Epigenetics	None	Actually earlier, but much dispute over terminology	[29]
2003	Human genome project completed	Algorithms for sequence assembly		https://www.genome.gov/human-genome-project
2015	*Deep learning developed*			[30]
2022	*Large language models developed*			[31]

Most of these dates are approximate
Lines in italics indicate important developments in AI

function of a single gene could take 3 years or more. Currently, new genes are being identified and characterized on a routine, daily basis. I have a colleague who sequences and assigns a preliminary function to multiple genes on a fishing boat off the coast of Scotland.[5]

In the rest of this book various authors describe the use of AI in a range of biological fields. While these algorithms are rapidly changing the face of the field, there are a few caveats which must be borne in mind. One is the tendency of some algorithms, particularly large language models, to *hallucinate*, producing reasonable sounding but completely non-existent results in some cases. This problem is made worse by the ease of use of many AI algorithms. Users tend to assume that default parameter values are acceptable, and accept the results generated without really understanding the algorithms they are using. One of the aims of this book is to rectify this issue, by providing an overview of the algorithms, with examples of how they can be used.

Molecular biology is a complex subject, although the basics are straightforward. However, this complexity becomes evident when we consider diseases which arise from malfunctioning of the cell. AI can be used to further our understanding of the workings of cells in sickness and in health, but must be used with care and understanding.

References

1. Costello, M.J., Wilson, S., and Houlding, B.: 'Predicting total global species richness using rates of species description and estimates of taxonomic effort', Systematic Biology, 2012, 61, (5), pp. 871
2. Locey, K.J., and Lennon, J.T.: 'Scaling laws predict global microbial diversity', Proceedings of the National Academy of Sciences, 2016, 113, (21), pp. 5970–5975
3. Mora, C., Tittensor, D.P., Adl, S., Simpson, A.G., and Worm, B.: 'How many species are there on Earth and in the ocean?', PLoS Biology, 2011, 9(8), pp. e1001127
4. Costello, M.J., May, R.M., and Stork, N.E.: 'Can we name Earth's species before they go extinct?', Science, 2013, 339, (6118), pp. 413–416
5. Weiss, M.C., Sousa, F.L., Mrnjavac, N., Neukirchen, S., Roettger, M., Nelson-Sathi, S., and Martin, W.F.: 'The physiology and habitat of the last universal common ancestor', Nature microbiology, 2016, 1, (9), pp. 1–8
6. Margulis, L.: 'Five-kingdom classification and the origin and evolution of cells': 'Evolutionary Biology: Volume 7' (Springer, 1974), pp. 45–78
7. Woese, C.R., Magrum, L.J., and Fox, G.E.: 'Archaebacteria', Journal of Molecular Evolution, 1978, 11, pp. 245–252
8. Makarova, K.S., Aravind, L., Wolf, Y.I., Tatusov, R.L., Minton, K.W., Koonin, E.V., and Daly, M.J.: 'Genome of the extremely radiation-resistant bacterium *Deinococcus radiodurans* viewed from the perspective of comparative genomics', Microbiology and Molecular Biology Reviews, 2001, 65, (1), pp. 44–79
9. Li, Y.: 'Modern epigenetics methods in biological research', Methods, 2021, 187, pp. 104–113

[5] To the best of my knowledge, the gene for seasickness has not yet been identified.

10. Feinberg, A.P., and Levchenko, A.: 'Epigenetics as a mediator of plasticity in cancer', Science, 2023, 379, (6632), pp. eaaw3835
11. Migliore, L., and Coppedè, F.: 'Gene–environment interactions in Alzheimer disease: the emerging role of epigenetics', Nature Reviews Neurology, 2022, 18, (11), pp. 643–660
12. Mahmoud, A.M.: 'An overview of epigenetics in obesity: the role of lifestyle and therapeutic interventions', International Journal of Molecular Sciences, 2022, 23, (3), pp. 1341
13. Ntontsi, P., Photiades, A., Zervas, E., Xanthou, G., and Samitas, K.: 'Genetics and epigenetics in asthma', International Journal of Molecular Sciences, 2021, 22, (5), pp. 2412
14. Soto-Palma, C., Niedernhofer, L.J., Faulk, C.D., and Dong, X.: 'Epigenetics, DNA damage, and aging', The Journal of cCinical Investigation, 2022, 132, (16)
15. Planterose Jiménez, B., Liu, F., Caliebe, A., Montiel González, D., Bell, J.T., Kayser, M., and Vidaki, A.: 'Equivalent DNA methylation variation between monozygotic co-twins and unrelated individuals reveals universal epigenetic inter-individual dissimilarity', Genome Biology, 2021, 22, pp. 1–23
16. Cheng, M., Conley, D., Kuipers, T., Li, C., Ryan, C.P., Taeubert, M.J., Wang, S., Wang, T., Zhou, J., and Schmitz, L.L.: 'Accelerated biological aging six decades after prenatal famine exposure', Proceedings of the National Academy of Sciences, 2024, 121, (24), pp. e2319179121
17. Toledano, I., Supek, F., and Lehner, B.: 'Genome-scale quantification and prediction of pathogenic stop codon readthrough by small molecules', Nature Genetics, 2024, 56, (9), pp. 1914–1924
18. Nemeth, K., Bayraktar, R., Ferracin, M., and Calin, G.A.: 'Non-coding RNAs in disease: from mechanisms to therapeutics', Nature Reviews Genetics, 2024, 25, (3), pp. 211–232
19. Watson, J.D., and Crick, F.H.C.: 'Molecular structure of nucleic acids: A structure for Deoxyribose Nucleic Acid', Nature, 1953, 171, (4356), pp. 737–738
20. Crick, F.H.: 'On protein synthesis', Symposium of the Society for Experimental Biology, 1958, 12, (138–63), pp. 8
21. Hoagland, M.B., Stephenson, M.L., Scott, J.F., Hecht, L.I., and Zamecnik, P.C.: 'A soluble ribonucleic acid intermediate in protein synthesis', Journal of Biological Chemistry, 1958, 231, (1), pp. 241–257
22. Rosenblatt, F.: 'The perceptron: a probabilistic model for information storage and organization in the brain', Psychological Review, 1958, 65, (6), pp. 386
23. Holland, J.: 'Adaptation in natural and artificial systems' (MIT Press, 1975. 1975)
24. Crick, F.H.C., Barnett, L., Brenner, S., and Watts-Tobin, R.J.: 'General nature of the genetic code for proteins', Nature, 1961, 4809, pp. 1227–1232
25. Holley, R.W., Apgar, J., Everett, G.A., Madison, J.T., Marquisee, M., Merrill, S.H., Penswick, J.R., and Zamir, A.: 'Structure of a ribonucleic acid', Science, 1965, 147, (3664), pp. 1462–1465
26. Linnainmaa, S.: 'The representation of the cumulative rounding error of an algorithm as a Taylor expansion of the local rounding errors', University of Helsinki, 1970
27. Anfinsen, C.B.: 'Principles that govern the folding of protein chains', Science, 1973, 181, (4096), pp. 223–230
28. Berget, S.M., Moore, C., and Sharp, P.A.: 'Spliced segments at the 5′ terminus of adenovirus 2 late mRNA', Proceedings of the National Academy of Sciences, 1977, 74, (8), pp. 3171–3175
29. Riggs, A.D., and Porter, T.N.: 'Overview of epigenetic mechanisms', in Russo, V.E.A., Martienssen, R., and Riggs, A.D. (Eds.): 'Epigenetic Mechanisms of Gene Regulation' (Cold Spring Harbor Laboratory Press, 1996), pp. 29–45
30. LeCun, Y., Bengio, Y., and Hinton, G.: 'Deep learning', Nature, 2015, 521, pp. 436–444
31. Wei, J., Tay, Y., Bommasani, R., Raffel, C., Zoph, B., Borgeaud, S., Yogatama, D., Bosma, M., Zhou, D., and Metzler, D.: 'Emergent abilities of large language models', arXiv preprint arXiv:2206.07682, 2022

Chapter 3
Natural Language Understanding, Large Language Models and Application to Genetic Diseases and Healthcare

Sonika Tyagi

Abstract Natural Language Processing (NLP), is revolutionizing healthcare and genetic research by enabling machines to comprehend and analyze English text generated from diverse sources. Recent advancements in large language models (LLMs), such as BioGPT and BioBERT, have significantly enhanced the ability to extract, interpret, and synthesize information from vast biomedical datasets. These models excel at tasks such as named entity recognition, information retrieval, relationship extraction, and summarization, making them invaluable for applications in healthcare and genetic diseases.

In genetic research, LLMs facilitate the identification of gene-disease associations, interpretation of genomic variants, and the integration of data from scientific literature with clinical databases. In healthcare, they support personalized medicine by linking genetic information with electronic health records, aiding in disease diagnosis, risk prediction, and treatment planning.

LLMs can process unstructured data from diverse sources, accelerate discoveries in genomics and healthcare, and improve patient outcomes. However, challenges such as model interpretability, bias or imbalance in training data, hallucination, large computing requirements, lack of standardized benchmarks, and the ensuring of data privacy persist. Ethical considerations must guide the integration of these models into clinical practice.

The aim of this chapter is to:

1. Explain the basic principles of NLP and its relevance in processing and analyzing unstructured text in healthcare and genetics.
2. Understand the application of NLP in the biology and healthcare domains.
3. Explore a pipeline to process unstructured text into structured ones for downstream applications.
4. Explore state-of-the-art NLP techniques (e.g., named entity recognition, relationship extraction, and deep learning models) in the context of genetic and clinical research.

S. Tyagi (✉)
School of Computing Technologies, RMIT University, Melbourne, VIC, Australia
e-mail: sonika.tyagi@rmit.edu.au

M. Chetty, J. Hallinan (eds.), *From Algorithms to Ailments*,
https://doi.org/10.1007/978-3-032-11023-7_3

Introduction to NLP in Healthcare

Overview of NLP, NLU and NLG and Their Evolution

Natural Language Processing (NLP), is a field intersecting artificial intelligence (AI) and 'linguistics' and is devoted to making computers understand statements or words written in human language. NLP can be classified into two parts: Natural Language Understanding (NLU), and Natural Language Generation (NLG), dealing with the tasks of understanding and generating a text, respectively. NLP's key applications are in the area of text classification [36–39], tokenization and lemmatization [39, 40], named entity recognition (NER) [1–3], speech-to-text and text-to-speech systems [41–43], relation extraction [4–7], and information retrieval [8, 9]. NLU is a subset of NLP that focuses specifically on interpreting the meaning and intent behind text or speech. NLU involves understanding context, semantics, and syntactical relationships to extract actionable insights. NLU is applied to tasks such as sentiment and emotion analysis, chatbots and virtual assistants (e.g., understanding user queries), semantic search and question-answering systems, automatic summarization, and context-aware machine translation. NLG focuses on the creation of human-like text from structured or unstructured data. It aims to generate coherent, contextually relevant, and linguistically accurate text outputs. NLG is frequently used for generating reports, articles, and summaries, conversational agents and personalized responses, data-to-text systems such as transforming numerical data into narratives, and creative writing.

Evolution of NLP, NLU, and NLG

Early NLP approaches (1950s–1980s) relied on rule-based approaches; for example: ELIZA, a rule-based chatbot (1966) [10], linguistic theories, and symbolic AI [44]. These systems used dictionaries, grammar rules, and expert knowledge. They were structured, transparent, and effective in domain-specific tasks, with the added advantage of not requiring large datasets. However, they struggled with handling ambiguity, adapting to variability, and scaling to broader or more complex language contexts. In the late 1980s statistical methods like Hidden Markov Models (HMMs) and n-grams introduced probabilistic approaches [45], improving language modeling and text classification. The Machine Learning (ML) era (1990s–2010s) introduced algorithms that could learn and improve from experience. NLP tasks began leveraging labeled datasets and ML algorithms such as Support Vector Machines (SVMs) and decision trees for tasks like text classification and NER. Models like Word2Vec [11] and GloVe [12] revolutionized NLP by introducing vector-based word representations and capturing semantic relationships. Context-free grammar parsing and early sentiment analysis systems also emerged during this period, driving advancements in understanding language intent. Early NLG systems generated text through template-based methods, but these lacked flexibility and generalization. The deep learning revolution (2010s–present) introduced the application of neural networks (NN) for NLP. NN architectures such as RNNs [13], LSTMs [13], and CNNs [14] allowed for better sequence modeling, enabling breakthroughs in various NLP applications. The invention of the Transformer architecture [15] introduced models like BERT [16], GPT [17], and T5 [18]. These models use self-attention mechanisms to process long-range context across sentences and documents, significantly improving NLU and NLG capabilities [28–31].

Pre-training on massive corpora followed by fine-tuning for specific tasks soon became the dominant paradigm, leading to state-of-the-art performance in NLP. Modern NLG systems such as GPT-3 and ChatGPT generate coherent and contextually appropriate text, enabling creative, context-sensitive applications. Models like GPT-4 and PaLM integrate NLP, NLU, and NLG capabilities in a seamless framework, improving multi-task and multi-modal performance. Pre-trained models now handle new tasks with minimal or no additional training, reducing dependence on labeled data.

Thus, the evolution of NLP, NLU, and NLG reflects a transition from rule-based approaches to sophisticated, data-driven systems capable of understanding and generating human-like language with unprecedented accuracy and fluency. Current efforts focused on making AI systems more interpretable are helping to address ethical and transparency challenges. Applications in the healthcare, legal, and financial sectors have been driving advancements in domain-specific NLP systems [19]. The integration of language with vision, audio, and other modalities is further expanding the scope of NLP research and applications [46, 47].

Relevance of NLP in Healthcare and Genetic Research

The application of NLP in healthcare and genetic research involves the analysis and extraction of valuable insights from vast amounts of unstructured textual data. Its ability to process clinical narratives, research papers, and genetic annotations has the potential to drive new innovations in diagnostics, personalized medicine, and biomedical discovery.

NLP in Healthcare

NLP is being used in healthcare for extracting valuable insights from unstructured Electronic Health Records (EHRs), enabling the identification of symptoms, diagnoses, treatments, and disease trends. It supports population-level health analysis and enhances Clinical Decision Support Systems (CDSS) by summarizing patient histories and clinical guidelines, and providing real-time analytics [48, 49].

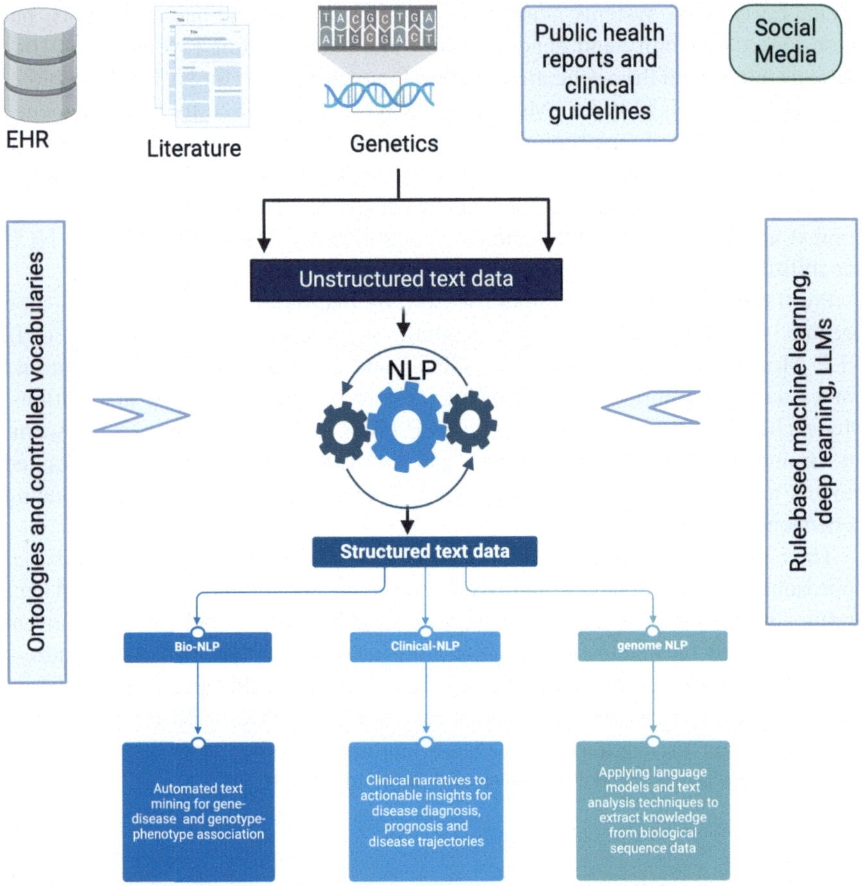

Fig. 3.1 Illustration of applications of NLP in genetic research and healthcare

Converting unstructured clinical narratives into a structured format suitable for AI applications can enhance diagnosis and decision-making by integrating them with other digital health data (Fig. 3.1). To achieve this aim, it is essential to accurately translate these narratives while maintaining the integrity of the medical vocabulary and underlying semantics.

NLP is also being used for disease surveillance by monitoring health trends through data from EHR, Telehealth platforms, wearable devices, environmental and social media, and identifying early epidemic signals from global reports [50, 51]. Recent advancements aim to enhance patient engagement by simplifying complex medical language into patient-friendly terms and automating responses through chatbots, improving communication. This approach also helps to save hours of waiting time and, in some cases, completely avoids hospital queues. NLP is also enhancing clinical trial management by extracting relevant data from trial registries and identifying eligible patients for studies through EHR mining [20–22]. This practice streamlines patient recruitment and ensures more efficient trial execution.

NLP in Genetic Research

The sheer volume of research articles makes it difficult to stay updated on new findings. Similarly, understanding the genetic basis of diseases involves linking genes to phenotypes, and is a complex task. NLP addresses these challenges in genetic research by efficiently extracting gene-disease associations from scientific articles, identifying biomarkers and therapeutic targets, and mapping gene-phenotype relationships through database and literature mining [52]. It is being used in prioritizing genes for research, parsing clinical narratives to extract ontology terms (HPO) for rare disease diagnosis, automating variant annotation, and enhancing precision in identifying pathogenic mutations.

Thus, NLP improves the efficiency and scalability of both healthcare and genetic research by automating labor-intensive processes such as manual curation and annotation and enabling large-scale analyses. Extracting actionable insights from combined unstructured and structured data accelerates discovery and innovation through holistic analysis. However, poor data quality, including variability, imbalance and noise in clinical and genetic data and the lack of transparency in NLP models poses challenges for sensitive applications [61]. Addressing biases in datasets that may lead to unfair outcomes and enhancing model interpretability for clinical trust is of utmost importance. Future work focuses on developing models tailored to healthcare and genetics and enabling real-time clinical and research insights. NLP has huge potential to unlock the value of unstructured data, advancing precision medicine, improving patient care, and accelerating biomedical discoveries.

Data and Information

Big Genomic Data

Advancements in technology have led to the generation of vast amounts of genetic and genomic data through various research and development activities. This data spans multiple omics types, including data from genes (genomics), RNA (transcriptomics), proteins (proteomics), and metabolites (metabolomics). Large-scale Genome-Wide Association Studies (GWAS) now provide insights into the association between genetic variants (genotypes) and disease phenotypes. Such data, available across diverse tissue types, disease conditions, and populations, is driving biomarker discovery and fostering innovation in precision medicine.

Genomic Databases and Ontologies

This explosion of genomic data from high-throughput sequencing technologies has necessitated organized repositories and tools for effective management, access, and analysis. Genomic databases and ontologies provide the infrastructure for storing, standardizing, and interpreting this data, enabling advancements in genomics research and biomarker discovery [53].

Genomic databases serve as centralized repositories for diverse types of genomic information, including sequences, annotations, variants, and functional data. They facilitate data sharing, large-scale analyses, and reproducibility in research. Specialized databases organize and store data from various omics fields and provide tools for searching, visualization, and analysis. Some common examples include GenBank and Ensembl (primary sequence repositories), dbSNP (a database for single nucleotide polymorphisms or SNPs), GTEx (Genotype-Tissue Expression) and ClinVar (a repository for clinically significant genetic variants) [81]. Matched data across multi-omics studies that enables integration across studies for a system level understanding of the biological system is being made available [58–60].

Ontologies in genomics provide structured controlled vocabularies and relationships to describe genes, phenotypes, biological processes, and diseases. They standardize terminology, facilitate interoperability, and enhance data integration and analysis. The ontologies help define concepts and their relationships in a machine-readable format, which in turn facilitates the semantic integration of data across databases to support computational analyses and knowledge discovery [54]. Some of the commonly used ones are: (1) Gene ontologies (GO), that provide structured controlled vocabularies for the annotation of gene products with respect to their molecular function, cellular component, and biological role; (2) International Statistical Classification of Diseases and Related Health Problems (ICD); (3) Human Phenotype Ontology (HPO); (4) The Systematized Nomenclature of Medicine Clinical Term (SNOMED); and (5) Medical Subject Headings (MeSH).

Over the years, genomic databases and ontologies have been instrumental in harmonizing data across studies, data types, and repositories. This melding enables integrative analysis, cross-validation of results from diverse data sources, and the standardization of interoperable ML processes. However, the adoption of ontologies remains slow, and automated batch processing of new data types continues to present challenges in data harmonization.

Genomic and Genetic Data Representations

Genomic and genetic data are represented in various forms to enable storage, analysis, and interpretation (https://genome.ucsc.edu/FAQ/FAQformat.html). These representations capture different levels of biological information, from raw sequences to complex annotations, relationships, and interactions. The most basic form of genetic data consists of nucleotide sequences. The primary sequences are stored as text files in one of the standard FASTA or FASTQ formats [55]. These primary sequences can be further processed by aligning to a reference genome and producing secondary formats such as BAM or SAM file formats. These are commonly used formats for identifying variants, structural changes, and gene expression levels. Another standard secondary format is the VCF or Variant Call Format that is used to represent differences in DNA, and structural variants. Further annotation of sequence data adds information about genes, regulatory elements, and functional regions. The GFF/GTF and BED file formats are used to represent such annotations.

Effective representation of genomic and genetic data is crucial for enabling precise analysis, fostering interoperability, and advancing research across genomics and personalized medicine. Multi-omics data integration requires the representation of information in standardized formats for combining genomics, transcriptomics, proteomics, and metabolomics data. This combination facilitates a system-level understanding of biological processes and disease mechanisms.

Healthcare Data and Electronic Health Records

An EHR contains a large amount of patient-related data, including both structured information (demographics, vital signs, lab results) and unstructured textual data (clinical notes, discharge summaries, referral letters). While structured data provides essential markers for tracking a patient's clinical progression, unstructured data in the form of free-text notes offers a wealth of detailed information about a patient's medical history, interventions, and lifestyle habits [56, 57]. This rich content has led to the development of advanced applications such as concept extraction, patient trajectory modeling, disease inference, and clinical decision support systems [62].

However, unstructured EHR data presents challenges due to its subjective nature and variability in documentation styles across institutions and individual preferences. Because EHRs are primarily designed for clinical care, not research, rigorous quality control procedures are required to ensure data accuracy and consistency for effective use of these data in research [68]. These efforts are crucial for generating reliable research outcomes. There are also several technical challenges related to analytics, cybersecurity, data infrastructure, and ethical and legal considerations that need to be resolved before EHR data can be utilized for research [61].

Technical Implementation of NLP in Biomedical Research

NLP is driving advancements and making a substantial impact across three key areas of research.

Bio-NLP

Bio-NLP facilitates genomic data retrieval and interpretation by mining the genetic literature, identifying variants and biomarkers, supporting gene-disease association studies, and analyzing genetic annotations (Fig. 3.1). NLP has demonstrated success in detecting rare diseases through text mining and automated analysis [64]. Ontologies like HPO and SNOMED are used to extract phenotypes, enabling case-based reasoning and aiding the diagnosis of rare and undiagnosed diseases.

Clinical NLP

Clinical NLP involves extracting valuable insights from unstructured textual data in EHRs, the medical literature, and patient-generated content (Fig. 3.1). Extracting psychosocial factors, comorbidities, and adherence patterns from narrative notes, when integrated with structured data, can be used for comprehensive modeling [69]. Predictive models leverage this data to forecast health outcomes, identify risks, and support proactive decision-making in healthcare. Successful application of clinical NLP involves predicting the likelihood of disease development based on an individual patient's history. This process extracts risk factors from clinical notes, discharge summaries, and lifestyle information, and, where possible, integrates social determinants of health from unstructured data [70, 71]. This information can also be used for analyzing temporal trends in clinical notes and lab reports and use it to identify early indicators of deterioration or improvement. Detecting mentions of allergies, side effects, or contraindications in clinical text enables proactive measures through real-time monitoring [73]. Identifying predictors of response based on personalized data can be used to predict and prevent potential adverse events or complications.

Clinical genetics also leverages NLP to extract valuable insights from unstructured clinical notes. Key applications include processing text to identify genetic information, extracting family history and pedigrees, linking phenotypic data to genetic conditions, and using NLP tools to support genetic counseling, enhancing precision and efficiency in genetic research and patient care.

Genome NLP

In recent years, NLP has been increasingly applied in genomics, leveraging DNA, RNA, and protein sequences, which can be represented as text (Fig. 3.1). Genome language modeling (GLM) is particularly promising, as it uses NLP techniques to process genomic sequences similarly to natural language [72]. GLM treats genetic sequences as a "language" with its own syntax and semantics, enabling the interpretation and prediction of genetic features directly from sequence data. While the "grammar" of genomics and the structure of its "words" are less obvious than those in natural language, this approach provides valuable insights. Despite these challenges, GLM has the potential to enhance our understanding of biological grammar and significantly advance genomic research.

Techniques Used in Clinical and Bio NLP for Predictive Modeling

Named Entity Recognition (NER)

Biomedical Named Entity Recognition (NER) is a key task in natural language processing, focusing on identifying and classifying entities such as diseases, genes, proteins, chemicals, and drugs in biomedical text. It identifies key entities such as diseases, medications and symptoms in unstructured text for use in models. Various techniques are used for biomedical NER, ranging from traditional rule-based methods to advanced deep learning approaches. Traditional dictionary-based and rule-based methods provide high precision, but are constrained by their dependence on exact string matching and predefined patterns, such as regular expressions and biomedical terminologies [76, 77]. In contrast, modern machine learning approaches overcome these limitations by leveraging feature learning models and classification algorithms such as Conditional Random Fields (CRFs), Hidden Markov Models (HMMs), and Support Vector Machines (SVMs). These approaches rely on handcrafted features, including word embeddings, part-of-speech tags, and lexical information, and require labeled datasets for effective training. More recently, LSTM and CNN architectures combined with softmax or CRF layers became popular. However, the introduction of large language models (LLM), built on the Transformer architecture and trained on extensive corpora, has significantly advanced the field. For example, SciBERT [23] is a pre-trained language model specifically designed for scientific text. It is based on the BERT (Bidirectional Encoder Representations from Transformers) architecture and is fine-tuned on a large corpus of scientific literature. NER can then be performed using the pretrained model.

Relation Extraction

Relation Extraction (RE) is a key task in NLP that focuses on identifying and extracting entities along with the relationships between them from textual data. Specifically, RE tasks often deal with binary relations, where the fundamental unit of analysis is represented as a triplet. This triplet consists of: Head entity (the first entity in the relationship), Relationship (the type of relation connecting the entities), and Tail entity (the second entity in the relationship). The importance of RE lies in its ability to transform vast amounts of unstructured textual information into structured data, thereby enabling efficient analysis and knowledge discovery. By uncovering structured insights, RE plays a crucial role in numerous downstream applications. One is Knowledge Graph construction [74], which involves automatically building and enriching KnowledgeBases [74, 75]. Another one is question answering systems that are able to derive contextually accurate answers by linking entities and their relationships [24]. The next is information retrieval, in which the relevance of search results is determined identifying relations within texts. Finally, healthcare and biomedical research is applied to extracting relationships between genes, diseases, and treatments from research articles [24].

Topic Modeling and Clustering

Data mining is a powerful process for uncovering hidden knowledge and identifying unexpected patterns, such as optimal clusters and intriguing anomalies within large, unstructured datasets. Topic modeling, a key area of machine learning research, has become a widely used analytical tool for interpreting vast text datasets. In the biomedical field, it has significant applications in text mining [79], image retrieval [84], and grouping similar clinical concepts to reveal latent patterns in patient records or clinical notes [82, 83].

Deep Learning and Large Language Models

Developing the foundation model (FM) of LLMs for the biomedical field involves tailoring the model architecture and training process to address the unique demands of the medical domain (Fig. 3.2). The model is pre-trained on diverse and extensive datasets comprising clinical notes, biomedical literature, EHRs, and publicly available public health and clinical guidelines along with UMLS [66], and SNOMED CT [63]. To ensure domain specificity, the vocabulary is optimized for medical terminology, and additional pre-training would focus on tasks like NER, RE, and medical text summarization. These FM can then be fine-tuned on task-specific datasets, such as disease classification, drug interactions, or clinical trial matching for real-world healthcare problems [25–27, 32]. The resulting model could serve as a versatile tool for healthcare applications, ranging from clinical decision support and medical documentation to patient engagement and biomedical research, revolutionizing healthcare delivery and research (Fig. 3.2).

Transformer-based models such as BERT, ClinicalBERT, BioBERT and BioGPT are widely used to process complex medical text for predictive modeling. While much current AI discourse highlights generative models like ChatGPT, encoding models such as BERT and T5 continue to deliver near state-of-the-art performance

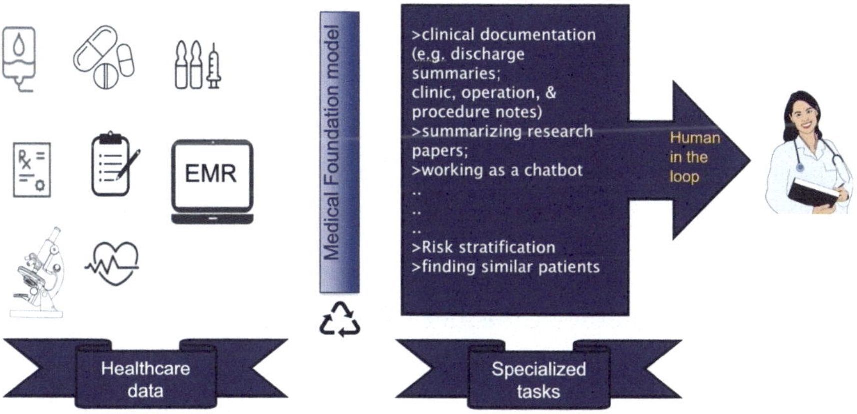

Fig. 3.2 Common applications of LLMs in healthcare

in non-question-answering tasks. Variants like ClinicalBERT, BioBERT, RoBERTa-PM, and clinical T5 further extend these capabilities. For example, ClinicalBERT and BioBERT have been fine-tuned for domain-specific applications like medical text classification. RoBERTa-PM and clinical T5 variants leverage multi-word masking for increased flexibility in training.

Curated reference corpuses (https://www.ncbi.nlm.nih.gov/research/bionlp/Data) and centralized repositories to access controlled vocabularies and ontologies [ref UMLS, Athena, Bioportal https://bioportal.bioontology.org/ontologies] make the development of domain-specific LLMs feasible.

Ontology Mapping

Standardizing clinical and biological terminology is crucial for harmonizing biomedical data. Analyzing and extracting biomedical entities from unstructured data poses significant challenges for NLP techniques, often resulting in errors and incomplete information. The use of inconsistent data further hinders the semantic understanding of relationships between biomedical concepts. These issues with data availability and quality have been major obstacles to the development and training of machine learning and AI models. Automating the standardization and conversion of biomedical concepts into structured ontologies and schemas is a crucial step toward addressing these challenges.

Controlled clinical vocabularies, often structured as ontologies, are vital for biomedical concept mapping, a resource-intensive process requiring extensive domain expertise. Medical concepts as entities refer to disease, diagnosis, symptoms, treatments, interventions, and procedures whereas the term "biological entities" refers to the names of genes, proteins, disease conditions etc. These methods often utilize resources like the Unified Medical Language System (UMLS), Athena, Medical

Subject Headings (MeSH), and PubChem. UMLS [66] and ATHENA [67] provide integrated platforms and tools with open-source repositories to access various international standardized medical terminologies, such as SNOMED CT [63], which is frequently used in the domain. Methods like BertMAP extends ClinicalBERT for ontology matching, performing well on SNOMED ontologies. Similarly, SapBERT [65] enhances embeddings through self-alignment training with UMLS data, improving vector distance adjustments for terminology alignment.

Ethical and Regulatory Considerations

Both genomic and clinical data processing poses significant privacy concerns, as the information is inherently identifiable and sensitive. Ensuring secure data handling, anonymization, and compliance with regulations like GDPR (https://gdpr-info.eu/) and HIPAA (https://www.hhs.gov/hipaa/index.html) is crucial to protect individuals from potential misuse. In genetic disease research, NLP models face challenges related to biases and fairness, as training data often underrepresent certain populations, potentially leading to disparities in diagnosis or treatment recommendations. The application of NLP in genetics and healthcare requires adherence to evolving legal and regulatory frameworks that balance innovation with accountability, addressing concerns like data sovereignty, intellectual property, and the transparent use of AI in healthcare decision-making. Together, these factors signify the need for a multidisciplinary approach to responsibly integrate NLP and genomic insights into medicine.

Future Directions and Emerging Trends

Multimodal approaches that combine text, images, and genomic data are revolutionizing genetic healthcare by enabling a holistic understanding of complex biological systems [80]. Integrating NLP with AI tools such as LLMs enhances the ability to extract meaningful insights from unstructured data like clinical notes, genomic sequences, and imaging reports. Real-time NLP applications in clinical genomics, such as variant interpretation and personalized treatment recommendations, are accelerating the pace of diagnosis and therapy. Collaborative platforms, in which researchers, clinicians, and AI developers can share resources and expertise, are pivotal in advancing the field. These platforms facilitate open data exchange, the development of standardized ontologies, and cross-disciplinary innovations, driving progress toward more precise and equitable genetic healthcare solutions.

Practical Implementations

The implementation of NLP tools in genetic research and healthcare faces several challenges, including data privacy concerns, the complexity of medical terminology, and the quality of training data [61]. The quality and diversity of training data is a major concern, as public genetic data banks are known to suffer from representation bias with the majority of the samples they include being of European origin [85]. Efforts are being made to close the diversity gap by deploying more regional efforts in collecting diverse data. Sustained funding and community support will be a key to closing the diversity gap. For analytics, the diversity and quality of the data can be enhanced by using annotated, high-quality datasets and applying techniques like data augmentation and transfer learning.

When using LLMs in healthcare, hallucination is a big problem [86]. This happens when a model generates answers that sound correct but contain factual mistakes. The answers may seem credible, but they are not always right. Using wrong information in healthcare can have a substantial impact on patient health. To avoid this, one should check the model's answers with trusted medical sources and use expert review before using the information. Integrating expert feedback into the training process, through mechanisms like "expert-in-the-loop" systems, can help refine the models and ensure the clinical relevance of their outputs. A technique called retrieval augmented generation (RAG) can also help reduce model hallucination by searching trusted medical sources before responding. For example, when a physician asks an AI system a question, the system can fetch data from trusted sources like the scientific literature before generating an answer.

LLM models are massive in size, with millions to billions of parameters to optimize, and therefore require a vast amount of computing power to operate. They usually need advanced hardware like GPUs, which are expensive to set up. To solve this issue, we can optimize the models by reducing their size. One approach is through distillation. Here, we create a smaller version of a big model without losing too much accuracy. We can also fine-tune these models for specific tasks so they become more efficient. For example, the LLM PMC-Llama [78] has only 13 billion parameters, yet it still beats Llama-2 (with 70 billion parameters) and GPT-3.5 (with 175 billion parameters) in certain medical question-answering tasks [78] (Table 3.1).

Table 3.1 Two NLP powered healthcare case study examples

1. AI Chatbots and Virtual Scribes
AI chatbots are conversational agents powered by artificial intelligence that simulate human-like interactions. They are designed to engage users in real time through text or voice, providing responses based on pre-trained algorithms, NLP, and machine learning models. Similarly, AI-based scribes help in documenting conversations, taking notes, and summarizing interactions
A virtual scribe supports physicians by transcribing clinical conversations in real-time, enabling them to concentrate on patient care instead of administrative documentation
Availability: Offers continuous support and information, 24/7
Cost-Effective: Lowers the need for extra administrative personnel
Improved Patient Engagement: Elevates the patient experience with instant responses and support
2. Clinical Trial Matching
A highly sought-after application of NLP is in clinical trial matching. By automating the process of identifying suitable participants, NLP enhances the efficiency of recruitment. It analyzes patient records to pinpoint individuals who meet the trial criteria, accelerating the matching process and ensuring that trials are paired with the most appropriate candidates
Benefits:
Enhanced Matching: Improves the accuracy of pairing patients with the right clinical trials
Increased Efficiency: Accelerates the recruitment process for trials
Tailored Approaches: Boosts the chances of successful trial outcomes by aligning patients with relevant studies

Conclusions

In conclusion, the integration of NLP into genetic research and healthcare has led to significant advancements, particularly in enhancing the interpretation of complex genetic data and improving clinical decision-making. Key developments, such as domain-specific LLMs foundation models (like BioBERT and ClinicalBERT) and applications like clinical documentation automation, disease progress prediction, fraud detection, and medical literature review have harnessed NLP in streamlining genetic diagnostics and delivering personalized healthcare.

However, realizing this potential requires addressing challenges such as data privacy, bias, and the need for high-quality training datasets. Despite these challenges, continuous collaboration between researchers, clinicians, and AI developers, combined with advancements in AI technologies, is leading to effective and scalable NLP solutions in genetic healthcare. To fully harness the power of NLP in genetics, it is essential for researchers, clinicians, and AI developers to collaborate across disciplines, creating solutions that are both scientifically rigorous and ethically sound. By fostering interdisciplinary partnerships and continuing to refine these technologies, we can ensure that NLP-driven innovations significantly impact genetic healthcare, providing personalized, accessible, and effective treatment options for patients worldwide.

Acknowledgements The authors thanks Aashish Bhandari and Navya Tyagi for their help in reviewing the document.

References

1. NER: dictionary and graph-based approaches https://pubmed.ncbi.nlm.nih.gov/25810767/
2. NER in the biomed domain https://pubmed.ncbi.nlm.nih.gov/16420734/
3. NER using DL https://bmcbioinformatics.biomedcentral.com/articles/10.1186/s12859-019-3321-4
4. RE review https://dl.acm.org/doi/10.1145/3674501
5. Zhang, J., Wibert, M., Zhou, H., Peng, X., Chen, Q., Keloth, V. K., ... & Raja, K. (2024). A Study of Biomedical Relation Extraction Using GPT Models. AMIA Summits on Translational Science Proceedings, 2024, 391.
6. Zhang, J., Wibert, M., Zhou, H., Peng, X., Chen, Q., Keloth, V. K., ... & Raja, K. (2024). A study of biomedical relation extraction using GPT Models. AMIA Summits on Translational Science Proceedings, 2024, 391.
7. Su, J., Wu, Y., Ting, H. F., Lam, T. W., & Luo, R. (2021). RENET2: high-performance full-text gene–disease relation extraction with iterative training data expansion. NAR Genomics and Bioinformatics, 3(3), lqab062.
8. Goel, A., Gueta, A., Gilon, O., Liu, C., Erell, S., Nguyen, L. H., ... & Feder, A. (2023, December). LLMs accelerate annotation for medical information extraction. In Machine Learning for Health (ML4H) (pp. 82–100). PMLR.
9. Ensemble pretrained language models to extract biomedical knowledge from literature https://academic.oup.com/jamia/article/31/9/1904/7634192.
10. ELIZA—a computer program for the study of natural language communication between man and machine https://dl.acm.org/doi/10.1145/365153.365168
11. Efficient estimation of word representations in vector space https://arxiv.org/abs/1301.3781
12. Glove: Global Vectors for Word Representation https://aclanthology.org/D14-1162/
13. Fundamentals of Recurrent Neural Network (RNN) and Long Short-Term Memory (LSTM) Network https://arxiv.org/abs/1808.03314
14. An Introduction to Convolutional Neural Networks https://arxiv.org/abs/1511.08458
15. Attention Is All You Need https://arxiv.org/abs/1706.03762
16. BERT: Pre-training of Deep Bidirectional Transformers for Language Understanding https://arxiv.org/abs/1810.04805
17. GPT-4 Technical Report: http://arxiv.org/abs/2303.08774
18. Exploring the Limits of Transfer Learning with a Unified Text-to-Text Transformer https://arxiv.org/abs/1910.10683
19. LLM in healthcare review https://www.medrxiv.org/content/10.1101/2024.04.15.24305869v1.full
20. Clinical trial https://pmc.ncbi.nlm.nih.gov/articles/PMC11500892/
21. https://www.ajmc.com/view/using-nlp-to-find-hidden-patients-for-clinical-trials
22. https://clinicaltrialsalliance.org.au/resource/novel-technologies-for-clinical-trial-recruitment-in-australia/
23. SciBERT: Pretrained Language Model for Scientific Text, http://arxiv.org/abs/1903.10676
24. Domain Specific Language Model Pretraining for Biomedical Natural Language Processing http://arxiv.org/abs/2007.15779
25. ClinicalBERT: Modeling Clinical Notes and Predicting Hospital Readmission https://arxiv.org/abs/1904.05342
26. BioGPT: Generative Pre-trained Transformer for Biomedical Text Generation and Mining https://arxiv.org/abs/2210.10341
27. BioBERT: a pre-trained biomedical language representation model for biomedical text mining https://academic.oup.com/bioinformatics/article/36/4/1234/5566506
28. https://watermark.silverchair.com/ocae061.pdf
29. https://pubmed.ncbi.nlm.nih.gov/16420734/
30. https://watermark.silverchair.com/357.pdf
31. https://pubmed.ncbi.nlm.nih.gov/25810767/

32. EHR representation using LLMs https://www.sciencedirect.com/science/article/pii/S1532046420302653#appA
33. EHR+omics https://www.nature.com/articles/s42256-024-00974-9
34. EHR + genomics for precision medicine https://pubmed.ncbi.nlm.nih.gov/38935958/
35. Jindal, J.A., et al. (2024). Ensuring useful adoption of generative artificial intelligence in healthcare. Journal of the American Medical Informatics Association, 31(6), 1441–1444. https://academic.oup.com/jamia/article/31/6/1441/7624147
36. Zhang, M. (2021). Applications of deep learning in news text classification. Scientific Programming, 2021(1), 6095354.
37. Li, Z., Wang, X., Yang, W., Wu, J., Zhang, Z., Liu, Z., … & Liu, S. (2022). A unified understanding of deep NLP models for text classification. IEEE Transactions on Visualization and Computer Graphics, 28(12), 4980–4994.
38. Jin, G. (2022, September). Application optimization of NLP system under deep learning technology in text semantics and text classification. In 2022 International Conference on Education, Network and Information Technology (ICENIT) (pp. 279–283). IEEE.
39. Tabassum, A., & Patil, R. R. (2020). A survey on text pre-processing & feature extraction techniques in natural language processing. International Research Journal of Engineering and Technology (IRJET), 7(06), 4864–4867.
40. Liu, H., Christiansen, T., Baumgartner, W. A., & Verspoor, K. (2012). BioLemmatizer: a lemmatization tool for morphological processing of biomedical text. Journal of biomedical semantics, 3, 1–29.
41. Chadha, N., Gangwar, R. C., & Bedi, R. (2015). Current Challenges and Application of Speech Recognition Process using Natural Language Processing: A Survey. Int. J. Comput. Appl, 131(11), 28–31.
42. Vinnarasu, A., & Jose, D. V. (2019). Speech to text conversion and summarization for effective understanding and documentation. International Journal of Electrical and Computer Engineering (IJECE), 9(5), 3642–3648.
43. Inupakutika, D., Nadim, M., Gunnam, G. R., Kaghyan, S., Akopian, D., Chalela, P., & Ramirez, A. G. (2021). Integration of NLP and Speech-to-text Applications with Chatbots. Electronic Imaging, 33, 1–6.
44. Maruyama, Y. (2021). The categorical integration of symbolic and statistical AI: quantum NLP and applications to cognitive and machine bias problems. In Intelligent Systems Design and Applications: 19th International Conference on Intelligent Systems Design and Applications (ISDA 2019) held December 3–5, 2019 19 (pp. 466–476). Springer International Publishing.
45. Riis, S. K. (1999). Hidden Markov models and neural networks for speech recognition.
46. Wang, J., Jiang, H., Liu, Y., Ma, C., Zhang, X., Pan, Y., … & Zhang, S. (2024). A comprehensive review of multimodal large language models: Performance and challenges across different tasks. arXiv:2408.01319.
47. Mogadala, A., Kalimuthu, M., & Klakow, D. (2021). Trends in integration of vision and language research: A survey of tasks, datasets, and methods. Journal of Artificial Intelligence Research, 71, 1183–1317.
48. Oladele, O. K. (2024). Natural Language Processing in Healthcare: Transforming Electronic Health Records and Clinical Decision Support.
49. Upadhyaya, N., Joshi, H., & Agrawal, C. (2025). Examining NLP for Smarter, Data-Driven Healthcare Solutions. In Intelligent Systems and IoT Applications in Clinical Health (pp. 393–420). IGI Global.
50. Munro, R., Gunasekara, L., Nevins, S., Polepeddi, L., & Rosen, E. (2012, March). Tracking epidemics with natural language processing and crowdsourcing. In 2012 AAAI Spring Symposium Series.
51. Rees, E., Ng, V., Gachon, P., Mawudeku, A., McKenney, D., Pedlar, J., … & Knox, J. (2019). Early detection and prediction of infectious disease outbreaks. CCDR, 45(5).

52. Manoharan, S., & Iyyappan, O. R. (2022). A hybrid protocol for finding novel gene targets for various diseases using microarray expression data analysis and text mining. In Biomedical text mining (pp. 41–70). New York, NY: Springer US.
53. Clark, A. J., & Lillard Jr, J. W. (2024). A comprehensive review of bioinformatics tools for genomic biomarker discovery driving precision oncology. Genes, 15(8), 1036.
54. Lim, E. H., Liu, J. N., & Lee, R. S. (2009, August). Knowledge discovery from text learning for ontology modeling. In 2009 Sixth International Conference on Fuzzy Systems and Knowledge Discovery (Vol. 7, pp. 227–231). IEEE.
55. Shen, W., Le, S., Li, Y., & Hu, F. (2016). SeqKit: a cross-platform and ultrafast toolkit for FASTA/Q file manipulation. PloS one, 11(10), e0163962.
56. Wang, Y. (2024). NLP Applications—Clinical Documents. In Natural Language Processing in Biomedicine: A Practical Guide (pp. 325–349). Cham: Springer International Publishing.
57. Nagamine, T., Gillette, B., Pakhomov, A., Kahoun, J., Mayer, H., Burghaus, R., ... & Saxena, M. (2020). Multiscale classification of heart failure phenotypes by unsupervised clustering of unstructured electronic medical record data. Scientific reports, 10(1), 21340.
58. https://www.nature.com/articles/s41467-023-37200-w;
59. https://academic.oup.com/bib/article/22/6/bbab185/6279836;
60. https://academic.oup.com/gigascience/article/9/6/giaa064/5858063
61. https://www.taylorfrancis.com/chapters/edit/10.1201/9781003262152-4/technical-issues-implementing-ai-healthcare-sonika-tyagi]
62. Ahmed, A., Xi, R., Hou, M., Shah, S. A., & Hameed, S. (2023). Harnessing big data analytics for healthcare: A comprehensive review of frameworks, implications, applications, and impacts. IEEE Access.
63. https://bmcmedinformdecismak.biomedcentral.com/articles/10.1186/s12911-018-0651-5
64. Dong, H., Suárez-Paniagua, V., Zhang, H., Wang, M., Casey, A., Davidson, E., ... & Wu, H. (2023). Ontology-driven and weakly supervised rare disease identification from clinical notes. BMC Medical Informatics and Decision Making, 23(1), 86.
65. SapBERT: https://aclanthology.org/2021.naacl-main.334/
66. UMLS https://pubmed.ncbi.nlm.nih.gov/14681409/
67. ATHENA: https://dl.acm.org/doi/10.14778/2994509.2994536
68. EHR-QC: https://pubmed.ncbi.nlm.nih.gov/37827477/
69. Tayefi, M., Ngo, P., Chomutare, T., Dalianis, H., Salvi, E., Budrionis, A., & Godtliebsen, F. (2021). Challenges and opportunities beyond structured data in analysis of electronic health records. Wiley Interdisciplinary Reviews: Computational Statistics, 13(6), e1549.
70. Patra, B. G., Sharma, M. M., Vekaria, V., Adekkanattu, P., Patterson, O. V., Glicksberg, B., ... & Pathak, J. (2021). Extracting social determinants of health from electronic health records using natural language processing: a systematic review. Journal of the American Medical Informatics Association, 28(12), 2716–2727.
71. Agnikula, K. S., & Balls-BerryJoyce Joy, E. (2021). Social and behavioral determinants of health in the era of artificial intelligence with electronic health records: a scoping review. Health Data Science.
72. GLM https://www.preprints.org/manuscript/202411.0285/v1
73. Janowski, A. (2023). Natural language processing techniques for clinical text analysis in healthcare. Journal of Advanced Analytics in Healthcare Management, 7(1), 51–76.
74. https://www.nature.com/articles/s41597-023-01960-3
75. BioBIKE https://pmc.ncbi.nlm.nih.gov/articles/PMC2703918/
76. Phan, R. (2020). Robust Biomedical Name Entity Recognition Based on Deep Machine Learning (Doctoral dissertation, University of Canberra).
77. Li, J., Sun, A., Han, J., & Li, C. (2020). A survey on deep learning for named entity recognition. IEEE transactions on knowledge and data engineering, 34(1), 50–70.
78. PMCllama: https://academic.oup.com/jamia/article/31/9/1833/7645318
79. Rashid, J., Shah, S. M. A., Irtaza, A., Mahmood, T., Nisar, M. W., Shafiq, M., & Gardezi, A. (2019). Topic modeling technique for text mining over biomedical text corpora through

hybrid inverse documents frequency and fuzzy k-means clustering. IEEE Access, 7, 146070–146080.
80. https://www.medrxiv.org/content/10.1101/2024.03.21.24304655v2
81. https://www.nature.com/articles/nrg3932
82. Howes, C., Purver, M., & McCabe, R. (2013). Investigating topic modelling for therapy dialogue analysis. Association for Computational Linguistics.
83. Li, D. C., Thermeau, T., Chute, C., & Liu, H. (2014). Discovering associations among diagnosis groups using topic modeling. AMIA Summits on Translational Science Proceedings, 2014, 43.
84. https://www.sciencedirect.com/science/article/pii/S1532046419300309
85. https://pmc.ncbi.nlm.nih.gov/articles/PMC7614889/
86. Hallucination https://arxiv.org/abs/2311.05232

Chapter 4
Reconstructing Genetic Networks

Madhu Chetty, Hasini Nakulugamuwa Gamage, and Jennifer Hallinan

Abstract Mathematical modelling in computational systems biology has become essential for comprehending intricate biological processes, and particularly the regulatory mechanisms that govern these biological systems. Among the computational paradigms, gene regulatory network (GRN) inference plays a vital role in unravelling gene-gene interactions and elucidating the regulatory architecture of living organisms. By reconstructing and analyzing the way in which genes influence one another, GRN inference provides valuable insights into the key biological interactions amongst various genes, including those involved in development, disease progression, and response to environmental stimuli. However, GRN inference using computational approaches is challenging due to the complexity of gene interactions and factors such as noise in gene expression data, the presence of indirect regulatory relationships, and the high dimensionality of biological data. In this chapter we review key computational methodologies employed in GRN inference, highlighting their strengths and limitations. We also describe the way in which these methods can address the challenges faced in GRN inference, including data noise, scalability, and biological complexity. We demonstrate that ensemble methods are effective, particularly our GRAMP approach, which has significantly outperformed key individual inference methods, showcasing its effectiveness in improving the accuracy and efficiency of inferred genetic networks. Thus, the development of GRN inference approaches can pave the way for advances in computational systems biology toward creating predictive models of cellular behavior, facilitating personalized medicine, innovative therapeutic strategies, and synthetic biological designs.

M. Chetty (✉) · H. N. Gamage
Institute of Innovation, Science and Sustainability, Federation University, Churchill, VIC, Australia

J. Hallinan
BioThink Pty Ltd, Redcliffe, QLD, Australia

M. Chetty, J. Hallinan (eds.), *From Algorithms to Ailments*,
https://doi.org/10.1007/978-3-032-11023-7_4

Algorithms Used

The algorithms summarized here are an overview of those discussed in the chapters. For further information, read the chapter!

Linear Differential Equations (LDEs)

Linear differential equations are one of the foundational approaches for modelling GRN dynamics. In these models, a complex biological system is represented by a set of linear relationships between genes. The general form of a linear differential equation is as follows:

$$\frac{dx_i}{dt} = \sum_{j=1}^{n} w_{ij} x_j, \text{ where } n = 1, 2, \ldots, n \tag{4.1}$$

Here, w_{ij} represents the *ij*-th entry of the interaction matrix *W*, which defines the effect of gene *j* on the expression value of gene *i*.

Non-linear Differential Equations (NLDEs)

Non-linear differential equations (NLDEs) provide a more detailed and realistic approach for modeling GRNs. These models are better suited to represent the transcriptional and translational processes of gene regulation but come with greater computational complexity. The general form of a non-linear ODE for gene *j* at time *t* is:

$$\frac{dx_j(t)}{dt} = -c_j x_j(t) + f_j\left(x^{-j}(t)\right) \tag{4.2}$$

where $x^{-j}(t)$ represents the expression levels of regulatory genes at time *t*, f_j is a non-linear function that describes the transcription rate of gene *j*, and c_j is the decay rate parameter.

S-System Models

Among non-linear ODE models, S-system models have gained popularity for their precise representation of GRN dynamics. These models are based on a power-law formalism and are described by the following equation:

$$\frac{dX_i}{dt} = \alpha_i \prod_{j=1}^{n} X_j^{g_{ij}} - \beta_i \prod_{j=1}^{n} X_j^{h_{ij}} \tag{4.3}$$

In this equation, X_i and X_j represent the expression levels of genes i and j, respectively. The exponents g_{ij} and h_{ij} denote the interaction type (activation or repression) between genes, while α_i and β_i are the rate constants for synthesis and degradation.

Regression-Based Methods

Regression methods are widely used for GRN inference because they model the relationship between gene expression levels and potential regulators. These methods have shown strong performance in inferring regulatory relationships in gene networks, addressing challenges such as high dimensionality and noise. One of the most straightforward approaches is linear regression, in which the slope of the regression line represents the strength of the relationship between the variables and the target gene. In the context of GRNs, this slope is used to quantify the connection strength between candidate regulatory genes and a target gene. For every gene v, its expression level x_{vi} in sample i, can be estimated by:

$$x_{vi} = \sum_{j \neq n} w_j x_{ji} + \varepsilon_i \tag{4.4}$$

where ε_i is a noise term and w_j denotes the weight associated with the network edge between gene j and gene n. In nature, Regression models give a direction to the network and capture high-order conditional dependencies.

Fuzzy Concept-Based Methods

Fuzzy logic theory serves as a knowledge-based problem-solving framework that operates through three main stages: fuzzification, inference, and defuzzification. In the fuzzification stage, precise numerical values are converted into discrete descriptors (e.g., low, medium, or high) according to fuzzy membership functions (Fig. 4.5). During the inference phase, an inference engine applies fuzzy rules structured as "IF-THEN" statements to generate fuzzy outputs. Fuzzy set logical operations, such as AND, OR, and NOT, are employed to evaluate and combine these rules.

Introduction

Gene Regulatory Networks

Since the establishment of the field of systems biology, it has been recognized that biological systems are intrinsically complex, characterized by numerous subsystems whose interactions and functions are not yet fully elucidated. This complexity presents a significant challenge to researchers, who endeavor to explore and define these poorly understood systems. Consequently, continuous efforts to investigate these elusive interactions have led to considerable advancements and innovations within the field. Computational systems biology has emerged as a pivotal discipline within data science, providing a framework for comprehensive analysis by uncovering the principles governing entire biological systems. The complex interactions within biological systems are determined by examining them holistically, rather than in isolation. A biological system can be conceptualized as a network of multiple interrelated processes. Biological processes are organized into distinct layers of complexity, from DNA through proteins and RNAs, to structural and functional complexes which interact with metabolites and the environment. Interactions occur within individual layers and between processes across different layers, highlighting the intricate and interconnected nature of these systems [1, 2].

In most of these interactions, genes are crucial to the execution of complex biochemical mechanisms. Gene regulatory networks (GRNs) (Fig. 4.1) therefore play a critical role in elucidating the underlying biological processes of living organisms. Models of GRNs are instrumental in advancing our understanding of the molecular basis of complex diseases and in the development of novel therapeutic strategies. These networks represent the functional circuitry of an organism, illustrating the regulatory relationships among genes within a cellular context [3].

Gene activity is typically represented through gene expression profiles, which are captured using technologies such as DNA microarrays and sequencing. Recent

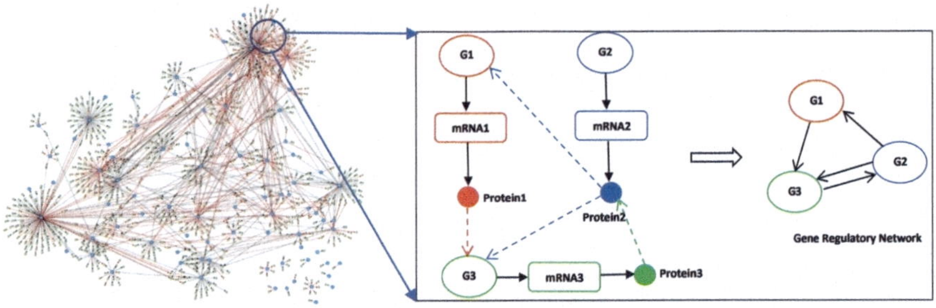

Fig. 4.1 A structured overview of gene regulatory networks and their formation, based on the interactions between genes and their resulting products, including mRNA and proteins. (Source [4])

advancements in RNA sequencing technologies have facilitated the study of gene expression profiles, allowing researchers to monitor temporal changes in gene activity. The expression level of a particular gene is influenced by the regulatory effects exerted by other genes and metabolites, with the pattern of gene expression being a product of these regulatory interactions [5].

GRNs are the biological blueprints of cellular function, orchestrating the behavior of genes through complex regulatory mechanisms. GRNs consist of nodes representing genes or transcription factors and edges symbolizing regulatory interactions. Regulatory interactions can involve activation, whereby one gene promotes the expression of another, or repression, whereby one gene inhibits the expression of another. However, accurately reconstructing a network of regulatory interactions poses a significant challenge due to the inherent fluctuations and noise in gene expression data, the high dimensionality of datasets, and low sample size. Addressing these challenges requires sophisticated methodologies to accurately decipher the underlying regulatory mechanisms (Fig. 4.2) [6, 7].

Significance of GRN Inference

GRN inference is a critical aspect of systems biology that provides profound insights into the regulatory mechanisms governing biological processes. By elucidating the way in which genes interact and regulate one another, GRN inference facilitates a deeper understanding of various biological phenomena. Recent advancements in computational tools and high-throughput technologies have highlighted the significance of GRN inference in several key areas of biological research.

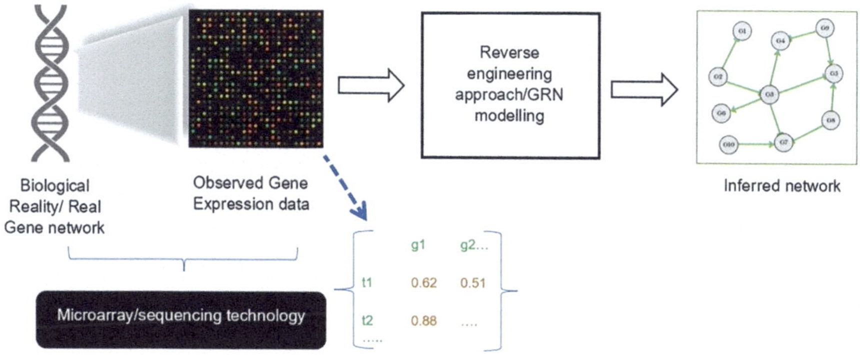

Fig. 4.2 Reconstructing a gene regulatory network involves applying GRN inference methods to gene expression data obtained from an actual gene network, resulting in an inferred network. (Source [4])

Cancer Research

In cancer the disruption of GRNs is a prevalent feature, often leading to aberrant cellular behaviors such as uncontrolled proliferation and metastasis. Cancer-specific GRN reconstruction enables the identification of crucial regulatory nodes and pathways involved in tumorigenesis. Studies have demonstrated that oncogenes and tumor suppressor genes significantly alter GRNs, contributing to cancer progression [8, 9]. Recent research has used GRN inference to uncover novel biomarkers and therapeutic targets in cancer [10]. For example, one study utilized GRN models to identify key regulators in breast cancer, revealing potential targets for improved treatment strategies [11]. Additionally, integrative GRN approaches combining transcriptomic and proteomic data have enhanced our understanding of the way in which specific genetic alterations drive oncogenic processes [12].

Developmental Biology

GRNs are fundamental to understanding the complex process of cellular differentiation and tissue development during embryogenesis. These networks orchestrate the transition of stem cells into various specialized cell types by regulating gene expression in a spatial and temporal manner. By analyzing GRNs, researchers can identify critical genes and regulatory interactions that drive developmental processes. For example, the GRN underlying *Drosophila* embryogenesis has been extensively studied to elucidate the regulatory mechanisms governing segmentation and pattern formation [13]. Similarly, GRN inference has been applied to study human developmental disorders, providing insights into congenital diseases and potential therapeutic interventions [14].

Synthetic Biology

In synthetic biology, GRN inference plays a crucial role in designing and engineering novel biological circuits for diverse applications, ranging from industrial biotechnology to therapeutic interventions. By reconstructing and manipulating GRNs, synthetic biologists can create engineered gene networks with specific functions, enabling the production of valuable compounds or the modulation of cellular behaviors. For instance, recent advancements in synthetic biology have utilized GRN models to construct synthetic gene circuits that can produce biofuels or pharmaceuticals. One study [15] demonstrated that synthetic GRNs offer innovative solutions across a wide range of fields, including agriculture, pharmaceuticals, environmental management, industrial processes, and energy-related biotechnologies. GRN inference has been instrumental in developing gene therapies by designing networks that can correct genetic defects or modulate immune responses [16].

Data Sources for GRN Inference

The process of inferring GRNs relies on a range of different high-throughput experimental techniques, which generate large amounts of biological data. These datasets provide crucial insights into gene interactions and regulatory mechanisms at multiple levels. Below are the primary sources used in GRN inference, each of which contributes unique information that helps map out complex gene regulation.

Gene Expression Data

Gene expression data serves as the foundation for most GRN inference studies. This data is typically obtained through RNA-sequencing (RNA-seq) or microarray technologies, both of which measure the abundance of messenger RNA (mRNA) transcripts in cells under specific conditions. By quantifying mRNA levels, researchers can assess the activity of genes and explore their roles in regulating cellular functions. RNA-seq has emerged as the gold standard for gene expression analysis due to its high sensitivity and ability to capture a broad range of transcripts, including rare and novel RNA species. This method generates precise quantitative data on gene expression, enabling the identification of differentially expressed genes and the reconstruction of GRNs by modelling the relationships between gene expression profiles [17]. Microarrays, although less precise, are still widely used for large-scale studies due to their cost-effectiveness and high throughput [18].

Gene expression data from these techniques provides a snapshot of transcriptional activity, offering indirect evidence of regulatory interactions. For example, co-expression analysis can reveal correlated patterns of gene activity, which may suggest regulatory relationships between genes. However, gene expression alone often lacks the resolution needed to directly infer regulatory connections, leading researchers to integrate additional data types.

Chromatin Immunoprecipitation Sequencing (ChIP-Seq)

Chromatin immunoprecipitation sequencing is a powerful technique that identifies regions of the genome bound by transcription factors (TFs) and other DNA-binding proteins. This method provides direct evidence of regulatory interactions, as it reveals the specific genomic locations where TFs bind to DNA and exert control over gene expression.

In ChIP-seq, specific antibodies are used to target and isolate DNA-protein complexes, followed by sequencing to identify the bound DNA fragments. The resulting data highlights the regulatory regions, such as promoters and enhancers, that transcription factors bind *in vivo* [19]. By mapping these binding events to specific genes, ChIP-seq data enables the reconstruction of TF-target regulatory interactions, thus enhancing the accuracy of GRN inference [20]. For instance, ChIP-seq has been instrumental in identifying key regulatory elements in cancer, such as the binding sites of oncogenic transcription factors, which can then be incorporated into GRN models to explore the transcriptional programs driving tumorigenesis [21].

Proteomic Data

While gene expression data provides insights into the transcriptome, proteomic data offers a complementary perspective by capturing information about the abundance and activity of proteins, which are the functional molecules responsible for most biological processes. Proteins, particularly transcription factors, play a critical role in regulating gene expression by binding to DNA or interacting with other regulatory proteins.

Proteomic approaches, such as mass spectrometry, allow researchers to quantify protein levels and identify post-translational modifications, which can modulate protein activity and, consequently, regulatory interactions. For example, phosphorylation or ubiquitination can alter the activity of transcription factors, impacting their ability to regulate target genes [22]. Proteomic data can thus refine GRN models by providing information on the way in which transcription factor activity changes in response to various signals and conditions [23]. Incorporating proteomic data into GRN inference helps to bridge the gap between transcriptomics and protein activity, leading to more accurate and dynamic models of gene regulation.

Single-Cell RNA-Seq (scRNA-Seq)

Single-cell RNA sequencing (scRNA-seq) is a transformative technology that enables gene expression profiling at the resolution of individual cells. This technique is especially valuable for studying cellular heterogeneity within complex tissues, as it captures the gene expression profiles of thousands of individual cells simultaneously. Unlike bulk RNA-seq, which averages gene expression across a population of cells, scRNA-seq reveals the diversity of gene expression within different cell types and states. This granularity allows researchers to infer cell-type-specific GRNs, providing insights into how regulatory networks vary between distinct cellular subpopulations [24]. scRNA-seq has been widely used in developmental biology to map the GRNs that govern cell differentiation. By analyzing the gene expression dynamics of single cells as they progress through different developmental stages, researchers can identify the key transcription factors and regulatory pathways that determine cell fate [25].

scRNA-seq has also been instrumental in studying disease heterogeneity, such as in cancer, in which different subpopulations of tumor cells may exhibit distinct regulatory programs that contribute to drug resistance or metastasis. The ability to reconstruct GRNs at the single-cell level provides a deeper understanding of how gene regulation varies across different cellular contexts.

Challenges in GRN Inference

Reconstructing GRNs is a critical task in systems biology, as these networks provide valuable insights into the regulatory mechanisms governing gene expression. Despite advances in computational methodologies and high-throughput technologies, accurately inferring GRNs remains a complex and challenging problem. Several factors contribute to the difficulty of reconstructing GRNs, including the high dimensionality of biological data, the inherent noise and sparsity of gene expression datasets, the dynamic nature of regulatory interactions, and the challenge of distinguishing direct from indirect gene associations.

One of the primary challenges in GRN reconstruction is the high dimensionality of gene expression data. High-throughput technologies such as RNA sequencing and microarrays can measure the expression levels of thousands of genes simultaneously. However, the number of samples or conditions under which these measurements are taken is often limited, resulting in a classic "curse of dimensionality" problem, in which the number of variables (genes) far exceeds the number of observations (samples) [26]. Gene expression datasets are inherently noisy due to various technical and biological factors. Measurement errors, batch effects, and environmental variability can introduce significant noise into the data, making it difficult to infer reliable gene regulatory interactions. Moreover, gene expression data is often sparse, meaning that many genes are either not expressed or are expressed at very low levels in a given dataset, further complicating the network inference process [27].

GRNs are inherently dynamic, with gene-gene interactions changing over time in response to different conditions, developmental stages, or cellular environments. However, most GRN inference methods are designed to infer static networks, which provide a snapshot of gene regulatory interactions at a single time point or condition. This static approach fails to capture the temporal and conditional changes in gene regulation, leading to incomplete or inaccurate representations of the true network [28].

One of the most significant challenges in GRN inference is distinguishing between direct and indirect regulatory interactions. Direct interactions occur when one gene directly influences the expression of another, typically through mechanisms such as transcription factor binding. In contrast, indirect interactions can arise from various pathways, in which the regulation of one gene affects another through intermediate genes or regulatory elements. This distinction is crucial because the accurate inference of direct interactions is essential for understanding the precise regulatory mechanisms within the network [29].

Computational Approaches for GRN Inference

The computational approaches for GRN inference can be broadly divided into two key categories: model-based methods and information theory-based methods. Model-based methods can further be subdivided into five major categories: Boolean model-based methods, Bayesian model-based methods, differential equation model-based methods, machine learning-based methods, and fuzzy concept-based methods [30, 31]. Model-based methods for gene regulatory network inference use mathematical or computational models to represent the dynamic behavior and interactions of genes within a biological system. Information theory-based methods focus on identifying statistical dependencies between gene pairs, often through measures like mutual information, allowing for the detection of complex, non-linear relationships. Each category brings unique strengths to GRN inference, with model-based approaches offering structured frameworks to simulate regulatory networks, while information theory-based methods capture diverse interactions between genes, aiding in our understanding of biological systems [30].

Model-Based Methods

Boolean Network-Based Models

Boolean networks are a widely used approach for reverse engineering GRNs, due to their simplicity [32]. In these models, genes are represented as nodes, while Boolean functions $F = \{f_A, f_B, f_C\}$ define the state transitions of each gene based on the input from its regulators (Fig. 4.3).

Directed edges in the network indicate interactions between genes, and update rules determine whether the states of all genes are updated synchronously or asynchronously. For instance, the state of a gene C, at time $t + 1$, is influenced by the states of genes A and B at the previous time t, with the Boolean function f_C governing the interaction:

$$C_{t+1} = f_y\left(A_t, B_t\right)$$

This model provides a simple binary representation of gene expression as "on" or "off." However, early Boolean models struggled with computational efficiency, especially for genes with numerous incoming regulatory connections.

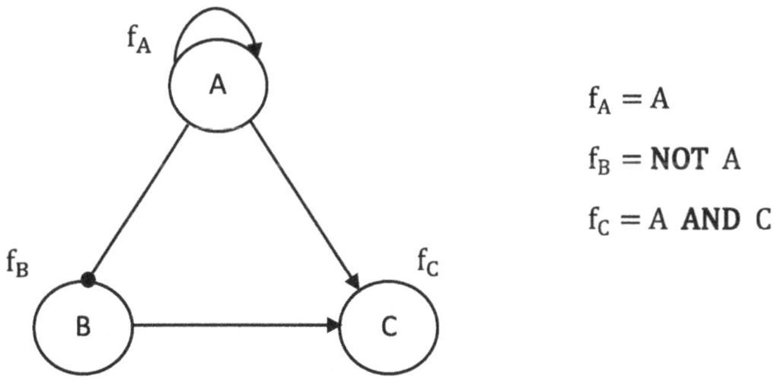

Fig. 4.3 Small Boolean network consisting of three variables (genes), A, B and C. The Boolean network is represented as a graph and the Boolean functions associated with each variable are f_A, f_B and f_C

Several extensions of the Boolean network approach have been proposed to enhance the inference of gene interactions and regulatory functions. One such method is the Best-Fit algorithm [33], which conducts an exhaustive search of all potential combinations of transcriptional regulators for each gene to identify the optimal set of regulators and the best-fitting Boolean function. Another approach, Bayesian Inference for Boolean Networks (BIBN) [34], is effective but limited to small networks with fewer regulatory interactions. The REVEAL method [35], a pioneering Boolean network-based technique, suffers from poor performance when faced with networks that have a high maximum in-degree. Conversely, the CST model [36], which leverages pairwise mutual information, is computationally efficient, but can only infer network topology, not regulatory dynamics. The Mutual Information Based Boolean Network Inference (MIBNI) method [37] introduced several advancements over previous models, but its application is restricted to small-scale networks due to the considerable time required to select an optimal regulatory rule from a vast set of possibilities. Additionally, the WAveS Analysis Based Inference (WASABI) model [38] is accurate when inferring network topology from single-cell data, though it cannot deduce regulatory functions. Finally, the And/Or Tree Ensemble Algorithm (ATEN) [39] struggles with scalability and introduces unnecessary iterations, limiting its overall efficiency. Later methods such as GABNI [40] introduced exhaustive search strategies to find the optimal set of regulators and Boolean functions for each gene. NNBNI is a hybrid method that combines a genetic algorithm (GA) with a supervised neural network (NN) model to infer a Boolean network from time-series gene expression data [41]. Another recent study [42] presented a simple, scalable Boolean network model-based approach for efficient inference of GRNs, capturing both the network structure and its dynamic behavior. This approach has been improved, incorporating feature selection methods to enhance accuracy by Gamage et al. [43]. Despite these improvements, challenges remain, such as discretizing gene expression into binary states, which can lead to information loss [43, 44].

Recent advancements in Boolean-based approaches for GRN inference have focused on addressing the limitations of early models, particularly in terms of scalability, computational efficiency, and biological realism. One significant improvement is the development of Probabilistic Boolean Networks (PBNs), which incorporate stochasticity to account for the inherent noise in gene expression data. PBNs offer a probabilistic framework in which the state transitions of genes are not strictly deterministic, allowing for more biologically plausible modelling [45]. More recently, Probabilistic Boolean Threshold Networks (PBTNs) have been proposed, which combine probabilistic and threshold-based logic to enhance the robustness and accuracy of GRN inference. These methods have shown good performance in identifying key gene interactions, even in noisy datasets [46].

Another notable advancement is the use of Dynamic Boolean Networks (DBNs), which account for time-series data and allow for asynchronous updates of gene states. This asynchronous approach is more realistic compared to earlier synchronous models, better reflecting the non-instantaneous nature of gene regulation in biological systems [47]. Additionally, Boolean Satisfiability (SAT)-based methods have emerged, leveraging SAT solvers to efficiently infer GRNs by transforming the inference problem into a satisfiability problem, allowing for faster and more scalable computations [48].

These recent methods demonstrate the ongoing evolution of Boolean-based GRN inference techniques, making them more suitable for large-scale, noisy biological datasets while maintaining their computational efficiency and interpretability. However, these inference methods oversimplify gene expression into binary states, a shortcut which can obscure important continuous dynamics and complex interactions. These models often lack temporal dynamics, making it difficult to capture time-dependent regulatory processes. They are also sensitive to noise, leading to potential inaccuracies in inferred relationships, and their parameterization can introduce bias due to reliance on prior knowledge. As the number of genes increases, the computational complexity escalates, posing scalability challenges. Additionally, these models risk overfitting the data, which can diminish their predictive power in real-world applications.

Bayesian Networks

Bayesian networks have been extensively used for inferring GRNs, due to their ability to model probabilistic relationships between genes and capture the uncertainty inherent in biological systems. A Bayesian network represents genes as nodes and directed edges between them as probabilistic dependencies, which are quantified using conditional probability distributions. These networks enable the prediction of the likelihood of gene regulation events, allowing for the inference of regulatory interactions from experimental data [49, 50]. In a Bayesian network, the structure of a GRN is inferred by estimating the joint probability distribution of gene expression levels. The inference process involves two primary tasks: learning the structure of the network (that is identifying the regulatory relationships between genes) and learning the parameters (that is the conditional probability distributions that quantify these relationships). Structure learning can be approached in two ways: score-based methods and constraint-based methods.

Score-based methods assign a score to each possible network structure based on how well it explains the observed data, with common scoring functions being the Bayesian Information Criterion (BIC) or Bayesian Dirichlet equivalent (BDe) score. A search algorithm, such as hill climbing or simulated annealing, is then used to find the structure that maximizes the score [51].

Constraint-based methods use conditional independence tests to detect dependencies between genes, constructing the network based on the relationships identified in these tests. Bayesian networks excel in their ability to model causal relationships and handle noisy or incomplete data, making them a valuable tool for GRN inference [52].

Dynamic Bayesian Networks (DBNs)

Dynamic Bayesian Networks (DBNs) extend traditional Bayesian networks by modelling the temporal evolution of gene expression data. In a DBN, each gene is represented as a node, and the directed edges reflect not only regulatory relationships at the current time point but also dependencies between gene states across consecutive time points. This temporal aspect allows DBNs to capture dynamic regulatory interactions that change over time, a process which is essential for understanding time-dependent biological processes such as cell differentiation, circadian rhythms, and disease progression.

In DBNs, the state of a gene at time $t + 1$ is influenced by its own state and those of its regulators at time t (Fig. 4.4). As shown in Eq. (4.5), the random variables $X = X_1, X_2, \ldots, X_n$ represent genes in a gene regulatory network.

$$P\left(X_1, X_2, \ldots, X_{t+1}\right) = P\left(X_1\right) P\left(X_2 | X_1\right) \ldots P\left(X_{t+1} | X_t\right) \tag{4.5}$$

The learning process involves optimizing the network structure and parameters to best explain the time-series gene expression data. Early applications of DBNs in GRN inference include those by Murphy and Mian [54], which introduced DBNs for gene expression modelling, and Zou and Conzen [55], who applied DBNs to time-course data for cancer research.

Recent advancements in Bayesian network-based approaches for GRN inference include more sophisticated algorithms that improve the scalability and accuracy of these methods. Grzegorczyk and Husmeier introduced a Markov Chain Monte Carlo (MCMC) approach to efficiently explore possible network structures, improving accuracy in large datasets [56]. Song et al. developed time-varying Dynamic

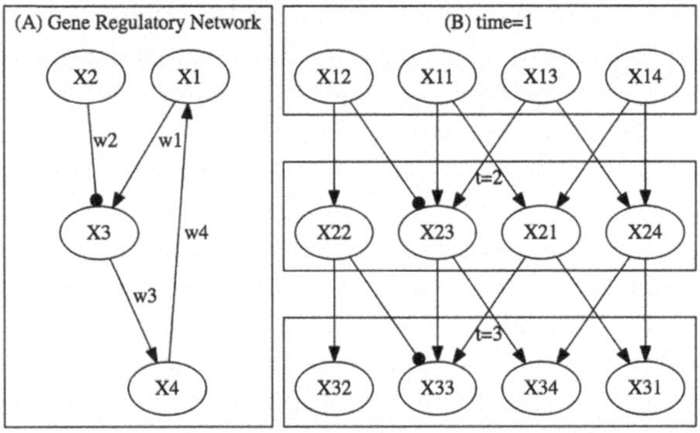

Fig. 4.4 (**a**) Gene regulatory network and (**b**) Dynamic Bayesian network representation. The gene regulatory network consists of a feedback loop X1 → X3 → X4 → X1. (Source [53])

Bayesian Networks, which model time-varying regulatory interactions and can better capture the dynamic nature of biological systems [57].

A more recent advancement is the integration of Markov Chain Monte Carlo (MCMC) methods with Bayesian networks to improve the efficiency of structure learning. Researchers applied MCMC-based structure learning to large-scale gene expression data, achieving higher accuracy in the inference of complex GRNs [58]. The development of continuous Bayesian networks, which allow for more nuanced modelling of gene expression as continuous rather than discrete values, has further enhanced the applicability of Bayesian networks in GRN inference [59].

However, Bayesian network-based methods for GRN inference have limitations that can impact their effectiveness. These include high data requirements for accurate inference, computational complexity, and reliance on assumptions of conditional independence, which may not hold true in biological contexts [60]. Parameter estimation can be challenging, especially with limited or noisy datasets, leading to potential overfitting [49]. While these methods can incorporate prior knowledge, integrating expert input remains difficult, and the resulting networks can lack biological interpretability [61]. The scalability issues associated with larger networks and sensitivity to initial conditions further complicate their application in diverse biological settings [62, 63]. Overall, while Bayesian networks are powerful tools and researchers must navigate these limitations to achieve reliable GRN inferences.

Differential Equation Models

Differential equations (DE) have long been used in computational biology as a deterministic modelling technique for capturing the dynamic behavior of GRNs and their regulatory interactions. These models are particularly effective in providing accurate representations of gene regulation over time. In recent years, numerous variants of DE models have been developed to address the complexity of GRNs, including stochastic differential equations (SDEs), which incorporate randomness to account for the inherent stochasticity in gene expression. Differential equation models can be divided into two main categories: linear and non-linear models.

Linear Differential Equations (LDEs)

Linear differential equations are one of the foundational approaches for modelling GRN dynamics. In these models, a complex biological system is represented by a set of linear relationships between genes. The general form of a linear differential equation is as follows:

$$\frac{dx_i}{dt} = \sum_{j=1}^{n} w_{ij} x_j, \text{where } n = 1, 2, \ldots, n \tag{4.1}$$

Here, w_{ij} represents the *ij*-th entry of the interaction matrix *W*, which defines the effect of gene *j* on the expression value of gene *i*. Several GRN inference algorithms, such as Network Identification by Multiple Regression (NIR) [64], Microarray Network Identification (MNI) [65], and Time-Series Network Identification (TSNI) [66], have been developed using this linear framework. Although linear models provide a simplified view of gene interactions, they may not always capture the complexity of biological systems, particularly when non-linear interactions are present.

Non-linear Differential Equations (NLDEs)

Non-linear differential equations (NLDEs) provide a more detailed and realistic approach to modeling GRNs. These models are better suited to represent the transcriptional and translational processes of gene regulation but come with greater computational complexity. The general form of a non-linear ODE for gene *j* at time *t* is:

$$\frac{dx_j(t)}{dt} = -c_j x_j(t) + f_j\left(x^{-j}(t)\right) \tag{4.2}$$

where $x^{-j}(t)$ represents the expression levels of regulatory genes at time *t*, f_j is a non-linear function that describes the transcription rate of gene *j*, and c_j is the decay rate parameter. Non-linear ODE models, while more computationally demanding, are capable of accurately simulating the complex gene regulatory processes that occur in cells [4, 5].

S-System Models

Among non-linear ODE models, S-system models have gained popularity for their precise representation of GRN dynamics. These models are based on a power-law formalism and are described by the following equation:

$$\frac{dX_i}{dt} = \alpha_i \prod_{j=1}^{n} X_j^{g_{ij}} - \beta_i \prod_{j=1}^{n} X_j^{h_{ij}} \tag{4.3}$$

In this equation, X_i and X_j represent the expression levels of genes i and j, respectively. The exponents g_{ij} and h_{ij} denote the interaction type (activation or repression) between genes, while α_i and β_i are the rate constants for synthesis and degradation. S-system models are further categorized into canonical S-system and decoupled S-system models. The latter reduces computational complexity by dividing the canonical system into subproblems, allowing for more efficient inference of gene networks [67–69].

In recent years, S-system models have been integrated with optimization algorithms such as Evolutionary Algorithms to enhance the accuracy of GRN inference [69]. These optimization techniques help overcome the challenge of parameter estimation, which is difficult due to the noisy and sparse nature of time-series gene expression data.

Recent developments in differential equation-based methods for GRN inference have significantly enhanced the accuracy, scalability, and robustness of these models. By integrating techniques such as machine learning, stochastic processes, and optimization, these models are now better equipped to handle the complexities of gene regulation in large-scale, noisy biological data. However, challenges remain in scaling these models to genome-wide networks and in biologically interpreting the inferred interactions.

Machine Learning Methods

Machine learning (ML) methods have become a key component in inferring GRNs due to their ability to handle complex, high-dimensional biological data. These approaches range from traditional supervised and unsupervised learning techniques to more advanced methods that leverage deep learning and ensemble approaches. The evolution of ML methods for GRN inference reflects the increasing complexity and scale of the datasets used in modern biological research. The widely used ML based reconstruction methods are primarily based on regression, while recent approaches utilize deep learning techniques.

Regression-Based Methods

Regression methods are widely used for GRN inference because they model the relationship between gene expression levels and potential regulators. These methods have shown strong performance in inferring regulatory relationships in gene networks [70, 71], addressing challenges such as high dimensionality and noise. One of the most straightforward approaches is linear regression [72], in which the slope of the regression line represents the strength of the relationship between the variables and the target gene. In the context of GRNs, this slope is used to quantify the connection strength between candidate regulatory genes and a target gene. For every gene v, its expression level x_{vi} in sample i, can be estimated by:

$$x_{vi} = \sum_{j \neq n} w_j x_{ji} + \varepsilon_i \tag{4.4}$$

where ε_i is a noise term and w_j denotes the weight associated with the network edge between gene j and gene n. In nature, Regression models give direction to the network and capture high-order conditional dependencies.

GENIE3 [73] is a widely recognized method that applies regression trees to infer GRNs. It decomposes the inference task into that of predicting the expression of each gene from the expression of other genes. The algorithm uses Random Forests, a machine learning method, to rank genes based on their importance in predicting the expression of each target gene. TIGRESS [74] is a linear regression-based method that employs Lasso (L1-penalized regression) combined with stability selection to infer GRNs. It uses bootstrapping to assess the robustness of the selected gene regulatory interactions, which makes it more reliable in identifying stable regulatory networks. GRNBoost2 [75] is an advanced method for GRN inference designed for single-cell transcriptomic data. It is based on a gradient boosting algorithm and provides a scalable and robust approach for large datasets. GRNBoost2 is part of the Arboreto framework and has been successfully applied to scRNA-seq datasets for building regulatory networks.

SCENIC [76] is a comprehensive pipeline that uses regression-based approaches to infer GRNs specifically from single-cell RNA-seq data. It integrates methods such as GENIE3 and RcisTarget for identifying gene modules and their regulators. SCENIC is widely used for clustering cells based on inferred regulatory networks. ENNET [77] is a gradient boosting algorithm with a regression stumps-based method, and was developed to infer dynamic GRNs from time-series data. By integrating both L1 and L2 regularization, ENNET can handle noisy time-series expression data and infer temporal regulatory interactions. It is useful for understanding the way in which gene regulation evolves over time under different biological conditions. Recent enhancements of regression methods [78, 79] incorporate ensemble techniques in aggregating diverse model learning techniques to address data overfitting and multicollinearity issues in regression-based inference methods.

However, these methods still struggle with data overfitting issues and reduced accuracy when the number of genes exceeds that of available samples. Additionally, these methods often assume that relationships between genes are linear, an approach which may fail to capture the complex, non-linear interactions present in biological systems [80].

Deep Learning-Based Methods

Deep learning approaches have recently emerged as powerful tools for GRN inference, capable of modeling complex non-linear relationships and capturing higher-order interactions between genes. DeepSEM [81] combines deep learning with structural equation models to infer causal relationships in GRNs, leveraging the feature extraction capabilities of deep neural networks. DeepDRIM is a supervised deep neural network-based GRN inference method which aims to capture complex gene-gene interactions by effectively eliminating false positives. DeepFGRN [82] is another recent method that builds a node bidirectional module to capture the embedding representation of the directed graph structure in a GRN.

Despite the aforementioned advances, many machine learning approaches lack interpretability, making it challenging for researchers to derive meaningful biological insights from the inferred networks [83]. The integration of diverse data types, such as transcriptomic and epigenomic data, adds another layer of complexity, as aligning and harmonizing these datasets for training remains a critical hurdle [84]. Overall, while machine learning offers promising avenues for GRN inference, these challenges must be addressed to enhance the reliability and applicability of the resulting models.

Fuzzy Concept-Based Methods

Fuzzy logic theory serves as a knowledge-based problem-solving framework that involves three main stages: fuzzification, inference, and defuzzification. In the fuzzification stage, precise numerical values are converted into discrete descriptors (e.g., low, medium, or high) according to fuzzy membership functions (Fig. 4.5). During the inference phase, an inference engine applies fuzzy rules structured as "IF-THEN" statements to generate fuzzy outputs. Fuzzy set logical operations, such as AND, OR, and NOT, are employed to evaluate and combine these rules.

These heuristic fuzzy rules are often informed by existing expert knowledge and the established activator/repressor regulatory principles (Fig. 4.6) [85, 86]. For instance, a typical fuzzy rule might state:

> *If an activator's expression is Low AND the repressor's expression is High, then the target gene's expression will be Low.*

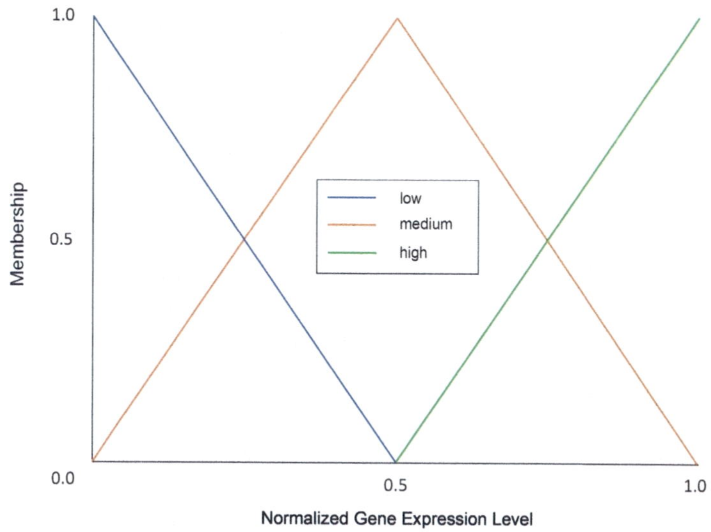

Fig. 4.5 Fuzzy membership function for the expression level of a target gene, categorized into three distinct levels: low; medium; and high. (Source [4])

Fig. 4.6 A fuzzy decision rule matrix as used to predict the expression level of a target gene based on the expression levels of paired activator and repressor genes

If Activator is \ If Repressor is	HI	MED	LO
HI	Target is MED	Target is HI	Target is HI
MED	Target is LO	Target is MED	Target is HI
LO	Target is LO	Target is LO	Target is MED

After assessing each fuzzy rule's output using selected fuzzy set operations, the results are aggregated through various accumulation techniques, such as maximum, bounded sum, or normalized sum, to derive a final output. The defuzzification stage then converts this fuzzy output back into a crisp value using methods like the centroid approach, weighted average, or maxima techniques [87].

Fuzzy logic theory is particularly effective for GRN inference. The expression levels of activator and repressor genes are translated into linguistic values (High, Medium, Low) based on corresponding fuzzy membership functions. In the inference stage, paired activator and repressor interactions predict the expression level of a target gene using predefined fuzzy rules. The overlap of predictions generates a fuzzified score for the target variable. The aggregation of results from each fuzzy rule is typically accomplished using bounded sum methods, with the final predictions transformed back to gene expression values through defuzzification techniques, in which the centroid method is commonly employed [87, 88].

Recent advancements have introduced various adaptations of traditional fuzzy methods tailored for GRN inference. For example, Gamage et al. proposed a hybrid fuzzy inference system that integrates maximal information content-based techniques to improve the accuracy of GRN reconstruction. This approach utilizes fuzzy logic to handle uncertainty in gene expression data while incorporating information theory concepts to refine the selection of genes [89]. Another method is the fuzzy cognitive map (FCM) approach [90] which combines fuzzy logic with graph theory to model complex regulatory interactions among genes. This method allows for a dynamic representation of gene relationships and their regulatory effects, making it particularly useful for exploring nonlinear interactions in GRNs.

These advancements illustrate the ongoing evolution of fuzzy logic in GRN inference, highlighting its versatility and effectiveness in addressing the complexities of gene regulation. While fuzzy logic methods offer advantages for GRN inference, they also have several limitations. The reliance on expert-defined rules introduces subjectivity, which can lead to biases and inconsistencies. Managing and updating these rules becomes complex as the number of genes and interactions increases, hindering scalability in large datasets. The results may be hard to interpret, making it difficult to extract meaningful biological insights. Fuzzy methods are also sensitive to data quality, and poor-quality inputs can yield inaccurate inferences. Traditional fuzzy approaches may struggle to capture nonlinear relationships and dynamic biological processes. The computational demands can increase significantly with model complexity, and there is a risk of overfitting when too many rules are applied to limited data [87]. Addressing these challenges is crucial to enhancing the effectiveness of fuzzy logic in GRN inference.

Information Theory-Based Methods

Information theory-based methods play a crucial role in reconstructing GRNs by assessing the bidirectional correlations between genes. These methods are popular due to their efficiency in handling GRN reconstruction, despite the complexity of regulatory interactions. By evaluating mutual dependencies, they infer the underlying structure of GRNs, often represented as undirected networks (skeletons). These methods have been successfully applied to a wide range of GRN problems because of their simplicity and effectiveness in capturing both linear and nonlinear gene relationships [91].

The reconstruction of GRNs using information theory-based methods typically involves the following steps (Fig. 4.7):

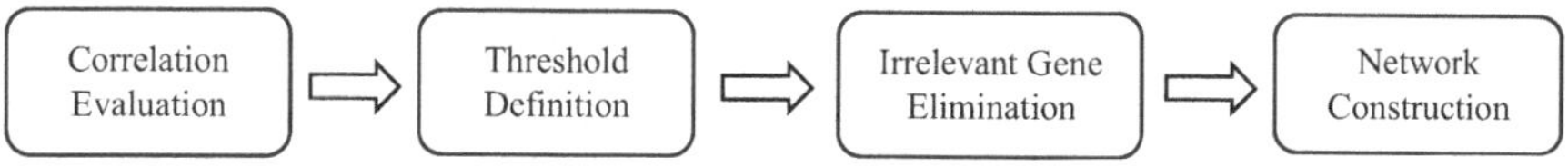

Fig. 4.7 GRN reconstruction using information theory-based methods

(a) Correlation Evaluation:
Correlations between genes are initially evaluated, and for each target gene, a regulatory gene set is established based on the highest correlations.
(b) Threshold Definition:
A predefined threshold is used to select the most informative genes. Only genes with a dependency score greater than this threshold are retained.
(c) Irrelevant Gene Elimination:
Genes that show indirect or irrelevant regulatory interactions are excluded from further analysis to refine the set of potential regulators.
(d) Network Construction:
Regulatory interactions are ranked by their correlation scores, and the inferred network is constructed by linking genes with high-ranked associations.

Various information theory-based metrics, such as entropy, mutual information (MI), conditional mutual information (CMI) [92]. and maximal information coefficient (MIC) [93], are used to evaluate the dependency between genes.

Entropy and Mutual Information

Mutual information (MI) [94] is a widely used metric for quantifying the dependency between two genes. Its non-linear nature makes it particularly suitable for capturing complex regulatory relationships that may not be adequately described by linear measures like the Pearson correlation coefficient. In GRN reconstruction, the entropy of each gene is first computed to assess the uncertainty of its expression levels. Entropy is calculated as:

$$H(X) = \sum_{x \in X} P(x) \log \frac{1}{P(x)} \tag{4.6}$$

where $P(x)$ represents the probability of gene X taking a particular expression level.

Next, the mutual information between two genes (random variables X and Y) is calculated to measure their pairwise association:

$$I(X;Y) = \sum_{y \in Y} \sum_{x \in X} P(x,y) \log \frac{P(x,y)}{P(x)P(y)} \tag{4.7}$$

Where $(x,)$ is the joint probability distribution of X and Y, and (x) and (y) are their marginal distributions.

Conditional Mutual Information (CMI)

In the context of GRN inference, conditional mutual information (CMI) is a valuable tool for understanding the relationships between variables/genes. CMI assesses the statistical dependence between two variables/genes while accounting for the influence of a third variable/gene. By quantifying the information gained about one gene when the expression level of another is known, CMI helps to identify direct regulatory interactions amidst the complex background of gene expression data. The CMI of random variables *X* and *Y* given *Z* is defined as:

$$I(X,|Y,|Z) = \sum_{x \in X} \sum_{y \in Y} \sum_{z \in Z} P(x,y,z) \log \frac{P(x,|y,|z)}{P(x|z)P(y|z)} \tag{4.8}$$

where $P(x, y, z)$ is the cross-time joint probability, $P(x, y| z)$ is the conditional cross-time joint probability, and $P(x| z)$ and $P(y| z)$ represent conditional marginal probabilities. In the context of entropy, CMI can alternatively be expressed as:

$$I(X,|Y,|Z) = H(X,Z) + H(Y,Z) - H(Z) - H(X,Y,Z) \tag{4.9}$$

This approach allows researchers to construct GRNs by determining which genes interact directly and which relationships are confounded by other variables. By focusing on the unique information provided by each pair of genes, conditioned on additional genes, CMI enhances the accuracy of inferred regulatory connections. Ultimately, this method aids in unravelling the intricate regulatory mechanisms that govern cellular processes.

Maximal Information Coefficient (MIC)

Maximal information coefficient (MIC) is a powerful metric used to capture relationships of varying complexity in datasets, whether they are functional or non-functional. MIC has two main features: generality and approximate equitability. Generality enables MIC to identify both functional and non-functional relationships in data, provided there is an adequate sample size, without bias towards any specific type of relationship. Approximate equitability ensures that MIC assigns similar scores to relationships with equivalent levels of noise, regardless of the nature of the relationship. This characteristic ensures fairness, allowing MIC to act as an unbiased tool in detecting intricate dependencies in datasets [95]. The MIC of a set of two-variable (*X* and *Y*) data pairs, *D* can be defined as follows:

$$MIC(D) = \max_{XY<B(n)} \left\{ \frac{I^*(D,X,Y)}{\log_2(\min(X,Y))} \right\} \quad (4.10)$$

where D consists of pair of values $<x, y>$, $x \in X$, $y \in Y$ with sample size n. The grid size is $XY < B(n)$, where the function of sample size, $B(n) = n^{0.6}$ is the default setting to achieve high performance. The term, $I^*(D, x, y)$ is the maximum mutual information taken over an x and y pair. We use $log_2(min(x, y))$ to normalize the maximum mutual information [93, 95]. MIC has been found to be effective in quantifying the strength of associations in two-variable relationships, as reported in [95, 96].

In recent years, information theory-based methods have advanced significantly, leading to improved accuracy in GRN inference, particularly in handling large-scale datasets and noisy data [97]. Some of the most prominent methods include ARACNE: Algorithm for the Reconstruction of Accurate Cellular Networks [98], which applies the data processing inequality (DPI) to reduce false positives, removing indirect relationships between genes and retaining only the most direct regulatory interactions. CLR: Context Likelihood of Relatedness [99] enhances traditional mutual information methods by normalizing MI scores through their local statistical distributions, thereby reducing the effect of noise and improving robustness in the presence of large-scale data.

MRNET [100] a uses the maximum relevance minimum redundancy (mRMR) criterion to identify relevant gene interactions. It ranks potential regulators based on MI scores, aiming to find a balance between high relevance to the target gene and minimal redundancy with other genes. Context-Specific Thresholding, CST [36] focuses on pairwise interactions and implements context-dependent thresholds to improve accuracy in identifying regulatory relationships. This approach is computationally efficient, making it suitable for large datasets. MIBNI: Mutual Information-Based Boolean Network Inference [37] is a Boolean network inference method that employs mutual information to reconstruct regulatory networks. It incorporates Boolean logic to handle the binary nature of gene states, making it highly applicable for inferring discrete regulatory interactions.

As further enhancements, the MICRAT method employs the MIC to infer GRNs by constructing undirected graphs. These graphs depict gene interactions based on time series gene expression data. This approach allows for the identification of relationships between genes without assuming a specific directionality. Then, a hybrid fuzzy method called MICFuzzy [89], integrates a distinctive fuzzy approach with information theory-based techniques. This method utilizes the MIC for preprocessing and quantifying the strength of gene regulatory relationships.

A recent reverse engineering approach [101] uses Partial Information Decomposition (PID): a novel method that extends mutual information by decomposing the shared information between a set of genes into unique, shared, and synergistic components. This approach allows researchers to distinguish between direct regulatory interactions and co-regulated genes. PID has demonstrated strong performance in reducing redundancy and improving the specificity of inferred networks.

Despite the progress made in recent years, information theory-based methods still face several challenges: one of the primary limitations is the high rate of falsely predicted regulatory interactions, especially when applied to large-scale GRNs. This problem can arise from the symmetric nature of mutual information, which cannot capture the directional aspect of gene regulation. These methods are also highly sensitive to noise in gene expression data. Noisy measurements can distort the MI or correlation estimates, leading to inaccurate inference of gene regulatory relationships. Information theory-based methods typically produce undirected networks due to the bidirectional nature of correlation and mutual information measures, which means they cannot naturally capture the direction of gene regulation (i.e., which gene regulates another) [102].

The reverse engineering approaches for GRNs mentioned above differ in their foundational concepts, carry inherent biases, and produce varying outcomes depending on the specific context of the problem. There are a large number of publications on each of these methods. Due to the scope of the chapter and page restrictions, it is not possible to go into the depths of any of these methods for inferring a GRN, and we direct the readers to explore these methods from the references provided earlier. Selecting the most suitable reverse engineering method for reconstructing a particular GRN is complicated by the biological variability found in living organisms and the diverse gene expression datasets available. Consequently, it is crucial to understand that no single method can effectively tackle every GRN inference challenge or deliver optimal results across all dataset types. Achieving "robustness" and reducing issues in GRN reconstruction is challenging when trying to identify the best method for a given problem. A promising strategy is to develop ensemble methods that integrate the results from multiple techniques, rather than relying on just one algorithm [61, 103, 104].

Ensemble Modelling

The concept of ensemble methods has proven effective across various real-world applications, with notable prominence in computational biology, particularly in GRN inference [105]. To enhance the robustness and reliability of GRN inference, many recent reverse engineering strategies have adopted techniques to develop ensemble models. These models integrate diverse outputs generated by multiple GRN modelling approaches (Fig. 4.8), effectively using the strengths of each method to create a comprehensive solution [106–110].

Several methods have been developed which take individual algorithms and create ensemble variants by averaging their results after applying them to resampled datasets. For example, the GENEI3 [111] method employs the random forest algorithm, running it multiple times on resampled training datasets and subsequently combining the resulting GRNs to improve accuracy. An advanced variant, known as dynGENEI3 [112], builds upon GENEI3, while BTNET [113], is another well-regarded method that utilizes a boosted-tree algorithm for ensemble GRN

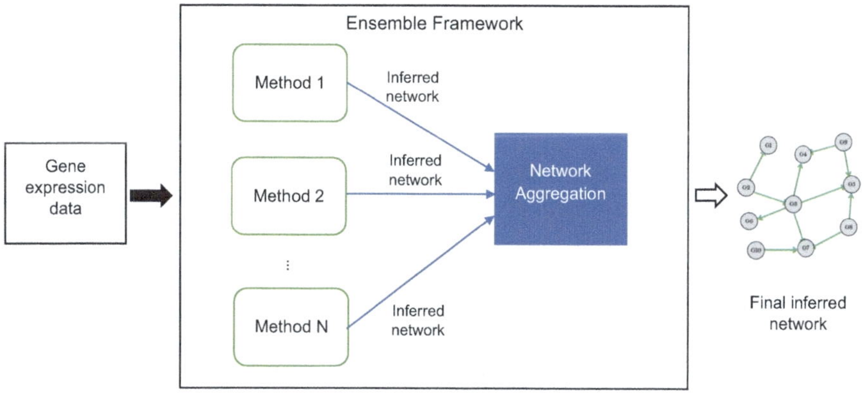

Fig. 4.8 The fundamental framework of the ensemble method for a gene regulatory network

inference. Despite their advantages, these ensemble methods can still be subject to limitations when applied to various inference challenges, primarily due to inherent biases and errors associated with the single method they employ. To address these shortcomings, Marbach introduced the concept of community networks, an approach which involves aggregating networks inferred through different methods. This approach aims to mitigate the limitations of single methods by harnessing the collective insights from multiple sources [61, 103, 114].

Marbach's framework categorizes the selected inference methods into six distinct qualitative categories, demonstrating that combining inferred networks from these diverse categories leads to enhanced accuracy. Initially, interactions inferred from each method were aggregated using an unweighted rank-averaging technique, often referred to as the Borda count. However, further research indicated improved performance with a weighted voting approach, in which predictions from high-performing methods are prioritized in the consensus-building process. Although the enhancements achieved through weighted voting were only marginally better than those obtained with unweighted rank averaging, this method highlights the importance of leveraging high-quality predictions [61]. It is important to note, however, that Marbach's approach does not provide a specific strategy for identifying the most suitable methods when inferring the structure of an entirely unknown network. Recent advancements are beginning to address this problem by integrating machine learning techniques to assess method performance dynamically, allowing for more adaptive ensemble strategies. By continually refining the selection process and incorporating additional sources of data, future ensemble models have the potential to further improve the accuracy and reliability of GRN inference.

Ensemble methods have become increasingly popular in GRN inference due to their robustness and ability to improve prediction accuracy by combining multiple inference models. Many recent reverse engineering approaches now focus on ensemble model construction, using the strengths of diverse algorithms. For instance, ComHub [115] employs a community-based strategy to identify hub genes, providing insight into key regulatory elements within the network. Another innovative approach, developed by Peignier and colleauges [106] integrates genetic algorithms and frequent itemset mining to optimize the selection of methods for designing compact yet effective ensembles, primarily targeting machine learning-based techniques. These strategies are particularly effective for large-scale networks, where single-model predictions often falter due to data complexity.

Traditional aggregation methods like rank average (Borda count), scaleSum, and scaleLSum [116] continue to be widely used in ensemble approaches to GRN inference. However, recent developments have introduced more sophisticated techniques. EnGRaiN, for example, is the first supervised ensemble network learning approach designed specifically for inferring precise regulatory interactions. EnGRaiN [116] outperforms traditional methods such as rank average and scaleLSum under specific conditions, offering improved prediction accuracy by leveraging prior biological knowledge. However, its reliance on known interactions makes it less suitable for entirely novel networks, highlighting a limitation when dealing with unknown regulatory systems.

A critical challenge in ensemble approaches lies in selecting the appropriate aggregation method for combining networks. Recent advancements in Top*k*Net [104] have introduced a consensus-based approach to GRN inference. Top*k*Net identifies the optimal algorithms for a dataset by measuring its similarity to datasets associated with known regulatory networks. The assumption is that if the dataset of a known network is highly similar to that of an unknown network, the optimal algorithms for the known case will also work for the unknown one. Top*k*Net's strength lies in integrating predictions from selected algorithms to form a consensus network. However, its reliance on dataset similarity, algorithm diversity, and confidence level differences can lead to inconsistencies across gene-gene interactions, especially in heterogeneous datasets. This issue highlights the need for more reliable approaches that can prioritize high-performing methods in complex scenarios.

EnsInfer [117] is an ensemble method that combines predictions from multiple cutting-edge GRN inference algorithms using a simple Naive Bayes model, which treats the outputs of each algorithm as priors for determining the likelihood of regulatory connections. This approach allows for the seamless integration of diverse data types, such as bulk and single-cell RNA sequencing, and is flexible enough to incorporate new inference methods, enhancing its adaptability and accuracy in reconstructing gene regulatory networks.

As ensemble approaches gain popularity, researchers are increasingly exploring the use of Evolutionary Algorithms (EAs) to enhance ensemble model building [118]. EAs help to identify the optimal combination of methods for constructing efficient ensembles. One such method integrates genetic algorithms and frequent itemset mining techniques to select the best combination of machine learning-based methods for GRN inference. While these methods improve accuracy, their fitness functions can struggle to detect novel interactions in real-world biological networks [119]. GENECI (GEne NEtwork Consensus Inference), an evolutionary machine learning approach, organizes ensembles by analyzing outcomes from multiple reverse engineering methods. GENECI optimizes consensus networks using genetic algorithms, considering both confidence levels and topological features. However, its focus on machine learning and information theory-based methods limits the diversity in the ensemble model [118].

While many ensemble approaches aggregate a large number of models to improve performance, recent research suggests that using a few high-performing methods may yield better results [31]. For example, GRAMP, a modelling framework recently proposed by us, employs a small but highly optimized set of methods to construct accurate and robust GRNs [31]. GRAMP identifies the importance of inference methods for a particular problem context and prioritizes the most effective algorithms for consensus network construction, rather than relying on sheer quantity. These methods offer new strategies for combining multiple algorithms but also underscore the need for further refinement in selecting and aggregating models, particularly in terms of balancing performance, scalability, and data complexity.

Experimental Valuation of Ensemble Modelling

Numerous experimental studies have demonstrated that ensemble models significantly outperform individual methods for GRN inference [61]. For instance, comparative analyses have shown that recent ensemble approaches, such as GRAMP, produce higher accuracy and specificity than traditional single-method inference techniques. We considered GRAMP as a case study in this chapter and the following results demonstrate the effectiveness and reliability of GRAMP in reconstructing GRNs through ensemble approaches, highlighting its performance metrics and comparative advantages over individual inference methods. The data and findings illustrated in this chapter provide insights into the capabilities of ensemble modelling in addressing the complexities of gene regulatory interactions.

First, the performance of GRAMP was assessed using simulated datasets created with the gene expression simulator GeneNetWeaver [120]. These datasets varied in size, from 20 to 100 genes, with each network size comprising 50 datasets derived from five distinct networks. The first three networks were based on the *Escherichia coli* network, while the latter two were sourced from the *Saccharomyces cerevisiae* cell-cycle network. As shown in Fig. 4.9, the performance of GRAMP was evaluated by comparing its True Positive Rate (TPR), False Positive Rate (FPR), and Structural Accuracy (SA) against existing individual inference strategies, including the Boolean network-based method [43], a regression based method [79], and a fuzzy method (MICFuzzy) [89].

GRAMP consistently achieved a Structural Accuracy of more than 0.8 across all network inference challenges examined. It surpassed the performance of individual inference methods in terms of TPR, FPR, and SA. These results indicate the effectiveness of the ensemble approach over the individual methods in GRN inference [31].

The performance of GRAMP was evaluated against that of several methods: ARACNE, GABNI NABNI, Boolean, Regression, and Fuzzy (MICFuzzy) and established ensemble methods, including GENEI3, dynGENEI3, and BTNET, along with key inference approaches outlined in the study [31, 41] (Table 4.1) on

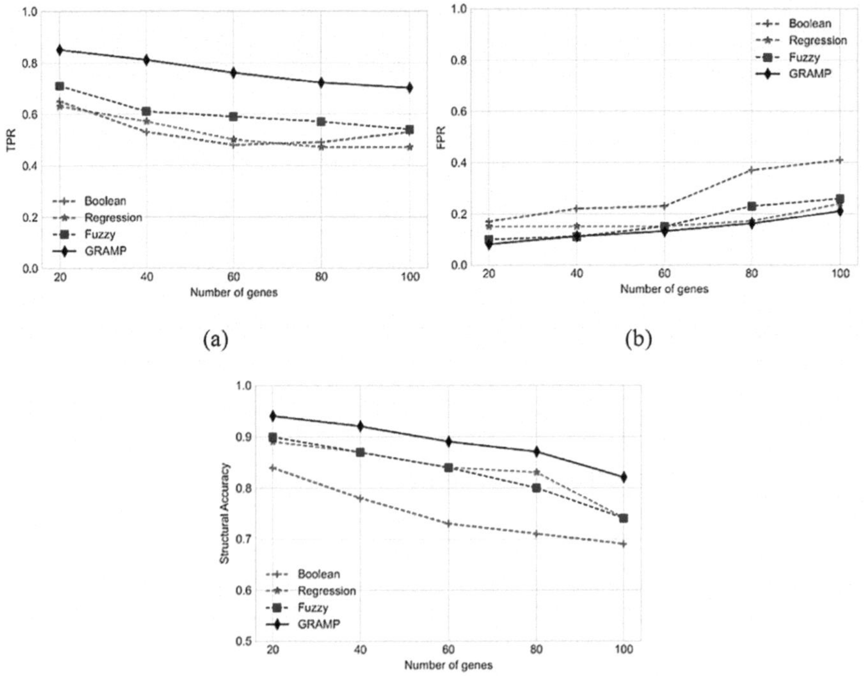

(a) (b)

(c)

Fig. 4.9 Analysis of the performance of individual methods: Boolean, Regression, Fuzzy (MICFuzzy) and GRAMP includes a comparison of (**a**) True Positive Rate, (**b**) False Positive Rate, and (**c**) Structural Accuracy of various algorithms on simulated gene expression datasets observed from GRNs, with the number of genes varying from 20 to 100

Table 4.1 Structural Accuracies of the inference of small-scale real gene networks, CDC-15, CDC-28 and *S. cerevisiae*

Method	CDC-15	CDC-28	*S. cerevisiae*
ARACNE	0.66	0.55	0.67
GABNI	0.72	0.71	0.74
NNBNI	0.78	0.77	0.77
GENIE3	0.61	0.54	0.67
Boolean	0.54	0.59	0.69
Regression	0.70	0.80	0.74
Fuzzy	0.74	0.77	0.76
dynGENIE3	0.61	0.56	0.67
BTNET	0.58	0.57	0.69
GRAMP	**0.81**	**0.94**	**0.90**

three simulated datasets derived from two different networks. The first network was the *S. cerevisiae* cell-cycle network, which consists of nine genes and 17 interactions, and includes two expression datasets, CDC-15 and CDC-28, featuring 24 and 17 time samples, respectively [121]. The second network was the *S. cerevisiae* G1 cell-cycle network [122], comprising 11 genes and 22 interactions across 18 time points.

Even the ensemble versions of regression methods, such as GENEI3, dynGENEI3, and BTNET, exhibited lower performance than the individual methods considered. This observation underscores the significance of aggregating diverse methods and employing effective aggregation techniques. The SA of the aggregation approach used in GRAMP surpassed those of both individual methods and other ensemble methods.

Next, the performance of GRAMP was assessed using a real eight-gene network derived from the SOS DNArepair network of *Escherichia coliv* [123]. This network includes the genes uvrD, lexA, umuD, recA, uvrA, uvrY, ruvA, and polB (Fig. 4.10a). The SOS DNA dataset was collected from four different experiments conducted under various UV light conditions, with gene expression measured at 50 time points, evenly spaced at six-minute intervals. Since the true structure of the network is unknown, conventional performance metrics could not be used for evaluation. Instead, the performance of GRAMP was evaluated based on the nine documented regulatory interactions among the eight genes. The performance of GRAMP was evaluated against various state-of-the-art techniques, including Perrin's method

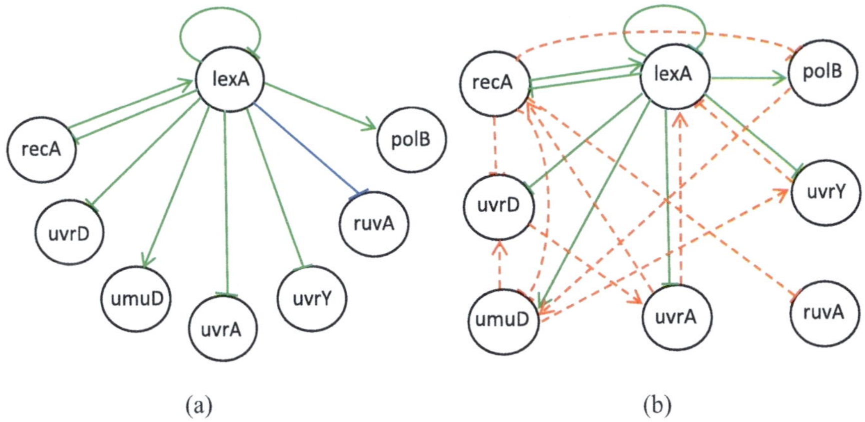

Fig. 4.10 The structure of the SOS DNArepair network inferred using GRAMP. (**a**) In this depiction, blue lines signify true regulatory interactions that were not predicted by the method, while green lines indicate the regulations that were accurately inferred along with their corresponding regulation types. (**b**) True and false regulatory interactions identified by the proposed method, with green lines denoting correctly inferred regulations and red dashed lines indicating false predictions. In the figure, arrows represent positive interactions, while barred lines indicate negative interactions. (Source [31])

Table 4.2 Comparison of the true regulations inferred by GRAMP with those identified by other methods in the SOS DNA repair network

Regulation	Perrin	Banjo	GlobalMIT	Morshed	Boolean	Regression	Fuzzy	GRAMP
lexA ➔ uvrD				y	y	y		y
lexA ➔ lexA	y				y	y		y
lexA ➔ umuD			y	y	y		y	y
lexA ➔ recA	y		y	y		y	y	y
lexA ➔ uvrA	y	y	y	y	y	y	y	y
lexA ➔ uvrY			y		y		y	y
lexA ➔ ruvA								
lexA ➔ polB			y			y	y	y
recA ➔ lexA	y	y					y	y

[124], Banjo [125], Morshed's approach [126], and GlobalMIT [127], a Boolean method, a regression method and a fuzzy method (MICFuzzy) (Table 4.2) [31].

The ensemble method demonstrated superior performance compared to all existing methods, correctly inferring eight regulatory interactions, including the types of regulation (activation or inhibition) for five. While it produced 11 false regulations, many algorithms in this study failed to identify regulation types or quantify false regulations (Fig. 4.10b). GRAMP successfully inferred self-regulation for lexA and incorporated unique regulations identified by individual methods, such as recA → lexA from the fuzzy approach and lexA → uvrD from the Boolean and regression methods (Table 4.2). The fuzzy model-based approach accurately inferred six regulations, outperforming methods like Perrin, Banjo, GlobalMIT, and Morshed, while the regression and Boolean methods each identified five. Overall, GRAMP showed its effectiveness in aggregating diverse capabilities from various methods, leading to enhanced inference of the SOS DNA repair network. This finding further underscores the effectiveness of ensemble methods over individual modelling approaches, as GRAMP demonstrated superior performance in inferring gene regulatory networks, exhibiting both high accuracy and efficiency in experiments conducted on simulated datasets and a real-world gene expression dataset [31].

Applications of Inferred Gene Regulatory Networks

Inferred GRNs have emerged as a powerful tool in modern biological research, offering profound insights into the intricate web of gene interactions that govern cellular functions. Their applications span a diverse array of fields (Fig. 4.11), each contributing to our understanding of complex biological systems and paving the way for identification of the causes of diseases and designing innovative solutions in real-world challenges [128].

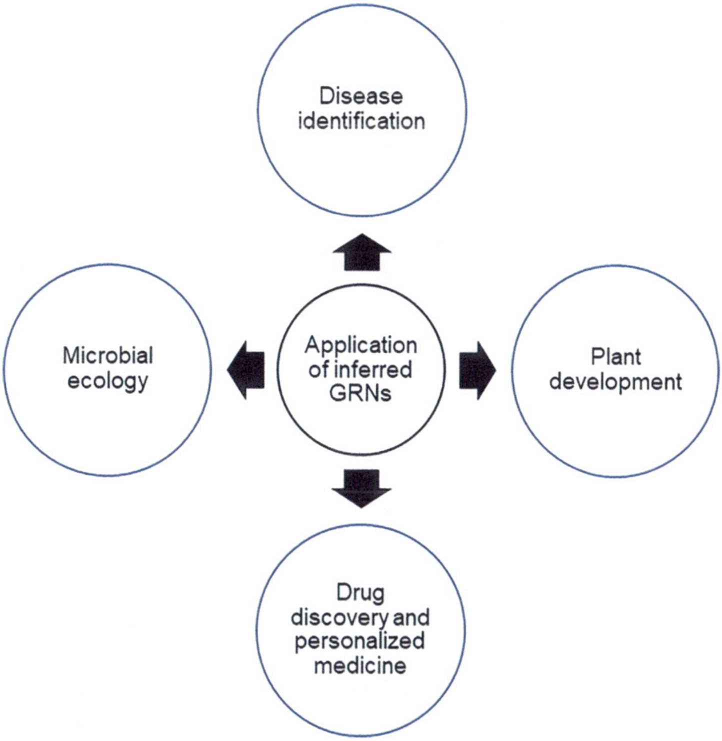

Fig. 4.11 Some applications of inferred gene regulatory networks. The applications of GRNs in four key domains: disease identification, plant development, microbial ecology, and drug discovery and personalized medicine

Disease Identification

One of the most significant applications of inferred GRNs is in cancer research. By elucidating the regulatory pathways involved in tumorigenesis, researchers can identify key players that drive cancer progression. For instance, one study [129] focused on breast cancer, in which GRN inference was utilized to uncover critical transcription factors and their target genes that facilitate tumor growth and metastasis. This work not only enhanced the understanding of the molecular underpinnings of breast cancer but also highlighted potential therapeutic targets for intervention, aiming to disrupt the regulatory networks that sustain malignancy.

The application of inferred GRNs extends to metabolic diseases such as type 2 diabetes, in which they help illuminate the regulatory mechanisms behind insulin resistance. Researchers employed GRN inference to map the interactions among genes associated with insulin signaling pathways. By identifying critical nodes within these networks, the study revealed potential targets for therapeutic intervention aimed at enhancing insulin sensitivity, which is vital for diabetes management [130].

In the realm of cardiovascular research, inferred GRNs have been instrumental in unravelling the regulatory mechanisms underlying heart development and disease progression. A recent study [131] utilized GRN inference to examine the role of specific transcription factors in cardiac hypertrophy.

Inferred GRNs have proven invaluable in the study of neurodegenerative diseases [132], such as Alzheimer's disease. Research conducted by Bai et al. [133] employed GRN inferenceto investigate the regulatory changes associated with neuronal cell death. By analyzing transcriptomic data from Alzheimer's patients, the researchers identified dysregulated pathways that contribute to the disease's progression. This knowledge has implications for early diagnosis, offering hope for effective interventions that could slow or halt the progression of neurodegenerative disorders.

Plant Development and Stress Response

The field of plant biology has also greatly benefited from inferred GRNs, particularly in understanding the way in which plants respond to environmental stressors. A notable example was reported in [134], in which the inferred GRNs in *Arabidopsis thaliana* were used to explore the response of plants to drought stress. Through this analysis, the researchers uncovered key regulatory interactions that govern stress tolerance mechanisms. These insights are critical for developing crops that can withstand drought conditions, thereby enhancing agricultural resilience in the face of climate change.

Microbial Ecology

Inferred GRNs are also valuable in the exploration of microbial ecosystems. Researchers have investigated the regulatory networks of soil bacteria in response to nutrient variations to provide insights into the way in which microbial communities adapt to environmental changes, thereby contributing to soil health and agricultural productivity. Understanding these interactions is crucial for developing strategies to maintain ecosystem balance and enhance soil fertility [135].

Drug Discovery and Personalized Medicine

Inferred GRNs are increasingly recognized as valuable tools in drug discovery and personalized medicine. By providing insights into the complex interactions between genes and their regulatory elements, GRNs enable researchers and clinicians to identify potential therapeutic targets, predict drug responses, and tailor treatments to individual patient profiles [136, 137]. Here, we explore how GRNs can be effectively utilized in these areas, along with illustrative examples.

Drug Discovery

The drug discovery process traditionally relies on the identification of biological targets, which are often proteins involved in disease pathways. Inferred GRNs enhance this process by revealing key regulatory nodes and interactions that might be overlooked by conventional methods [138]. GRNs contribute to drug discovery in several ways:

Target Identification

By analyzing GRNs associated with specific diseases, researchers can identify critical transcription factors and signaling pathways that drive disease progression. For instance, inferred GRNs were utilized to identify key regulatory genes involved in the development of lung cancer [139]. This research led to the discovery of novel targets for drug development, which were further validated in preclinical models. Another study [140] utilized GRNs to identify key regulatory changes associated with bipolar disorder. By analyzing the complex interactions between genes, GRNs provided a deeper understanding of the way in which gene expression patterns are altered in bipolar disorder. The network-based signatures derived from these GRNs were then used to explore potential drug repurposing opportunities. This approach allowed the identification of drugs that could potentially reverse or modulate the dysregulated gene interactions specific to bipolar disorder, offering a novel strategy for discovering therapeutic interventions.

Pathway Analysis

GRNs help in understanding the pathways through which drugs exert their effects. By mapping the way in which a drug influences gene expression within a GRN, researchers can better predict its therapeutic efficacy and potential side effects. For example, Cheng et al. [141] used GRN inference to analyze the effects of a new anti-inflammatory drug on rheumatoid arthritis. Their findings revealed the impact of drugs on multiple regulatory pathways, guiding further optimization of the compound for enhanced efficacy.

Compound Screening

GRNs can also aid in the high-throughput screening of compounds. By integrating GRN data with compound libraries, researchers can prioritize candidates based on their predicted interactions with key regulatory genes. This approach was exemplified in several studies [142, 143], which used GRNs to screen for small molecules that could modulate the activity of critical transcription factors involved in cardiac hypertrophy, leading to the identification of several promising candidates.

Personalized Medicine

Personalized medicine aims to tailor treatment strategies to individual patients based on their genetic profiles, and inferred GRNs play a crucial role in this endeavor [144, 145]:

Biomarker Identification

GRNs can help to identify biomarkers associated with drug response. By analyzing the regulatory networks in patient samples, researchers can determine which genetic variations correlate with treatment efficacy or adverse effects. For example, Wang et al. [146] used GRN inference to identify a set of biomarkers in breast cancer patients that predicted responses to specific chemotherapy agents, enabling more personalized treatment plans.

Predicting Drug Responses

By integrating patient-specific genomic data with inferred GRNs, clinicians can predict how individual patients are likely to respond to certain therapies. This approach was demonstrated in different studies [144, 147] in which GRN analysis was used to predict treatment outcomes in patients with colorectal cancer. One study [147] identified patients likely to respond to targeted therapies based on the specific regulatory interactions in their tumor samples.

Tailoring Treatment Regimes

In addition to predicting responses, GRNs can inform the design of personalized treatment regimens. By understanding the regulatory mechanisms that govern drug metabolism and efficacy, clinicians can adjust dosages or combinations of therapies to optimize outcomes [137]. One study revealed that using GRNs to guide combination therapies for patients with metastatic melanoma led to improved survival rates through tailored treatment strategies [145].

The applications of inferred gene regulatory networks are many and varied, demonstrating their versatility as a tool for advancing biological research. From elucidating the mechanisms of cancer and neurodegenerative diseases to enhancing agricultural resilience and informing therapeutic strategies, inferred GRNs are paving the way for innovative solutions to pressing challenges in health, agriculture, and environmental sustainability. Additionally, their integration into drug discovery and personalized medicine holds the promise of enhancing the efficacy and safety of therapeutic interventions, ultimately improving patient outcomes, and revolutionizing modern medicine. As technology and methodologies continue to evolve, the potential of GRNs in these fields will only expand, offering exciting avenues for future research and application.

Conclusions

Gene regulatory network (GRN) inference stands at the forefront of modern computational biology, illuminating the intricacies of the regulatory mechanisms that govern biological processes. Understanding this field is essential not only for advancing our understanding of fundamental biological processes, such as development and cellular differentiation, but also for providing critical insights into complex diseases, including cancer. The ability to accurately infer GRNs allows researchers to decode the genetic regulatory landscape, paving the way for targeted therapies and precision medicine. As high-throughput technologies continue to produce vast amounts of biological data, the methods for GRN inference must evolve to meet the challenges posed by this deluge of information. Recent advancements in computational techniques including ensemble approaches have significantly enhanced the accuracy and applicability of GRN inference methods. Key areas for future development include the integration of multi-omics data, which combines information from genomics, transcriptomics, proteomics, and metabolomics to provide a more comprehensive view of gene regulation. There is also a pressing need for scalable algorithms that can handle the increasing complexity of biological data, alongside the refinement of experimental validation techniques to confirm computational predictions. Among the various approaches to GRN inference, ensemble models have emerged as a particularly promising strategy. By integrating multiple models or methods, ensemble techniques enhance predictive accuracy and robustness, leveraging the strengths of individual models while mitigating their weaknesses. This synergy allows for more reliable estimations of gene interactions, making ensemble models indispensable in the quest for accurate GRN inference. The need for GRN inference, driven by technological innovations and methodological advancements, is evident. The continued exploration of ensemble models, in particular, will play a pivotal role in refining our understanding of gene regulatory networks and their implications in health and disease, ultimately contributing to the development of more effective therapeutic strategies.

References

1. S. Kesić, "Systems biology, emergence and antireductionism," *Saudi Journal of Biological Sciences,* pp. 584–591, 2016.
2. I. S. Peter, "Chapter Nine—The function of architecture and logic in developmental gene regulatory networks," *Current Topics in Developmental Biology,* vol. 139, pp. 267–295, 2020.
3. M. Flores, T.-H. Hsiao, Y.-C. Chiu, E. Y. Chuang, Y. Huang and Y. Chen, "Gene Regulation, Modulation, and Their Applications in Gene Expression Data Analysis," *Advances in Bioinformatics,* 2013.
4. H. N. Gamage, "Ensemble Approaches for Robust Reconstruction of Gene Regulatory," Federation University Australia, 2024.
5. I. Androulakis, E. Yang and R. Almon, "Analysis of Time-Series Gene Expression Data: Methods, Challenges, and Opportunities," *Annual Review of Biomedical Engineering,* vol. 9, pp. 205–228, 2007.
6. F. Emmert-Streib, M. Dehmer and B. Haibe-Kains, "Gene regulatory networks and their applications: understanding biological and medical problems in terms of networks," *Frontiers in Cell and Developmental Biology,* vol. 2, no. 38, 2014.
7. M. A. Gaafar, N. A. Yousri and M. A. Ismail, "A novel ensemble selection method for cancer diagnosis using microarray datasets," in *IEEE 12th International Conference on Bioinformatics & Bioengineering (BIBE),* Larnaca, Cyprus, 2012.
8. Y. Chen, X.-F. Zhang and L. Ou-Yang, "Inferring cancer common and specific gene networks via multi-layer joint graphical model," *Computational and Structural Biotechnology Journal,* vol. 21, p. 974–990, 2023.
9. Y. Li, W. Vongsangnak, L. Chen and B. Shen, "Integrative analysis reveals disease-associated genes and biomarkers for prostate cancer progression," *BMC Medical Genomics,* vol. 7, 2014.
10. F. Aziz, A. Acharjee, J. A. Williams, D. Russ, L. Bravo-Merodio and G. V. Gkoutos, "Biomarker Prioritisation and Power Estimation Using Ensemble Gene Regulatory Network Inference," *International Journal of Molecular Sciences,* vol. 21, no. 21, 2020.
11. R. Lusby, Z. Zhang, A. Mahesh and V. K. Tiwari, "Decoding gene regulatory circuitry underlying TNBC chemoresistance reveals biomarkers for therapy response and therapeutic targets," *npj Precision Oncology,* vol. 8, no. 64, 2024.
12. A. Salehi, L. Wang, P. J. Coates, L. N. Spaak, X. Gu, N. Sgaramella and K. Nylander, "Reiterative modeling of combined transcriptomic and proteomic features refines and improves the prediction of early recurrence in squamous cell carcinoma of head and neck," *Computers in Biology and Medicine,* vol. 149, 2022.
13. Y.-C. Chen and C. Desplan, "Gene regulatory networks during the development of the *Drosophila* visual system," *Current Topics in Developmental Biology,* vol. 139, pp. 89–125, 2020.

14. C. Feigin, S. Li, J. Moreno and R. Mallarino, "The GRN concept as a guide for evolutionary developmental biology," *Journal of Experimental Zoology Part B,* vol. 340, no. 2, p. 92–104, 2023.
15. K. D. Bhalerao, "Synthetic gene networks: the next wave in biotechnology?," *Trends in Biotechnology,* vol. 27, no. 6, pp. 368–374, 2009.
16. J. S. Weinstock, M. M. Arce, J. W. Freimer, M. Ota, A. Marson, A. Battle and J. K. Pritchard, "Gene regulatory network inference from CRISPR perturbations in primary CD4+ T cells elucidates the genomic basis of immune disease," *bioRxiv [Preprint],* https://doi.org/10.1101/2023.09.17.557749, 2023.
17. D. Deshpande, K. Chhugani, Y. Chang, A. Karlsberg, C. Loeffler, J. Zhang, A. Muszy, V. Munteanu, H. Yang, J. Rotman, L. Tao, B. Balliu, E. Tseng, E. Eskin, F. Zhao and P. Mohammadi, "RNA-seq data science: From raw data to effective interpretation," *Frontiers in Genetics,* vol. 14, 2023.
18. A. L. Tarca, R. Romero and S. Draghici, "Analysis of microarray experiments of gene expression profiling," *American Journal of Obstetrics and Gynecology,* vol. 195, no. 2, p. 373–388, 2008.
19. P. J. Park, "ChIP-Seq: advantages and challenges of a maturing technology," *Nature Reviews Genetics,* vol. 10, no. 10, p. 669–680, 2009.
20. S. Heinz, C. Benner, N. Spann, E. Bertolino, Y. C. Lin, P. Laslo, J. X. Cheng, C. Murre, H. Singh and C. K. Glass, "Simple combinations of lineage-determining transcription factors prime cis-regulatory elements required for macrophage and B cell identities," *Molecular Cell,* vol. 38, no. 4, p. 576–589, 2010.
21. J. V. Shiah, D. E. Johnson and J. R. Grandis, "Transcription Factors and Cancer: Approaches to Targeting," *Cancer J,* vol. 29, no. 1, p. 38–46, 2023.
22. N. Zhang, J. Wu and Q. Zheng, "Chemical proteomics approaches for protein post-translational modification studies," *Biochimica et Biophysica Acta (BBA) - Proteins and Proteomics,* vol. 1872, no. 4, 2024.
23. J. Cox and M. Mann, "MaxQuant enables high peptide identification rates, individualized p.p.b.-range mass accuracies and proteome-wide protein quantification," *Nature Biotechnology,* vol. 26, p. 1367–1372, 2008.
24. C. J. Dragomirka Jovic, X. Liang, H. Zeng, L. Lin, F. Xu and Y. Luo, "Single-cell RNA sequencing technologies and applications: A brief overview," *Clinical and Translational Medicine,* vol. 12, no. 3, p. e694, 2022.
25. S. Petropoulos, D. Edsgärd, B. Reinius, Q. Deng, S. P. Panula, S. Codeluppi, A. P. Reyes, S. Linnarsson, R. Sandberg and F. Lanner, "Single-Cell RNA-Seq Reveals Lineage and X Chromosome Dynamics in Human Preimplantation Embryos," *Cell,* vol. 165, no. 4, pp. 1012–26, 2016.
26. M. Banf and S. Y. Rhee, "Computational inference of gene regulatory networks: Approaches, limitations and opportunities," *Biochimica et Biophysica Acta (BBA) - Gene Regulatory Mechanisms,* vol. 1860, no. 1, pp. 41–52, 2017.
27. I. Shmulevich, E. R. Dougherty, S. Kim and W. Zhang, "Probabilistic Boolean networks: a rule-based uncertainty model for gene regulatory networks," *Bioinformatics,* vol. 18, no. 2, p. 261–274, 2002.
28. C. Sima, J. Hua and S. Jung, "Inference of Gene Regulatory Networks Using Time-Series Data: A Survey," *Current Genomics,* vol. 10, no. 6, p. 416–429, 2009.
29. J. Schäfer and K. Strimmer, "An empirical Bayes approach to inferring large-scale gene association networks," *Bioinformatics,* vol. 21, no. 6, p. 754–764, 2005.
30. J. Lei, Z. Cai, X. He, W. Zheng and J. Liu, "An approach of gene regulatory network construction using mixed entropy optimizing context-related likelihood mutual information," *Bioinformatics,* vol. 39, no. 1, 2023.
31. H. N. Gamage, M. Chetty, S. Lim and J. Hallinan, "GRAMP: A gene ranking and model prioritisation framework for building consensus genetic networks," *Knowledge-Based Systems,* vol. 302, no. 112374, October 2024.

32. S. Kauffman, "Metabolic stability and epigenesis in randomly constructed genetic nets," *Journal of Theoretical Biology,* vol. 22, no. 3, pp. 437–467, 1969.
33. H. Lähdesmäki, I. Shmulevich and O. Yli-Harja, "On Learning Gene Regulatory Networks Under the Boolean Network Model," *Machine Learning,* vol. 52, p. pages147–167, 2003.
34. S. Han, R. K. W. Wong, T. C. M. Lee, L. Shen, S.-Y. R. Li and X. Fan, "A Full Bayesian Approach for Boolean Genetic Network Inference," *PLoS ONE,* vol. 9, no. 12, 2014.
35. S. Liang, S. Fuhrman and R. Somogyi, "REVEAL, a general reverse engineering algorithm for inference of genetic network architectures," *Pacific Symposium on Biocomputing,* pp. 18–29, 1998.
36. H. Kim, J. K. Lee and T. Park, "Boolean networks using the chi-square test for inferring large-scale gene regulatory networks," *BMC Bioinformatics,* vol. 8, no. 1, 2007.
37. S. Barman and Y.-K. Kwon, "A novel mutual information-based Boolean network inference method from time-series gene expression data," *PLoS ONE,* vol. 12, no. 2, 2017.
38. A. Bonnaffoux, U. Herbach, A. Richard, A. Guillemin, S. Gonin-Giraud, P.-A. Gros and O. Gandrillon, "WASABI: a dynamic iterative framework for gene regulatory network inference," *BMC Bioinformatics,* vol. 20, 2019.
39. N. Shi, Z. Zhu, K. Tang, D. Parker and S. He, "ATEN: And/Or tree ensemble for inferring accurate Boolean network topology and dynamics," *Bioinformatics,* vol. 36, no. 2, p. 578–585, 2020.
40. S. Barman and Y.-K. Kwon, "A Boolean network inference from time-series gene expression data using a genetic algorithm," *Bioinformatics,* vol. 34, no. 17, p. i927–i933, September 2018.
41. S. Barman and Y.-K. Kwon, "A neuro-evolution approach to infer a Boolean network from time-series gene expressions," *Bioinformatics,* vol. 36, no. Issue Supplement_2, p. i762–i769, December 2020.
42. H. N. Gamage, M. Chetty, A. Shatte and J. Hallinan, "An Efficient Boolean Modelling Approach for Genetic Network Inference," in *2021 IEEE Conference on Computational Intelligence in Bioinformatics and Computational Biology (CIBCB)*, Melbourne, Australia, 2021.
43. H. N. Gamage, M. Chetty, A. Shatte and J. Hallinan, "Filter feature selection based Boolean Modelling for Genetic Network Inference," *Biosystems,* vol. 221, 2022.
44. A. Saadatpour, "Boolean modeling of biological regulatory networks: A methodology tutorial," *Methods,* vol. 62, no. 1, pp. 3–12, 2013.
45. I. Shmulevich, E. Dougherty and W. Zhang, "From Boolean to probabilistic Boolean networks as models of genetic regulatory networks," *Proceedings of the IEEE,* vol. 90, no. 11, pp. 1778–1792, 2002.
46. L. Li, L. Sun, G. Chen, C.-W. Wong, W.-K. Ching and Z.-P. Liu, "LogBTF: gene regulatory network inference using Boolean threshold network model from single-cell gene expression data," *Bioinformatics,* vol. 39, no. 5, p. btad256, 2023.
47. C. M. David Murrugarra, A. Veliz-Cuba, B. Aguilar, S. Arat and R. Laubenbacher, "Modeling stochasticity and variability in gene regulatory networks," *EURASIP Journal on Bioinformatics and Systems Biology,* vol. 1, no. 5, 2012.
48. D. A. Rosenblueth, S. Muñoz, M. Carrillo and E. Azpeitia, "Inference of Boolean Networks from Gene Interaction Graphs Using a SAT Solver," *Algorithms for Computational Biology,* vol. 8542, p. 235–246, 2014.
49. N. Friedman, M. Linial, I. Nachman and D. Pe'er, "Using Bayesian networks to analyze expression data," *Journal of Computational Biology,* vol. 7, no. 3–4, pp. 601–20, 2000.
50. M. Sanchez-Castillo, D. Blanco, I. M. Tienda-Luna, M. C. Carrion and Y. Huang, "A Bayesian framework for the inference of gene regulatory networks from time and pseudo-time series data," *Bioinformatics,* vol. 34, no. 6, pp. 964–970, 2018.
51. D. Heckerman, D. Geiger and D. M. Chickering, "Learning Bayesian Networks: The Combination of Knowledge and Statistical Data," *Machine Learning,* vol. 20, p. 197–243, 1995.

52. H. d. Jong, "Modeling and simulation of genetic regulatory systems: a literature review," *Journal of Computational Biology,* vol. 9, no. 1, pp. 67–103, 2002.
53. H. Gong, J. Klinger, K. Damazyn, X. Li and S. Huang, "A novel procedure for statistical inference and verification of gene regulatory subnetwork," *BMC Bioinformatics,* vol. 16, no. 7, 2015.
54. K. Murphy and S. Mian, "Modelling Gene Expression Data using Dynamic Bayesian Networks," Computer Science Division, University of California, Berkeley, 1999.
55. M. Zou and S. D. Conzen, "A new dynamic Bayesian network (DBN) approach for identifying gene regulatory networks from time course microarray data," *Bioinformatics,* vol. 21, no. 1, p. 71–79, 2005.
56. M. Grzegorczyk and D. Husmeier, "Improvements in the reconstruction of time-varying gene regulatory networks: dynamic programming and regularization by information sharing among genes," *Bioinformatics,* vol. 27, no. 5, p. 693–699, 2011.
57. L. Song, M. Kolar and E. Xing, Time-Varying Dynamic Bayesian Networks, 2009.
58. Y. Ni, F. C. Stingo and V. Baladandayuthapani, "Bayesian Nonlinear Model Selection for Gene Regulatory Networks," *Biometrics,* vol. 71, no. 3, p. 585–595, 2015.
59. A. V. Werhli, M. Grzegorczyk and D. Husmeier, "Comparative evaluation of reverse engineering gene regulatory networks with relevance networks, graphical gaussian models and bayesian networks," *Bioinformatics,* vol. 22, no. 20, pp. 2523–31, 2006.
60. S. Barbosa, B. Niebel, S. Wolf, K. Mauch and R. Takors, "A guide to gene regulatory network inference for obtaining predictive solutions: Underlying assumptions and fundamental biological and data constraints," *Biosystems,* vol. 174, pp. 37–48, 2018.
61. D. Marbach, J. C. Costello, R. Küffner, N. M. Vega, R. J. Prill, D. M. Camacho, K. R. Allison, T. D. Consortium, M. Kellis, J. J. Collins and G. Stolovitzky, "Wisdom of crowds for robust gene network inference," *Nature Methods,* vol. 9, p. 796–804, 2012.
62. Z. Li, P. Li, A. Krishnan and J. Liu, "Large-scale dynamic gene regulatory network inference combining differential equation models with local dynamic Bayesian network analysis," *Bioinformatics,* vol. 27, no. 19, p. 2686–2691, 2011.
63. S. Sebastian, S. Roy and J. Kalita, "A generic parallel framework for inferring large-scale gene regulatory networks from expression profiles: application to Alzheimer's disease network," *Briefings in Bioinformatics,* vol. 24, no. 1, p. bbac482, 2023.
64. T. S. Gardner, D. d. Bernardo, D. Lorenz. and J. J. Collins, "Inferring genetic networks and identifying compound mode of action via expression profiling," *Science,* vol. 301, p. 102–105, 2003.
65. D. D. Bernardo, M. Thompson, T. Gardner, S. Chobot, E. Eastwood, A. Wojtovich, S. Elliott, S. Schaus and J. Collins, "Chemogenomic profiling on a genome-Wide scale using reverse-engineered gene networks," *Nature Biotechnology,* vol. 23, p. 377–383, 2005.
66. M. Bansal, G. D. Gatta and D. d. Bernardo, "Inference of gene regulatory networks and compound mode of action from time course gene expression profiles," *Bioinformatics,* vol. 22, p. 815–822, 2006.
67. N. Noman and H. Iba, "Inference of gene regulatory networks using S-system and Differential Evolution," in *Genetic and Evolutionary Computation Conference*, Washington DC, USA, 2005.
68. A. R. Chowdhury, M. Chetty and N. X. Vinh, "Adaptive regulatory genes cardinality for reconstructing genetic networks," in *2012 IEEE Congress on Evolutionary Computation*, Brisbane, QLD, Australia, 2012.
69. J. Gill, M. Chetty, A. Shatte and J. Hallinan, "Dynamically Regulated Initialization for S-system Modelling of Genetic Networks," in *2021 IEEE Conference on Computational Intelligence in Bioinformatics and Computational Biology (CIBCB)*, Melbourne, Australia, 2021.
70. M. Zhao, W. He, J. Tang, Q. Zou and F. Guo, "A comprehensive overview and critical evaluation of gene regulatory network inference technologies," *Briefings in Bioinformatics,* vol. 25, no. 5, pp. 1–15, 2021.

71. H. Kim, J. K. Lee and T. Park, "Inference of large-scale gene regulatory networks using regression-based network approach," *J Bioinform Comput Biol.,* vol. 7, no. 4, pp. 717–35, 2009.
72. F. H. M. Salleh, S. Zainudin and S. M. Arif, "Multiple Linear Regression for Reconstruction of Gene Regulatory Networks in Solving Cascade Error Problems," *Advances in Bioinformatics,* p. 14, 2017.
73. V. A. Huynh-Thu, A. Irrthum, L. Wehenkel and P. Geurts, "Inferring Regulatory Networks from Expression Data Using Tree-Based Methods," *PLoS ONE,* vol. 5, no. 9, 2010.
74. A.-C. Haury, F. Mordelet, P. Vera-Licona and J.-P. Vert, "TIGRESS: Trustful Inference of Gene Regulation using Stability Selection," *BMC Systems Biology,* vol. 6, no. 145, 2012.
75. T. Moerman, S. A. Santos, C. B. González-Blas, J. Simm, Y. Moreau, J. Aerts and S. Aerts, "GRNBoost2 and Arboreto: efficient and scalable inference of gene regulatory networks," *Bioinformatics,* vol. 35, no. 12, p. 2159–2161, 2019.
76. S. Aibar, C. B. González-Blas, T. Moerman, V. A. Huynh-Thu, H. Imrichova, G. Hulselmans, F. Rambow, J.-C. Marine, P. Geurts, J. Aerts, J. v. d. Oord, Z. K. Atak and J. Wo, "SCENIC: Single-cell regulatory network inference and clustering," *Nature Methods,* vol. 14, no. 11, p. 1083–1086, 2017.
77. J. Sławek and T. Arodź, "ENNET: inferring large gene regulatory networks from expression data using gradient boosting," *BMC Systems Biology,* vol. 7, no. 106, 2013.
78. H. N. Gamage, M. Chetty, A. Shatte and J. Hallinan, "Ensemble Regression Modelling for Genetic Network Inference," in *IEEE Conference on Computational Intelligence in Bioinformatics and Computational Biology (CIBCB)*, Ottawa, ON, Canada, 2022.
79. H. N. Gamage, M. Chetty, S. Lim, J. Hallinan and H. Nguyen, "A Robust Ensemble Regression Model for Reconstructing Genetic Networks," in *International Joint Conference on Neural Networks (IJCNN)*, Gold Coast, Australia, 2023.
80. M. Emadi, F. Z. Boroujeni and J. Pirgazi, "Gene regulatory network inference from gene expression data based on knowledge matrix and improved rotation forest," *Biomedical Signal Processing and Control,* vol. 92, 2024.
81. H. Shu, J. Zhou, Q. Lian, H. Li, D. Zhao, J. Zeng and J. Ma, "Modeling gene regulatory networks using neural network architectures," *Nature Computational Science,* vol. 1, p. 491–501, 2021.
82. Z. Gao, Y. Su, J. Xia, R.-F. Cao, Y. Ding, C.-H. Zheng and P.-J. Wei, "DeepFGRN: inference of gene regulatory network with regulation type based on directed graph embedding," *Briefings in Bioinformatics,* vol. 25, no. 3, p. bbae143, 2024.
83. R. Magnusson, J. N. Tegnér and M. Gustafsson, "Deep neural network prediction of genome-wide transcriptome signatures—beyond the Black-box," *npj Systems Biology and Applications volume,* vol. 8, no. 9, 2022.
84. H. G. Lim, K. Rychel, A. V. Sastry, G. J. Bentley, J. Mueller, H. S. Schindel, P. E. Larsen, P. D. Laible, A. M. Guss, W. Niu, C. W. Johnson, G. T. Beckham, A. M. Feist and B. O. Palsson, "Machine-learning from Pseudomonas putida KT2440 transcriptomes reveals its transcriptional regulatory network," *Metabolic Engineering,* vol. 72, pp. 297–310, 2022.
85. R. I. Hamed, S. I. Ahson and R. Parveen, "A New Approach for Modelling Gene Regulatory Networks Using Fuzzy Petri Nets," *Journal of Integrative Bioinformatics,* vol. 7, no. 1, 2010.
86. P. J. Woolf and Y. Wang, "A fuzzy logic approach to analyzing gene expression data," *Physiological Genomics,* vol. 3, no. 1, pp. 9–15, 2000.
87. K. Raza, "Fuzzy logic based approaches for gene regulatory network inference," *Artificial Intelligence in Medicine,* vol. 97, pp. 189–203, 2019.
88. J. Mendel, "Fuzzy logic systems for engineering: a tutorial," in *Proceedings of the IEEE,* 1995.
89. H. N. Gamage, M. Chetty, S. Lim and J. Hallinan, "MICFuzzy: A maximal information content based fuzzy approach for reconstructing genetic networks," *PLoS One,* vol. 18, no. 7, 2023.

90. J. Liu, Y. Chi and C. Zhu, "A Dynamic Multiagent Genetic Algorithm for Gene Regulatory Network Reconstruction Based on Fuzzy Cognitive Maps," *IEEE Transactions on Fuzzy Systems,* vol. 24, no. 2, pp. 419–431, 2016.
91. D. M. Budden and E. J. Crampin, "Information theoretic approaches for inference of biological networks from continuous-valued data," *BMC Syst Biol,* vol. 10, no. 89, 2016.
92. C. E. Shannon and W. Weaver, The Mathematical Theory, Urbana: The University of Illinois Press, 1964.
93. B. Yang, Y. Xu, A. Maxwell, W. Koh, P. Gong and C. Zhang, "MICRAT: a novel algorithm for inferring gene regulatory networks using time series gene expression data," *BMC Systems Biology,* vol. 12, no. 115, 2018.
94. C. E. Shannon and W. Weaver, Urbana: The University of Illinois Press, Urbana: The University of Illinois Press, 1964.
95. D. N. Reshef, Y. A. Reshef, H. K. Finucane, S. R. Grossman, G. McVean, P. J. Turnbaugh, E. S. Lander, M. Mitzenmacher and P. C. Sabeti, "Detecting Novel Associations in Large Datasets," *Science,* vol. 334, no. 6062, p. 1518–1524, 2011.
96. M. A. H. Akhand, R. N. Nandi, S. M. Amran and K. Murase, "Gene Regulatory Network Inference Using Maximal Information Coefficient," *International Journal of Bioscience, Biochemistry and Bioinformatics,* vol. 5, no. 5, pp. 296–310, 2015.
97. P. E. Meyer, F. Lafitte and G. Bontempi, "minet: A R/Bioconductor Package for Inferring Large Transcriptional Networks Using Mutual Information," *BMC Bioinformatics,* vol. 9, no. 461, October 2008.
98. A. A. Margolin, I. Nemenman, K. Basso, C. Wiggins, G. Stolovitzky, R. D. Favera and A. Califano, "ARACNE: An Algorithm for the Reconstruction of Gene Regulatory Networks in a Mammalian Cellular Context," *BMC Bioinformatics,* vol. 7, no. S7, 2006.
99. J. J. Faith, B. Hayete, J. T. Thaden, I. Mogno, J. Wierzbowski, G. Cottarel, S. Kasif, J. J. Collins and T. S. Gardner, "Large-Scale Mapping and Validation of *Escherichia coli* Transcriptional Regulation from a Compendium of Expression Profiles," *PLOS Biology,* vol. 5, no. 1, 2007.
100. P. E. Meyer, K. Kontos, F. Lafitte and G. Bontempi, "Information-theoretic inference of large transcriptional regulatory networks," *EURASIP J Bioinform Syst Biol,* vol. 1, 2007.
101. T. E. Chan, M. P. Stumpf and A. C. Babtie, "Gene Regulatory Network Inference from Single-Cell Data Using Multivariate Information Measures," *Cell Systems,* vol. 5, no. 3, p. 251–267, 2017.
102. M. Zhao, W. He, J. Tang, Q. Zou and F. Guo, "A comprehensive overview and critical evaluation of gene regulatory network inference technologies," *Briefings in Bioinformatics,* vol. 22, no. 5, p. bbab009, 2021.
103. D. Marbach, R. J. Prill, T. Schaffter, C. Mattiussi, D. Floreano and G. Stolovitzky, "Revealing strengths and weaknesses of methods for gene network inference," *Biophysics and Computational Biology,* vol. 107, no. 14, pp. 6286–6291, 2010.
104. T. Hase, S. Ghosh, R. Yamanaka and H. Kitano, "Harnessing Diversity Towards the Reconstructing of Large Scale Gene Regulatory Networks," *PLOS Computational Biology,* vol. 9, no. 11, 2013.
105. P. Yang, Y. H. Yang, B. B. Zhou and A. Y. Zomaya, "A review of ensemble methods in bioinformatics: Including stability of feature selection and ensemble feature selection methods," *Current Bioinformatics,* vol. 5, no. 4, 2010.
106. S. Peignier, B. Sorin and F. Calevro, "Ensemble Learning Based Gene Regulatory Network Inference," in *IEEE 33rd International Conference on Tools with Artificial Intelligence (ICTAI),* Washington, DC, USA, 2021.
107. R. Zheng, M. Li, X. Chen, S. Zhao, F.-X. Wu, Y. Pan and J. Wang, "An Ensemble Method to Reconstruct Gene Regulatory Networks Based on Multivariate Adaptive Regression Splines," *IEEE/ACM TRANSACTIONS ON COMPUTATIONAL BIOLOGY AND BIOINFORMATICS,* vol. 18, no. 1, 2021.

108. O. Sagi and L. Rokach, "Ensemble learning: A survey," *WIREs: Data Mining and Knowledge Discovery,* vol. 8, no. 4, 2018.
109. V. A. Huynh-Thu and G. Sanguinetti, "Combining tree-based and dynamical systems for the inference of gene regulatory networks," *Bioinformatics,* vol. 31, no. 10, p. 1614–1622, 2015.
110. X. Dong, Z. Yu, W. Cao, Y. Shi and Q. Ma, "A survey on ensemble learning," *Front. Comput. Sci.,* vol. 14, no. 12, p. 241–258, 2020.
111. V. A. Huynh-Thu and P. Geurts, "dynGENIE3: dynamical GENIE3 for the inference of gene networks from time series expression data," *Scientific Reports,* vol. 8, no. 3384, 2018.
112. S. Park, J. M. Kim, W. Shin, S. W. Han, M. Jeon, H. J. Jang, I.-S. Jang and J. Kang, "BTNET: boosted tree based gene regulatory network inference algorithm using time-course measurement data," *BMC Systems Biology,* vol. 12, no. 20, March 2018.
113. D. Marbach, T. Schaffter, C. Mattiussi and D. Floreano, "Generating realistic in silico gene networks for performance assessment of reverse engineering methods," *Journal of Computational Biology,* vol. 16, no. 2, pp. 229–239, 2009.
114. J. Åkesson, Z. Lubovac-Pilav, R. Magnusson and M. Gustafsson, "ComHub: Community predictions of hubs in gene regulatory networks," *BMC Bioinformatics,* vol. 22, no. 58, February 2021.
115. M. Aluru, H. Shrivastava, S. P. Chockalingam, S. Shivakumar and S. Aluru, "EnGRaiN: a supervised ensemble learning method for recovery of large-scale gene regulatory networks," *Bioinformatics,* vol. 38, no. 5, February 2022.
116. B. Shen, G. Coruzzi and D. Shasha, "EnsInfer: a simple ensemble approach to network inference outperforms any single method," *BMC Bioinformatics,* vol. 114, 2023.
117. A. Segura-Ortiz, J. García-Nieto, J. F. Aldana-Montes and I. Navas-Delgado, "GENECI: A novel evolutionary machine learning consensus-based approach for the inference of gene regulatory networks," *Computers in Biology and Medicine,* vol. 155, March 2023.
118. T. Schaffter, D. Marbach and G. Roulet, "GNW User Manual: GeneNetWeaver 3.0 Beta," 2010.
119. P. T. Spellman, G. Sherlock, M. Q. Zhang, V. R. Iyer, K. Anders, M. B. Eisen, P. O. Brown, D. Botstein and B. Futcher, "Comprehensive Identification of Cell Cycle–regulated Genes of the Yeast *Saccharomyces cerevisiae* by Microarray Hybridization," *Molecular Biology of the Cell,* vol. 9, no. 12, 2017.
120. M. Rubiolo, D. H. Milone and G. Stegmayer, "Extreme learning machines for reverse engineering of gene regulatory networks from expression time series," *Bioinformatics,* vol. 34, no. 7, p. 1253–1260, 2018.
121. M. Ronen, R. Rosenberg, B. I. Shraiman and U. Alon, "Assigning numbers to the arrows: Parameterizing a gene regulation network by using accurate expression kinetics," *Biological Sciences,* vol. 99, no. 16, pp. 10555–10560, 2002.
122. B.-E. Perrin, L. Ralaivola, A. Mazurie, S. Bottani, J. Mallet and F. d'Alché–Buc, "Gene networks inference using dynamic Bayesian networks," *Bioinformatics,* vol. 19, no. suppl 2, p. ii138–ii148, 2003.
123. J. Yu, V. A. Smith, P. P. Wang, A. J. Hartemink and E. D. Jarvis, "Advances to Bayesian network inference for generating causal networks from observational biological data," *Bioinformatics,* vol. 20, no. 18, 2004.
124. N. Morshed, M. Chetty and N. X. Vinh, "Simultaneous learning of instantaneous and time-delayed genetic interactions using novel information theoretic scoring technique," *BMC Systems Biology,* vol. 6, no. 62, 2012.
125. N. X. Vinh, M. Chetty, R. Coppel and P. P. Wangikar, "GlobalMIT: learning globally optimal dynamic Bayesian network with the mutual information test criterion," *Bioinformatics,* vol. 27, no. 19, p. 2765–2766, 2011.
126. L. Yuan, L.-H. Guo, C.-A. Yuan, Y.-H. Zhang, K. Han, A. Nand, B. Honig and D.-S. Huang, "Integration of Multi-omics Data for Gene Regulatory Network Inference and Application to Breast Cancer," *IEEE/ACM Transactions on Computational Biology and Bioinformatics,* 2018.

127. J. Liu, S. Liu, Z. Yu, X. Qiu, R. Jiang and W. Li, "Uncovering the gene regulatory network of type 2 diabetes through multi-omic data integration," *Journal of Translational Medicine,* vol. 20, no. 1, 2022.
128. G. Pepe, R. Appierdo, G. Ausiello, M. Helmer-Citterich and P. F. Gherardini, "A Meta-Analysis Approach to Gene Regulatory Network Inference Identifies Key Regulators of Cardiovascular Diseases," *International Journal of Molecular Sciences,* vol. 25, no. 8, 2024.
129. D. Li, Y.-P. Li, Y.-X. Li, X.-H. Zhu, X.-G. Du, M. Zhou, W.-B. Li and H.-Y. Deng, "Effect of Regulatory Network of Exosomes and microRNAs on Neurodegenerative Diseases," *Chinese Medical Journal,* 2018.
130. B. Bai, X. Wang, Y. Li, P.-C. Chen, K. Yu, K. K. Dey, J. M. Yarbro, X. Han, B. M. Lutz, S. Rao, Y. Jiao, J. M. Sifford, J. Han and Ming, "Deep Multilayer Brain Proteomics Identifies Molecular Networks in Alzheimer's Disease Progression," *NeuroResource,* vol. 105, no. 6, 2020.
131. P. Gupta and S. K. Singh, "Gene Regulatory Networks: Current Updates and Applications in Plant Biology," in *Molecular Approaches in Plant Biology and Environmental,* 2019, p. 395–417.
132. P. Trivedi, M. Delgado-Baquerizo, C. Trivedi, H. Hu, I. C. Anderson, T. C. Jeffries, J. Zhou and B. K. Singh, "Microbial regulation of the soil carbon cycle: evidence from gene–enzyme relationships," *The ISME Journal,* vol. 10, p. 2593–2604, 2016.
133. M. G. P. v. d. Wijst, D. H. d. Vries, H. Brugge, H.-J. Westra and L. Franke, "An integrative approach for building personalized gene regulatory networks for precision medicine," *Genome Medicine,* vol. 10, no. 96, 2018.
134. L. H. Goetz and Nicholas J. Schork, "Personalized Medicine: Motivation, Challenges and Progress," *Fertility and Sterility,* vol. 109, no. 6, p. 952–963, 2018.
135. S. Huang, "Rational drug discovery: what can we learn from regulatory networks?," *Drug Discovery Today,* vol. 7, no. 20, pp. s163–s169, 2002.
136. B. A. Otálora-Otálora, L. López-Kleine and A. Rojas, "Lung Cancer Gene Regulatory Network of Transcription Factors Related to the Hallmarks of Cancer," *Current Issues in Molecular Biology,* vol. 45, no. 1, p. 434–464, 2023.
137. T. T. T. Truong, Z. S. J. Liu, B. Panizzutti, O. M. Dean, M. Berk, J. H. Kim and K. Walder, "Use of gene regulatory network analysis to repurpose drugs to treat bipolar disorder," *Journal of Affective Disorders,* vol. 350, pp. 230–239, 2024.
138. B.-S. Chen, S.-K. Yang, C.-Y. Lan and Y.-J. Chuang, "A systems biology approach to construct the gene regulatory network of systemic inflammation via microarray and databases mining," *BMC Medical Genomics*, vol. 1, no. 46, 2008.
139. H. Akazawa and I. Komuro, "Roles of Cardiac Transcription Factors in Cardiac Hypertrophy," *Circulation Research,* vol. 92, no. 10, 2003.
140. S. Kohli, S. Ahuja and V. Rani, "Transcription Factors in Heart: Promising Therapeutic Targets in Cardiac Hypertrophy," *Current Cardiology Reviews,* vol. 7, no. 4, pp. 262–271, 2011.
141. R.-S. Wang, B. A. Maron and J. Loscalzo, "Multiomics Network Medicine Approaches to Precision Medicine and Therapeutics in Cardiovascular Diseases," *Arteriosclerosis, Thrombosis, and Vascular Biology,* vol. 43, no. 4, 2023.
142. L. Wang, L. Yu, J. Shi, F. Li, C. Zhang, H. Xu, X. Yin, L. Wang, S. Lin, A. Litvinova, Y. Ping, S. Ning and H. Zhao, "Functional regulations between genetic alteration-driven genes and drug target genes acting as prognostic biomarkers in breast cancer," *Scientific Reports,* vol. 12, no. 10641, 2022.
143. C. Lu, X. Zhang, J. Schardey, U. Wirth, K. Heinrich, L. Massiminio, G. M. Cavestro, J. Neumann, A. V. Bazhin, J. Werner and F. Kühn, "Molecular characteristics of microsatellite stable early-onset colorectal cancer as predictors of prognosis and immunotherapeutic response," *npj Precision Oncology,* vol. 7, no. 63, 2023.

144. L. Yan, J. Shi and J. Zhu, "Cellular and molecular events in colorectal cancer: biological mechanisms, cell death pathways, drug resistance and signalling network interactions," *Discover Oncology,* vol. 15, no. 294, 2024.
145. K. Grützmann, T. Kraft, M. Meinhardt, F. Meier, D. Westphal and M. Seifert, "Network-based analysis of heterogeneous patient-matched brain and extracranial melanoma metastasis pairs reveals three homogeneous subgroups," *Computational and Structural Biotechnology Journal,* p. 1036–1050, 2024.
146. L. Wang, L. Yu, J. Shi, F. Li, C. Zhang, H. Xu, X. Yin, L. Wang, S. Lin, A. Litvinova, Y. Ping, S. Ning and H. Zhao, "Functional regulations between genetic alteration-driven genes and drug target genes acting as prognostic biomarkers in breast cancer," *Scientific Reports*, vol. 12, no. 10641, 2022.
147. C. Lu, X. Zhang, J. Schardey, U. Wirth, K. Heinrich, L. Massiminio, G. M. Cavestro, J. Neumann, A. V. Bazhin, J. Werner and F. Kühn, "Molecular characteristics of microsatellite stable early-onset colorectal cancer as predictors of prognosis and immunotherapeutic response," *npj Precision Oncology*, vol. 7, no. 63, 2023.

Chapter 5
Protein Design and Synthetic Biology

Anil Wipat and Jennifer Hallinan

Abstract The ability to predict protein structure from a DNA sequence has been a major challenge for bioinformatics since the inception of the use of computers in biology. The advent of efficient AI a decade ago has largely solved this problem, paving the way for the design of proteins which can perform known functions or even completely novel functions. This research has several benefits: from a commercial point of view the ability to design novel proteins to perform functions of importance to the biotechnology industry allows for such proteins to be protected and sold, potentially earning a considerable amount; a deeper understanding of the relationship between sequence and structure can lead to an increased understanding of the biology of cells; and, most importantly for us, this understanding, together with the ability to design proteins, can facilitate individualized medicine. Synthetic biology builds upon this work to engineer complete, novel genetic circuits. Synthetic biology is currently not as commercially important as the design of individual enzymes, but applications are being developed, and the field is an active area of research.

Introduction

In Chap. 2 we looked at the mechanism of protein production, with the unspoken assumption that we are dealing with naturally evolved proteins. There is considerable interest in the development of novel proteins, for two main reasons. First, and perhaps most importantly, the ability to design new proteins to order allows the production of enzymes which are more efficient than existing proteins, those which perform entirely novel functions, unknown in nature, or any other application which may come to mind.

A. Wipat
School of Computing, Newcastle University, Newcastle upon Tyne, UK

J. Hallinan (✉)
BioThink Pty Ltd, Redcliffe, QLD, Australia

M. Chetty, J. Hallinan (eds.), *From Algorithms to Ailments*,
https://doi.org/10.1007/978-3-032-11023-7_5

The second reason is that novel proteins, even those who perform the same functions as existing proteins, can be patented by industrial companies, potentially generating considerable revenue. Enzymes are ubiquitous in industry, being used for everything from food preparation to bioremediation, with the market worth at least $US13.11 billion.[1] The ability to design and synthesize novel proteins is therefore an active area of research, although the involvement of industry means that technical details are often commercial-in-confidence.

The screening of proteins has previously been carried out using directed evolution, a process in which large numbers of proteins are generated at random and evaluated for their efficiency at performing a desired task [1]. However, this process is time-consuming, expensive, and requires skilled labor. The design of proteins *in silico* eliminates many of these problems and allows more proteins to be screened more cheaply than by directed evolution.

In this chapter we review some major aspects of the use of AI in the design of novel proteins, and its application to the field of synthetic biology. Because of the level of activity in this field, and the secrecy maintained by industrial players, it is not possible to cover this field exhaustively.

Protein Design

While considerable information can be gained from the analysis of genomes, particularly whole genomes, much of the structure and function of cells is dependent upon the proteins coded for by the genome. AI can be used to analyze the proteome from several different points of view. It can be used to investigate the functions of naturally occurring proteins, giving us a more complete understanding of the cell as a complex system. Alternatively, it can be used to design completely new proteins with desired functions.

The former issue has recently been successfully addressed using newly developed AI algorithms. While it is possible to sequence a genome relatively quickly and easily, the prediction of a protein's structure from its DNA sequence has long been a major aim of bioinformatics and molecular biology. A protein is a three-dimensional structure, and the parts of the underlying amino acid sequence which make up a specific domain may lie far from each other on the amino acid chain. To predict the function of a protein, it is essential to know its structure.

A major problem with protein design is the sheer size of protein space: the set of all proteins which could exist. The length of proteins varies enormously, but the National Institutes of Health estimate the average length at 300 amino acids.[2] Given that there are 20 naturally occurring amino acids (some researchers are working on developing novel amino acids, but we're not taking this into account), the number

[1] https://www.grandviewresearch.com/industry-analysis/enzymes-industry

[2] https://www.ncbi.nlm.nih.gov/books/NBK26830/

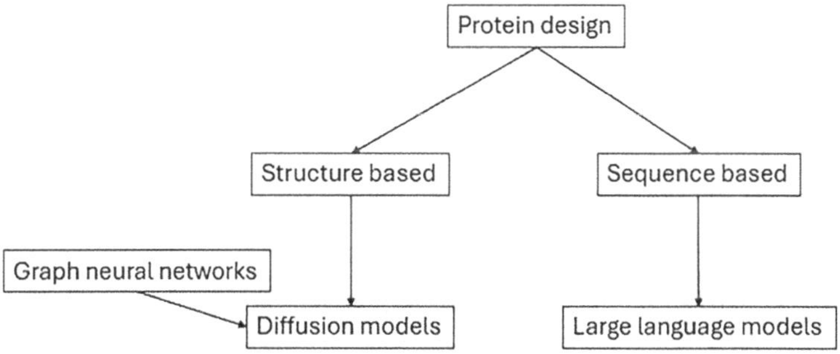

Fig. 5.1 A breakdown of approaches to protein design. Diffusion methods are strongly influenced by graph neural networks; large language models are the algorithms underlying programs such as ChatGPT

of possible proteins is around 20^{300}. Finding proteins to perform a given task is challenging, given the size of the protein space.

The application of learning algorithms to protein space is further complicated by its structure. The distance between proteins can be estimated from the difference between their amino acid sequences, and their fitness can be measured by their ability to perform the desired task, allowing the construction of a protein landscape. There is evidence that a rugged landscape, in which there are many peaks and troughs, is harder for evolution, and researchers, to navigate than a smooth landscape [2].

Many of the algorithms used for *de novo* protein design are generative algorithms: statistical models that learn a distribution over protein space. A generative model can take into account both the protein sequence and the fitness of that sequence, making it possible to sample proteins from regions of high fitness for a particular task. Winifrith and colleagues [3] divide these design approaches into sequence-based and structure-based approaches (Fig. 5.1).

These models, appropriately trained, can generalize beyond known proteins, and hence can explore completely novel areas of protein space.

Sequence-Based Algorithms

A major way to design proteins based on the known structure is to go straight to the underlying DNA sequence. Although we know a considerable amount about protein domains—which domains are binding sites for transcription factors, which are transmembrane sites, and so on—there may well be domains about which we are largely ignorant. Working from the DNA sequence eliminates this problem, while introducing problems of its own. Functional domains in a protein are not always at a single location on the chromosome but may be made up of multiple sites which are brought together in the tertiary, folded structures of the protein. This issue means that designed proteins must be similar to existing proteins for which the sequence is known.

Clearly, the more sequences available which code for proteins with a desired function, the better. Homologous proteins from different species can provide such a dataset. Vázquez and colleagues used multiple sequence alignment to produce inputs to an RFdiffusion algorithm, which produced a backbone structure. These backbones were input into a program called ProteinMPNN [4] followed by FastRelax [5] and AF2. The resulting libraries were filtered on the basis of the AF2 predicted aligned error. After considerable further processing, the result was a protein which neutralizes snake venom toxins [6], addressing an issue which is a significant problem in many parts of the world. At the time of writing this protein has only been tested in mice, but the prospects for its use in humans look promising. The code for this algorithm is freely available in GitHub.

A particularly valuable target for *de novo* protein design is the construction of antibodies. Fundamental to the workings of the immune system, antibodies, especially monoclonal antibodies, are widely used in medical treatments, for conditions such as cancers, autoimmune, metabolic, and infectious diseases. The global therapeutic monoclonal antibody market was valued at approximately US$115.2 billion in 2018, and therapeutic antibodies have become the predominant class of new drugs developed in recent years [7]. Conventionally, antibodies have been produced *in vivo* by injecting an antigen into a live animal and subsequently collecting its blood. Using computational design, antibodies can be developed with high levels of reagent reproducibility, stringent quality control, heightened target affinity and specificity, enhanced protein stability, and greater solubility than conventionally prepared molecules.

In order to function appropriately, synthetic antibodies must closely emulate the functions of their natural counterparts. Advances in technology have led to the rapid development of deep sequencing, whereby entire genomes and areas of interest such as antigen-selective sites in antibodies can be sequenced in parallel, rapidly and relatively cheaply [8, 9]. The data needed for training AI algorithms for the sequence-based design of antibodies is therefore readily available.

Lim and colleagues used convolutional neural networks to classify binder and non-binder antibody sequences for the cancer immunotherapy targets PD-1 and CTLA-4. They also constructed generative deep learning models using generative adversarial network models to produce synthetic antibodies against PD-1 and CTLA-4. The models were trained on 6003 non-binder and 1345 binder sequences for CTLA-4, and 6052 non-binder and 1719 binder sequences for PD-1, split into a training set containing 80% of the data and a test set of the remaining 20%. The models were tuned using a randomized search across various hyperparameters, including the number of filters, kernel size, dropout rate, and dense layer nodes, to determine the best hyperparameter combination for the final model architecture. The CTLA-4 and PD-1 models achieved a prediction accuracy of 91.2% and 92.6%, respectively. The areas under the ROC curves for the CTLA-4 and PD-1 models were 0.90 and 0.94, respectively. *In silico* mutagenesis analysis identified residues that were important for both the neural networks' binder classification and the antigen binding specificity.

Studies such as these suggest that AI-aided *in silico* design of a very delicately balanced system may provide a rapid, cost-effective way in which to not only replicate the function of a protein, but also to improve aspects of the functioning which would otherwise be difficult to optimize. As always, proteins designed *in silico* must be tested *in vitro*, but use of AI-driven approaches narrows the areas of protein space which should be evaluated.

Structure-Based Approaches

Because the size and shape of a protein determines its biological function, designing proteins on the basis of a desired structure appears to be an excellent approach to the problem, particularly when the aim is to design proteins which bind to a specific site on a chromosome, or perform a specific enzymic activity.

The first step in structure-based design is to accurately predict protein structure from an amino acid sequence. The ability to predict structure permits the identification of protein features such as binding sites, control regions, and the ability to function as transmembrane proteins, facilitating the assessment of probable protein function. As discussed in earlier chapters, this problem has been a significant issue until recently, but current AI algorithms have made the prediction of protein structure from sequence rapid and highly accurate.

The program AlphaFold [10] was developed by Google DeepMind in 2018. The program predicts the 3D structure of proteins with impressive accuracy and is discussed in more detail in Chaps. 1 and 2. AlphaFold has a novel neural network architecture which is trained using the evolutionary, physical and geometric constraints of protein structures. Multiple sequence alignments and pairwise features are included. The network predicts the 3D coordinates of all heavy atoms for a protein using the primary amino acid sequence and aligned sequences of homologues as inputs. The trunk of the network processes the inputs through repeated layers of a novel neural network block, and then a structure model produces an explicit 3D structure in the form of a rotation and translation for each residue of the protein. This process is iterative, and is a variant of a transformer [11]. AlphaFold has been extremely successful in addressing one of the key issues in bioinformatics: predicting protein structure from DNA sequence, as demonstrated by its performance in the CASP competition.

The current ultimate test for the accuracy of protein structure prediction is the CASP (Critical Assessment of Techniques for Protein Structure Prediction) competition [12].[3] Held annually since 1994, the competition brings together researchers from around the world to use novel algorithms to predict known protein structures (Fig. 5.2).

The CASP organizers have acknowledged the importance of AI in protein prediction [13]. Given the success of AI in protein design, several other competitions

[3] https://predictioncenter.org/

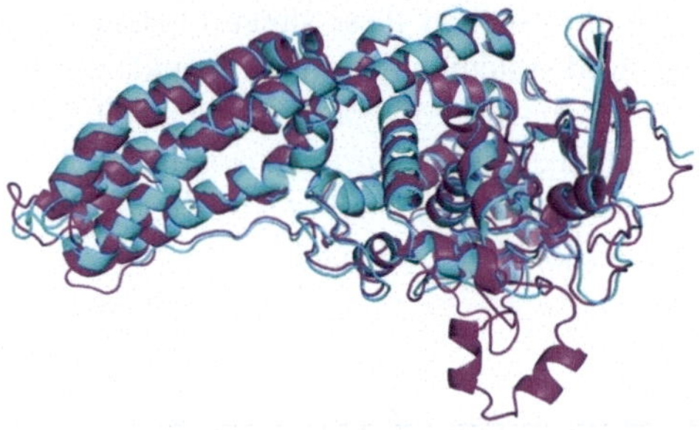

Fig. 5.2 Overlay of AlphaFold predicted protein structure (magenta or cyan) on known structure (magenta or cyan). From https://www.technologyreview.com/2020/11/30/1012712/deepmind-protein-folding-ai-solved-biology-science-drugs-disease/

have arisen, including, but not limited to, the Winter Protein Games,[4] the Adaptyv Bio Protein Design Competition,[5] the BioML Challenge,[6] and The Tournament.[7]

AlphaFold has been used to predict the structures of all amino acid sequences in the UniProt database, which contains over 200 million sequences. AlphaFold has a small error rate, meaning that not all sequences are accurate, and the data must be used with caution. However, the accuracy of the algorithm has been demonstrated to be very high, and most of these structures are correct [14, 15].

AlphaFold and is successors AlphaFold2 and AlphaFold3 have been so successful that several other successful deep learning-based protein structure prediction methods have been developed, including RoseTTAFold [16], a three-track network in which information at the one-dimensional (1D) sequence level, the 2D distance map level, and the 3D coordinate level is successively transformed and integrated; OmegaFold [17]; and ESMFold [18]. These methods can be used as the basis for the design of novel proteins for use in industry and medicine.

One example of this multi-layer approach is the development of denoising diffusion probabilistic models (DDPMs). These algorithms have been applied in several different fields but are primarily known for their success in generating synthetic images. They aim to learn the distribution of data in a data space and then generate new samples that closely resemble the original. Three main steps are involved. First, Gaussian noise is added to the input data, which is then randomly denoised to produce multiple, highly diverse outputs. The use of noise allows for uncertainty, which is important for assessing the results. Then there is an iterative generation step addressing specific design objectives, using conditioning information. Finally, to assess the likelihood of the new protein functioning as desired, it is important to model the 3D structure, in order to visualize structures such as binding sites and functional motifs.

[4] https://liberumbio.com/PDG24.htm

[5] https://design.adaptyvbio.com/

[6] https://www.biomlsociety.org/challenge

[7] https://alignbio.org/the-tournament-program

Watson and colleagues developed a DDPM system called RFdiffusion [19], using RoseTTAFold as the denoising step, and applied it to a number of problems in protein design. They found that it worked well, outperforming other state-of-the-art algorithms on issues including protein monomer generation, the design of higher order oligomers, functional motif scaffolding where the role of the scaffold is to hold a protein in precisely the right 3D structure for it to carry out binding or catalytic functions, scaffolding enzyme active sites, and the design of protein-binding proteins.

A different neural network based approach to *de novo* protein design was used by Dauparas and colleagues [4]. These researchers used a message-passing neural network (MPNN) [20] with three encoder and three decoder layers and 128 hidden dimensions, to predict protein sequences from the N to C terminus using protein backbone features as inputs. Once again, adding Gaussian noise to the protein backbones was found to improve the performance of the algorithm. They found that in cases where there was only a single backbone sequence available, their approach, dubbed ProteinMPNN, outperformed AlphaFold and RoseTTAFold, whereas the latter two algorithms worked better on multiple sequence alignments. The *de novo* proteins were tested by obtaining synthetic genes encoding the designs and expressing them in *Escherichia coli*. The proteins so obtained were monomers, cyclic oligomers, protein nanoparticles, and protein-protein interfaces, and were characterized biochemically and structurally. The novel proteins performed well.

Another neural network approach was used by Anishchenko and co-workers [21], who developed the trRosetta structure prediction network based on Rosetta [22], on randomly generated amino acid sequences to generate initial residue-residue distance maps. trRosetta is a web-based protein structure application which calculates the distance and orientations of pairs of residues and uses these as restraints to guide structure prediction via direct energy minimization. In this work, the initial distance maps were used as the restraints on Rosetta. trRosetta was found to be fast and accurate in the prediction of the structure of novel proteins.

The use of AI has facilitated the design of proteins *in silico*. However, the proteins designed in this way must be tested in the laboratory, and the success rate is still not great, hovering at around 20% [3]. Care must therefore be taken in evaluating the results of the computational design process. Despite this relatively low success rate, major industry players have found this approach to be worthwhile, and the field is an active area of research.

Synthetic Biology

A major application of novel protein design is in the field of synthetic biology: the application of engineering principles to biological systems to produce novel behaviors and organisms. The main differences between genetic engineering and synthetic biology are:

- *Scale*. Synthetic biology aims to build large-scale novel systems, and even completely novel cells. Genetic engineering generally focuses on single proteins or protein complexes.
- *Focus*. Whereas genetic engineering focuses largely on the development of commercially valuable enzymes and drugs, synthetic biology is largely concerned with the development of completely novel biological behaviours [23].
- *Implications*. The development of completely synthetic systems raises problems which are not easily addressed analytically [23]. Artificial intelligence can be used not only in the design of the components of a system, but also to address issues arising from the interactions between components in a complex system. These implications can be negative as well as positive, since large, unnatural systems can potentially cause unforeseen consequences, and ethical considerations have been incorporated into synthetic biology from its beginning [24].

The term synthetic biology was first used in 1910. However, at that time neither technology or molecular biology was sufficiently advanced to permit what we now consider to be synthetic biology; even the structure of DNA was not known. Early synthetic biology started in 1973 [25], but did not approach its modern form until 2000 [26, 27].

In 2003, Tom Knight designed BioBricks, standardized DNA parts, which formed the basis of the annual International Genetically Engineered Machines (iGEM) competition,[8] which featured genetic circuits designed and was implemented by university and high school students from all over the world. Students, with their active imaginations and lack of bias against "impossible" designs, produced a wide range of interesting and creative circuits. Although most of these designs were only developed to proof-of-concept status, several of them were picked up and further developed by various research teams [28]. These projects included a biosensor developed by the 2006 Edinburgh team [29]. The biosensor attaches to a smartphone and can detect arsenic in well water, a significant problem in Bangladesh and surrounding countries.

Today, synthetic biology approaches are applied in fields as diverse as materials design [30, 31], agriculture [32], the development of artificial life, and therapeutics such as vaccines, diagnostics and drugs [33–36], as well as the standard commercial enzymes [37, 38]. Recent developments in AI algorithms and computational power have led to an increasing use of AI in synthetic biology [39].

In the field of medicine, a combination of AI and synthetic biology has been applied to a plethora of issues, including: drug development; the prediction of host-pathogen interactions and their effects; clinical decision making, allowing for the development of personalized medicine; the prediction of prognoses; the selection of appropriate antigens; the prediction of drug resistance; finding new uses for previously approved drugs (an approach known as drug repurposing, which significantly reduces the cost and time required to develop new therapeutic approaches).

---

[8] https://competition.igem.org/

A powerful tool for the representation of disease systems is as a network, as previously described. A network consists of nodes with edges between them. The nodes may represent aspects of the system such as genes, gene products, cells, or individuals, while the edges can reflect any type of interaction between the nodes. There exists a considerable body or work on the properties and analysis of networks, which can inform the development and application of AI algorithms to the study of disease.

AI is well suited to synthetic biology–based diagnostics because of the high programmability of biological elements, the routine generation of large sequence-based datasets, and the ability of AI algorithms to extract valuable information from biomolecular networks of diseases [40].

Hallinan and colleagues [41] used evolutionary computation, an early form of AI, to investigate the role of stochasticity in genetic circuits. The circuit under study was the *Bacillus subtilis sin* operon, and the approach used was network analysis. Operons are sets of genes under the control of a single protein. While not a major feature of eukaryotic genomes, they are widespread in prokaryotic genomes. *B. subtilis* is non-pathogenic (in fact, it is used to ferment soybeans to make natto, a popular breakfast food in Japan), but the principles of the interaction between operons, stochasticity, and synthetic biology which apply to this bacterium apply to the design or modification of disease-causing bacteria.

The network used in this model was derived from the literature and is relatively small, to facilitate a deep understanding of the system. It is of interest because the control of gene expression is not only carried out by the binding of transcription factors to control regions on the genome, but also by competitive binding of the various proteins themselves (Fig. 5.3). The model was written in Java and SBML, a modelling language widely used in systems biology, and simulated using the COPASI biochemical network simulator Version 4.5 build 30 [42].

The model had 53 kinetic parameters, drawn from the literature, of which only those that could be modified *in vivo* were allowed to change. The change was achieved using an evolutionary algorithm, a long-established machine learning algorithm. Each parameterized network was run 100 times, with a different, small amount of noise, drawn from a normal distribution with mean 0 and variance 0.01, added to the parameter values each time to simulate biological stochasticity.

As can be seen from Fig. 5.3, a single input to the network can produce one of two possible outcomes. The input is phosphorylated Spo0A, a major transcription factor in *B. subtilis*. The possible outcomes are the production of a flagellum, which allows a bacterium to swim away from a potentially hazardous environment, or the production of a biofilm, a community of microorganisms which are embedded in a polysaccharide matrix, and which forms on living or nonliving surfaces. Biofilms are hard to remove and can be a major problem in a medical setting, contaminating catheters, causing the persistence of staphylococcal infections related to foreign bodies, and influencing chronic *Pseudomonas aeruginosa* lung infections in cystic fibrosis patients, to name just a few issues [43]. The bacteria in a biofilm are therefore also well protected from environmental hazards.

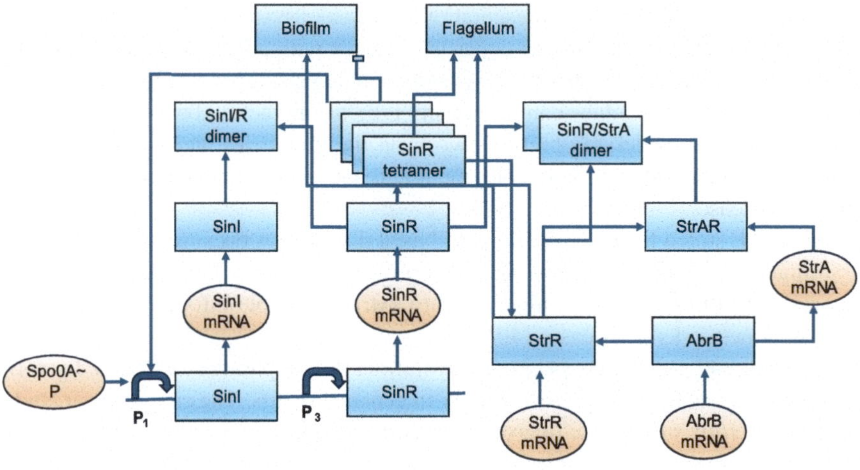

Fig. 5.3 The SinI/SinR model. The concentration of the SinI/R dimer, which controls the promoter P_1, is affected not only by the transcription rate of the genes, but also by the formation of dimers and tetramers between the proteins involved

The aim of the model was to identify parameter sets which produced flagellae 50% of the time and biofilms 50% of the time. Following evolution the effects of stochasticity were clear; different runs of the same network produced very different outcomes (Fig. 5.4).

Our model suggests that the *sin* operon switch can be evolved very easily to produce a large proportion of flagellated cells; less easily to produce an intermediate proportion; and only with difficulty to produce a large proportion of cells choosing the biofilm fate. This bias appears to make evolutionary sense, since the production of a flagellum, and subsequent motility and escape from difficult local conditions is likely to be less of an energy commitment for the cell than is biofilm formation. In a biological system not all of the cells involved in biofilm formation actually choose the biofilm phenotype; in fact, only a minority do so, and their contribution is sufficient to maintain the biofilm for the entire community [44].

It is important to understand the interplay between bacterial operons and biological stochasticity, and their implications for human disease. Operons are crucial to bacterial functioning and therefore are essential to an understanding of bacterial metabolism. Genes carried on operons have been implicated in human disease. For example, extraintestinal pathogenic *Escherichia coli* carry the gene *frz* which has been shown to be involved in adherence to and internalization in human type II pneumocytes and human enterocytes [45] in some pathogenic bacteria including group A and C streptococci. In some pathogenic bacteria, including group A and C streptococci, the synthesis of hyaluronic acid (HA) occurs in an operon (*has*) coding for enzymes involved in the production of HA precursors. HA is the capsule material of some pathogenic bacteria [46]. The *glpFKD* (*glp*) operon encodes proteins for the uptake and utilization of glycerol, a carbohydrate source, in *Borreliella*

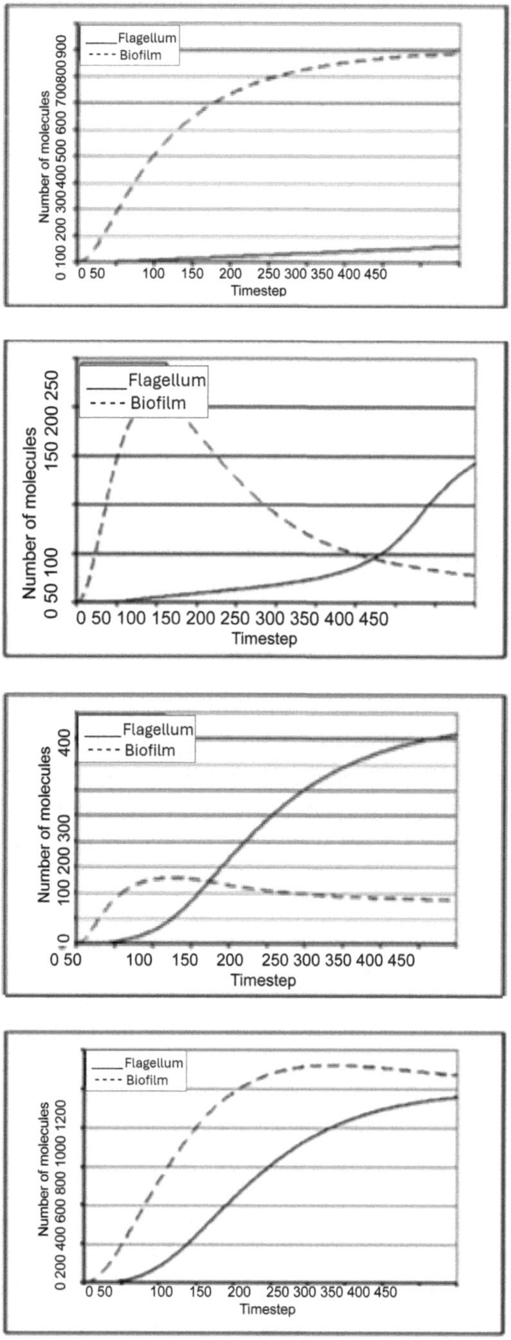

Fig. 5.4 The outcome of four runs of a network with the same parameter values and added noise

burgdorferi, the Lyme disease spirochete [47]. There are numerous other examples in the literature, and undoubtedly many of which we have no knowledge.

Synthetic biology is not as industrially important as engineered *de novo* proteins, particularly enzymes, but is still an active area of research, and holds considerable promise for the engineering of large-scale systems in the not-so-distant future.

Conclusions

There are several issues with the use of AI for synthetic biology. Most AI algorithms are trained on large amounts of data; the more the better. While biomedical datasets do tend to be very large, they are incomplete in ways which we often do not understand. The data are also frequently noisy, with unknown amounts of incorrect information. The problem of reproducibility of the results of biomedical experiments is significant, partly due to a general lack of sharing of protocols, data, and computer code, as well as the sensitivity of the results to even minor changes in the experimental equipment and environment, and errors in analysis. The effects of these problems can be wide-reaching; in 2010 there was widespread consternation when a cancer clinical trial was halted due to the irreproducibility of the results [48].

The foundation of all forms of life of which we are aware is DNA and the proteins and RNAs it produces. An understanding of this foundation is therefore crucial to our understanding of cells and cellular systems, in health and in sickness. The advent of AI has led to significant increases in our ability to understand the molecular basis of life, identify the genetic causes of and predispositions to a range of disease conditions, and predict previously unsuspected links between genotype and phenotype. Many deep learning algorithms use existing tools and build upon them, making the development of these sophisticated algorithms essentially a collaborative effort. Like all scientists, AI researchers stand on the shoulders of those who went before them.

The workhorses of the cell are proteins, although the contribution of noncoding RNAs must not be overlooked. The design of proteins which either mimic the behavior of naturally evolved proteins, or which perform completely novel functions is a significant challenge, which has not been addressed until the recent development of AI algorithms for the prediction of protein structure and for the design of proteins. Advances in such algorithms, along with the amount of computing power available, have meant that this is now a very active area of research.

Synthetic biology builds upon the basis of protein design to develop entire systems of interacting components, up to the scale of whole cells. This scaling up introduces its own issues related to understanding and manipulating protein and RNA interactions, some of which can be addressed using AI algorithms.

In this chapter we have provided a brief overview of the way in which AI has been used in protein design and construction, with an emphasis on its use for biomedical problems.

References

1. Xiong, W., Liu, B., Shen, Y., Jing, K., and Savage, T.R.: 'Protein engineering design from directed evolution to de novo synthesis', Biochemical Engineering Journal, 2021, 174, pp. 108096
2. Kauffman, S., and Levin, S.: 'Towards a general theory of adaptive walks on rugged landscapes', Journal of theoretical Biology, 1987, 128, (1), pp. 11–45
3. Winnifrith, A., Outeiral, C., and Hie, B.: 'Generative artificial intelligence for de novo protein design', arXiv preprint arXiv:2310.09685, 2023
4. Dauparas, J., Anishchenko, I., Bennett, N., Bai, H., Ragotte, R.J., Milles, L.F., Wicky, B.I., Courbet, A., de Haas, R.J., and Bethel, N.: 'Robust deep learning–based protein sequence design using ProteinMPNN', Science, 2022, 378, (6615), pp. 49–56
5. Tyka, M.D., Jung, K., and Baker, D.: 'Efficient sampling of protein conformational space using fast loop building and batch minimization on highly parallel computers', Journal of computational chemistry, 2012, 33, (31), pp. 2483–2491
6. Vázquez Torres, S., Benard Valle, M., Mackessy, S.P., Menzies, S.K., Casewell, N.R., Ahmadi, S., Burlet, N.J., Muratspahić, E., Sappington, I., and Overath, M.D.: 'De novo designed proteins neutralize lethal snake venom toxins', Nature, 2025, pp. 1–7
7. Lu, R.-M., Hwang, Y.-C., Liu, I.-J., Lee, C.-C., Tsai, H.-Z., Li, H.-J., and Wu, H.-C.: 'Development of therapeutic antibodies for the treatment of diseases', Journal of biomedical science, 2020, 27, pp. 1–30
8. Metzker, M.L.: 'Sequencing technologies—the next generation', Nature reviews genetics, 2010, 11, (1), pp. 31–46
9. Zhang, J., Chiodini, R., Badr, A., and Zhang, G.: 'The impact of next-generation sequencing on genomics', Journal of genetics and genomics, 2011, 38, (3), pp. 95–109
10. Potapenko, A.B., Meyer, C., Kohl, S.A., Ballard, A.J., Cowie, A., Romera-Paredes, B., Nikolov, S., Jain, R., and Hassabis, D.: 'Highly accurate protein structure prediction with AlphaFold', Nature, 2021, 596, pp. 583
11. Jumper, J., Evans, R., Pritzel, A., Green, T., Figurnov, M., Ronneberger, O., Tunyasuvunakool, K., Bates, R., Žídek, A., and Potapenko, A.: 'Highly accurate protein structure prediction with AlphaFold', nature, 2021, 596, (7873), pp. 583–589
12. Moult, J., Fidelis, K., Kryshtafovych, A., Schwede, T., and Topf, M.: 'Critical assessment of techniques for protein structure prediction, fourteenth round', CASP 14 Abstract Book, 2020
13. Ozden, B., Kryshtafovych, A., and Karaca, E.: 'The impact of AI-based modeling on the accuracy of protein assembly prediction: Insights from CASP15', Proteins: Structure, Function, and Bioinformatics, 2023, 91, (12), pp. 1636–1657
14. Varadi, M., Anyango, S., Deshpande, M., Nair, S., Natassia, C., Yordanova, G., Yuan, D., Stroe, O., Wood, G., Laydon, A., Žídek, A., Green, T., Tunyasuvunakool, K., Petersen, S., Jumper, J., Clancy, E., Green, R., Vora, A., Lutfi, M., Figurnov, M., Cowie, A., Hobbs, N., Kohli, P., Kleywegt, G., Birney, E., Hassabis, D., and Velankar, S.: 'AlphaFold Protein Structure Database: massively expanding the structural coverage of protein-sequence space with high-accuracy models', Nucleic Acids Research, 2021, 50, (D1), pp. D439–D444
15. Varadi, M., Bertoni, D., Magana, P., Paramval, U., Pidruchna, I., Radhakrishnan, M., Tsenkov, M., Nair, S., Mirdita, M., Yeo, J., Kovalevskiy, O., Tunyasuvunakool, K., Laydon, A., Žídek, A., Tomlinson, H., Hariharan, D., Abrahamson, J., Green, T., Jumper, J., Birney, E., Steinegger, M., Hassabis, D., and Velankar, S.: 'AlphaFold Protein Structure Database in 2024: providing structure coverage for over 214 million protein sequences', Nucleic Acids Research, 2023, 52, (D1), pp. D368–D375
16. Baek, M., DiMaio, F., Anishchenko, I., Dauparas, J., Ovchinnikov, S., Lee, G.R., Wang, J., Cong, Q., Kinch, L.N., and Schaeffer, R.D.: 'Accurate prediction of protein structures and interactions using a three-track neural network', Science, 2021, 373, (6557), pp. 871–876

17. Wu, R., Ding, F., Wang, R., Shen, R., Zhang, X., Luo, S., Su, C., Wu, Z., Xie, Q., and Berger, B.: 'High-resolution de novo structure prediction from primary sequence', BioRxiv, 2022, pp. 2022.2007. 2021.500999
18. Lin, Z., Akin, H., Rao, R., Hie, B., Zhu, Z., Lu, W., dos Santos Costa, A., Fazel-Zarandi, M., Sercu, T., and Candido, S.: 'Language models of protein sequences at the scale of evolution enable accurate structure prediction', BioRxiv, 2022, 2022, pp. 500902
19. Watson, J.L., Juergens, D., Bennett, N.R., Trippe, B.L., Yim, J., Eisenach, H.E., Ahern, W., Borst, A.J., Ragotte, R.J., and Milles, L.F.: 'De novo design of protein structure and function with RFdiffusion', Nature, 2023, 620, (7976), pp. 1089–1100
20. Gilmer, J., Schoenholz, S.S., Riley, P.F., Vinyals, O., and Dahl, G.E.: 'Message passing neural networks', Machine learning meets quantum physics, 2020, pp. 199–214
21. Anishchenko, I., Pellock, S.J., Chidyausiku, T.M., Ramelot, T.A., Ovchinnikov, S., Hao, J., Bafna, K., Norn, C., Kang, A., and Bera, A.K.: 'De novo protein design by deep network hallucination', Nature, 2021, 600, (7889), pp. 547–552
22. Löffler, P., Schmitz, S., Hupfeld, E., Sterner, R., and Merkl, R.: 'Rosetta: MSF: a modular framework for multi-state computational protein design', PLoS computational biology, 2017, 13, (6), pp. e1005600
23. Benner, S.A., and Sismour, A.M.: 'Synthetic Biology', Nature Reviews Genetics, 2005, 6, pp. 533–543
24. Bensaude Vincent, B.: 'Ethical perspectives on synthetic biology', Biological Theory, 2013, 8, (4), pp. 368–375
25. Cohen, S., Chang, A., Boyer, H., and Helling, R.: 'Construction of biological functional plasmids in vitro', Proceedings of the National Academy of Sciences, 1973, 70, pp. 3240–3244
26. Elowitz, M., and Leibler, S.: 'A synthetic oscillatory network of transcriptional regulators', Nature, 2000, 403, (6767), pp. 335–338
27. Gardner, T., Cantor, C., and Collins, J.: 'Construction of a genetic toggle switch in *Escherichia coli*', Nature, 2000, 403, (6767), pp. 339–342
28. Jainarayanan, A.K., Galanis, A., Sreejith, t., Suresh, S., Nakara, A.M., Kundltsch, G.E., and Rubio-Sanchez, R.: 'iGEM comes of age: trends in its research output', Nature Biotechnology, 2021, 39, pp. 1599–1601
29. Wan, X., Volpetti, F., French, C., Maerkl, S.J., and Wng, B.: 'Cascaded amplifying circuits enable ultrasensitive cellular sensors for toxic metals', Nature Chemical Biology, 2019, 15, pp. 540–548
30. Tzu-Chieh, T., An, B., Huang, Y., Vasikaran, S., Wang, Y., Jiang, X., Lu, T.K., and Zhong, C.: 'Materials design by synthetic biology', Nature Reviews Materials, 2021, 6, (4), pp. 332–350
31. Liu, A.P., Appel, E.A., Ashby, P.D., Baker, B.M., Franco, E., Gu, L., Haynes, K., Joshi, N.S., Kloxin, A.M., Kouwer, P.H., and Mittal, J.: 'The living interface between synthetic biology and biomaterial design', Nature Materials, 2022, 21, (4), pp. 390–397
32. Ke, J., Wang, B., and Yoshikuni, Y.: 'Microbiome engineering: synthetic biology of plant-associated microbiomes in sustainable agriculture', Trends in Biotechnology, 2021, 39, (3), pp. 244–261
33. Cubillos-Ruiz, A., Guo, T., Sokolovska, A., Miller, P.F., Collins, J.J., LuJose, T.K., and Lora, M.: 'Engineering living therapeutics with synthetic biology.', Nature Reviews Drug Discovery, 2021, 20, (12), pp. 941–960
34. Gurbatri, C.R., Arpaia, N., and Danino, T.: 'Engineering bacteria as interactive cancer therapies', Science, 2022, 378, (6622), pp. 858–864
35. Bashor, C.J., Hilton, I.B., Bandukwala, H., Smith, D.M., and Veiseh, O.: 'Engineering the next generation of cell-based therapeutics', Nature Reviews Drug Discovery, 2022, 21, (9), pp. 655–675
36. Wong, F., de la Fuente-Nunez, C., and Collins, J.J.: 'Leveraging artificial intelligence in the fight against infectious diseases', Science, 2023, 381, (6654), pp. 164–170

37. Wang, M., Chen, L., Zhang, Z., and Wang, Q.: 'Recent advances in genome mining and synthetic biology for discovery and biosynthesis of natural products', Critical Reviews in Biotechnology, 2025, 45, (1), pp. 236–256
38. Gurdo, N., Volke, D.C., McCloskey, D., and Nikel, P.I.: 'Automating the design-build-test-learn cycle towards next-generation bacterial cell factories', New Biotechnology, 2023, 74, pp. 1–15
39. García Martín, H., Mazurenko, S., and Zhao, H.: 'Special Issue on Artificial Intelligence for Synthetic Biology', ACS Synthetic Biology, 2024, 13, (2), pp. 408–410
40. Camacho, D.M., Collins, K.M., Powers, R.K., Costello, J.C., and Collins, J.J.: 'Next-generation machine learning for biological networks', Cell 2018, 173, pp. 1581–1592
41. Hallinan, J.S., Misirli, G., and Wipat, A.: 'Evolutionary computation for the design of a stochastic switch for synthetic genetic circuits', in Editor (Ed.)^(Eds.): 'Book Evolutionary computation for the design of a stochastic switch for synthetic genetic circuits' (IEEE, 2010, edn.), pp. 768–774
42. Hoops, S., Sahle, S., Gauges, R., Lee, C., Pahle, J., Simus, N., Singhal, M., Xu, L., Mendes, P., and Kummer, U.: 'COPASI—a complex pathway simulator', Bioinformatics, 2006, 22, (24), pp. 3067–3074
43. Høiby, N., Ciofu, O., Johansen, H.K., Song, Z.j., Moser, C., Jensen, P.Ø., Molin, S., Givskov, M., Tolker-Nielsen, T., and Bjarnsholt, T.: 'The clinical impact of bacterial biofilms', International journal of oral science, 2011, 3, (2), pp. 55–65
44. Chai, Y., Chu, F., Kolter, R., and Losick, R.: 'Bistability and biofilm formation in Bacillus subtilis', Molecular microbiology, 2008, 67, (2), pp. 254–263
45. Rouquet, G., Porcheron, G., Barra, C., Répérant, M., Chanteloup, N.K., Schouler, C., and Gilot, P.: 'A metabolic operon in extraintestinal pathogenic Escherichia coli promotes fitness under stressful conditions and invasion of eukaryotic cells', Journal of Bacteriology, 2009, 191, (13), pp. 4427–4440
46. Blank, L.M., Hugenholtz, P., and Nielsen, L.K.: 'Evolution of the hyaluronic acid synthesis (has) operon in Streptococcus zooepidemicus and other pathogenic streptococci', Journal of Molecular Evolution, 2008, 67, pp. 13–22
47. Zhang, J.-J., Raghunandanan, S., Wang, Q., Priya, R., Alanazi, F., Lou, Y., and Yang, X.F.: 'BadR directly represses the expression of the glycerol utilization operon in the Lyme disease pathogen', Journal of Bacteriology, 2024, 206, (2), pp. e00340–00323
48. Hutson, S.: 'Data handling errors spur debate over clinical trial', Nature Medicine, 2010, 16, (6), pp. 618

Chapter 6
AI-Driven Innovations in Cancer Care: A Comprehensive Overview

Jason Li, Han Aw Yeang, and Rashindrie Perera

Abstract This chapter explores the transformative potential of Artificial Intelligence (AI) in revolutionizing cancer care. It begins with an introduction to the fundamental motivation for AI in oncology, setting the stage for an in-depth exploration of its applications in cancer care. The chapter examines AI's role in cancer diagnosis and screening, including its use in medical imaging analysis, pathology, liquid biopsies and omics data integration. It then delves into AI applications in cancer treatment, covering personalized treatment planning, radiotherapy optimization, drug discovery, surgical oncology, and virtual health assistance. The discussion extends to AI's contributions to cancer care management and supportive care, encompassing predictive modelling, remote patient monitoring, and hospital administration. A critical analysis of the challenges associated with AI implementation in cancer care is presented, addressing issues such as data privacy, regulatory frameworks, algorithmic bias, and the need for transparency and interpretability in AI models. The chapter concludes by exploring future directions and opportunities, offering insights into the potential transformative impact of AI on cancer care. Throughout, the chapter emphasizes the interdisciplinary nature of AI in oncology and its potential to revolutionize patient outcomes, while also acknowledging the ethical and practical considerations that must be addressed for successful integration into clinical practice.

Jason Li, contributed equally to this work.

J. Li (✉) · H.A. Yeang · R. Perera
Cancer Research Division, Peter MacCallum Cancer Centre, Melbourne, VIC, Australia
e-mail: Jason.Li@petermac.org

M. Chetty, J. Hallinan (eds.), *From Algorithms to Ailments*,
https://doi.org/10.1007/978-3-032-11023-7_6

Introduction to Cancer Care

According to the World Health Organization's definition, "Cancer is a large group of diseases that can start in almost any organ or tissue of the body when abnormal cells grow uncontrollably, go beyond their usual boundaries to invade adjoining parts of the body and/or spread to other organs" [1]. Cancer is a genetic disease whereby the genes that control the normal proliferation of a cell are dysregulated, leading to uncontrolled proliferation and subsequent formation of a tissue mass (tumor). This situation can further lead to spreading of the cancer to various distant locations from the initial establishment of the primary tumor in a process termed metastasis [2]. Recently, it has been proposed that cancer be redefined as "a disease of uncontrolled proliferation by transformed cells subject to evolution by natural selection" [3]. Uncontrolled growth of cells, resulting in tumor mass has been recorded since prehistoric times, with the earliest recording of (breast) cancer was found in Edwin Smith Papyrus circa 3000 BC [4].

Globally, there were close to 20 million new cases of cancer in the year 2022 resulting in 9.7 million deaths from cancer [5]. For the year 2022, around one in 50 (1.8% or 456,200) people had cancer, with males slightly more likely than females to suffer from cancer (2.1% compared to 1.6%) [6]. There are historical records showing that the treatment of cancer has always involved topical medications or surgical intervention if the tumors were accessible and medical care available, commensurate with the century recorded in historical texts [4].

In modern times, the diagnosis of cancer has always involved the field of histology. Histology is a separate discipline from anatomy; the latter studies the gross physical structure and organization of the body, whilst the former examines the molecular and cellular level of the body organs [7, 8]. It wasn't until the invention of the light microscope in the sixteenth century by Jannsen and further refinement by Dutch scientist Anthony van Leeuwenhoek resulting in a microscope of higher magnification and better image quality in 1670 [8] that the field of histology took off. However, it took several more centuries for the discovery of histological stains (Prussian blue, 1774; hematoxylin and eosin (H&E stain) 1875–1878) along with paraffin wax for infiltration (and stabilization, 1893) of tissues before the use of histology for cancer diagnosis became more widespread [8].

Depending on the type of cancer, various types of treatments are available. These range from traditional treatment methods (surgery, chemotherapy, and radiotherapy) to modern modalities including hormone therapy, anti-angiogenic, stem cell therapies, and immunotherapy [9]. Currently, there are many types of routine tests and analyses, such as blood tests, cytogenetic screening, and liquid biopsy, that can be conducted to diagnose cancer [10]. Although there are some variances depending on the types of cancer being diagnosed, it is generally accepted that earlier diagnosis leads to better outcome and survival of the patient [11–13].

A very generic and simplified overview for a cancer diagnosis normally proceeds from a route that might be similar to that described by Jones [14]:

- Primary healthcare practitioner (or specialist) suspects potential tumour based on patient history and differential clinical diagnosis.
- The patient is referred to a cancer specialist who will request appropriate imaging (radiography-based) and/or tissue biopsy.
- If cancer is confirmed, treatment may consist of various modalities and can include, but is not limited to surgery, chemotherapy, radiotherapy, and immunotherapy.

Cancer care faces several significant challenges that hinder optimal outcomes for patients. Early detection remains a critical issue, as many cancers are diagnosed at advanced stages when treatment options are limited, reducing survival rates [15, 16]. Around 50% of cancers are only detected at an advanced stage [15]. Additionally, the complexity of cancer as a disease—varying across individuals in terms of genetic, environmental, and lifestyle factors—makes treatment personalization a daunting task. For example, gastric cancer has been found to be associated with genetic factors, high consumption of salty and smoked foods, smoking, and alcohol intake [16]. Managing the sheer volume of medical data, including imaging, genomics, and electronic health records, adds another layer of difficulty for clinicians striving to make timely and accurate decisions [17]. These factors cause delays during the patient consultation phase as well as in the downstream processes. Financial burdens, resource limitations in healthcare systems, and disparities in access to care further exacerbate the problem [18], emphasizing the urgent need for innovative solutions.

Artificial intelligence (AI) is emerging as a game-changer in addressing these challenges, offering tools to revolutionize cancer care across its continuum. By leveraging advanced machine learning algorithms, AI can analyze vast datasets, uncover hidden patterns, and provide precise insights that enable earlier and more accurate diagnoses. AI's ability to personalize treatment plans by integrating genomic, imaging, and clinical data offers new hope for tailored therapies [19]. Furthermore, AI-powered systems streamline workflows, enhance resource utilization, minimize overall costs, and reduce the time from diagnosis to treatment, improving both patient outcomes and the efficiency of healthcare delivery [20, 21]. Additionally, AI offers the potential to minimize the side effects of cancer treatments by identifying safer drug candidates and optimizing therapeutic designs through complex data analysis, predicting potential toxicities, and optimizing treatment designs to target tumors more precisely [22]. Through advanced predictive modeling, AI can help tailor therapies to individual patients, reducing off-target effects and improving overall treatment outcomes. AI is successfully being applied in different specialties including cardiology, surgery, gastroenterology, pneumology, nephrology, urology, dermatology, orthopedics, neurology, gynecology, ophthalmology, pediatrics, and hematology [23].

The foundation of AI in cancer research lies in the integration of diverse data sources, including genomic profiles, medical imaging, electronic health records, and clinical trial datasets, which provide a comprehensive understanding of cancer biology [24]. Key players in this field include technology companies, pharmaceutical giants, and academic institutions, while stakeholders include healthcare providers, policymakers, and patients, all working collaboratively to harness AI's transformative potential in oncology.

In this chapter, we explore the transformative role of AI in advancing the triage, diagnosis, treatment, and overall survival outcomes in cancer care. We present some of the examples of each aspect and discuss how AI has had an impact on each. We will also be looking at challenges that remain for effective integration into clinical workflows and explore potential future directions for advancing research and applications.

AI in Cancer Diagnosis and Screening

Medical Imaging Analysis

Medical imaging has revolutionized cancer diagnostics and treatment by providing detailed visualizations of internal structures. Technologies such as X-ray imaging, computed tomography (CT), magnetic resonance imaging (MRI), ultrasound, and positron emission tomography (PET) each offer unique capabilities. X-rays provide quick and efficient tools for identifying tumors, while CT scans produce high-resolution cross-sectional images of tissues and organs [25, 26]. MRI provides detailed soft-tissue imaging without the use of ionizing radiation, and ultrasounds enable real-time visualization, which is especially useful in guiding biopsies. This non-ionizing nature is important for individuals who require repeated imaging examinations or are concerned about radiation exposure [27]. PET scans assess metabolic activity through radiotracers and, when combined with CT, deliver comprehensive functional and structural insights. Recent innovations, including 4D imaging and total-body PET, have further enhanced diagnostic precision, providing dynamic, high-resolution views critical for cancer diagnosis and treatment planning [28].

AI tools can be used to analyze medical images, such as X-rays, CT scans, and MRIs, to identify abnormalities like tumors, fractures, or internal bleeding [17]. AI algorithms are transforming medical imaging by significantly enhancing tumor detection, characterization, and monitoring. These systems process large imaging datasets with exceptional speed and precision, improving diagnostic consistency by reducing subjectivity and variability in human interpretation.AI tools, such as the automated RANO and RECIST algorithms, have been shown to reduce interobserver variability in radiology, providing consistent and precise measurements of tumor volumes and treatment responses [29]. AI also delivers reproducible and quantitative analyses, allowing clinicians to rely on standardized results across different institutions. Frey et al., [30] demonstrated the use of AI in standardizing HER2 IHC scoring in breast cancer, producing high agreement rates across different institutions and scanners that enhanced consistency and efficiency in diagnostics.

Additionally, the APPRAISE-AI tool offers a standardized and quantitative method for assessing the robustness and clinical utility of AI models, addressing a key gap in existing AI reporting guidelines [31]. AI's advanced speed, supported by modern hardware and GPU accelerators, enables real-time predictions that reduce diagnostic delays and allow healthcare professionals to focus on patient care and complex decision-making.

AI techniques, particularly machine learning (ML) and deep learning (DL) models like convolutional neural networks (CNNs), are highly effective in medical imaging. For tumor detection, AI systems surpass traditional methods, achieving higher sensitivity and specificity. For instance, the use of a machine learning technique (Random Forest) was applied to the classification of nodules using conventional CT combined with PET/CT, achieving an accurate identification rate of 94.4% for malignant nodules. This result is 44.4% higher than that obtained by CT images alone and 11.1% higher than CT plus early PET images [32]. By identifying subtle patterns in imaging data, AI significantly improves the reliability and speed of cancer detection. AI also excels in tumor characterization, distinguishing between benign and malignant lesions and aiding in staging and treatment planning. EfficientNetB2, a deep learning architecture applied to brain tumor detection from MRI scans, achieved over 95% accuracy in identifying and classifying tumors, providing critical insights for clinicians [33]. Similarly, a large-scale breast cancer screening study involving 463,094 women showed that AI-assisted mammography improved detection rates to 6.7 per 1000 compared to 5.7 per 1000 in standard screenings, with no increase in false positives. The positive predictive value of follow-ups leading to biopsy was 64.5% with AI-assisted screening, compared to 59.2% with standard double reading [34]. These advancements highlight how AI enhances the precision of diagnosis and supports tailored treatment strategies.

AI's ability to monitor tumor growth and treatment response has further enabled personalized care. For instance, the Sybile AI model, developed at Massachusetts Institute of Technology (MIT), uses deep learning to analyze lung cancer imaging data. With an accuracy of 86–94%, Sybile identifies early signs of cancer, guiding clinicians to areas that require attention and facilitating regular monitoring for high-risk patients [35]. Additionally, some models trained on large datasets, such as the CAMELYON16 pathology dataset, demonstrated 92% sensitivity and 94% specificity in detecting breast cancer metastases in real time [36, 37]. This advance significantly expedites workflows in pathology labs, enabling faster diagnoses and treatment planning. Similarly, AI systems using deep CNNs and natural language processing (NLP) have been developed to automate the triaging of chest radiographs. The AI system identified normal chest radiographs with 71% sensitivity and 95% specificity, while reducing the average reporting delay from 11.2 days to 2.7 days [38]. These systems can prioritize radiographs based on urgency, significantly reducing reporting delays for critical findings. These examples underscore the transformative role of AI in modern oncology by improving workflows, enhancing diagnostic accuracy, and supporting real-time decision-making.

Digital Pathology

Digital pathology is being increasingly employed in cancer diagnostics, providing additional tools for faster, higher-quality, and more accurate diagnosis [39]. Digital pathology involves the digitization of glass slides into high-resolution images called Whole Slide Images (WSIs) that can be viewed, managed, and analyzed on computer systems. As a result of being captured at very high resolutions, a WSI scanned at the original 40x magnification would have a size greater than 1 GB, allowing it to be examined at very high detail comparable to light microscopy [40]. AI automates the analysis of whole slide images, reducing subjectivity and variability in pathological assessments and ensuring more reliable diagnoses [41]. This technology has revolutionized traditional microscopy-based practices, enabling pathologists to examine tissue samples remotely and collaborate more effectively [42]. AI systems can be trained on extensive datasets from past pathology reports, enabling them to identify patterns and abnormalities that may go unnoticed by the human eye [17].

The integration of AI into digital pathology has opened new possibilities for improved diagnostic accuracy, efficiency, and collaborations. AI algorithms have demonstrated remarkable capabilities in cancer detection and classification [39, 41]. For instance, an AI algorithm developed for prostate cancer diagnosis in whole slide images of core needle biopsies reported an area under the receiver operating characteristic curve (AUC) of 0.997 for cancer detection in the internal test set and 0·991 in an external validation set. The AI model was subsequently deployed in a clinical setting and run in parallel to the pathologists' routine workflow. Triggers were used to alert pathologists when discrepancies occurred between their diagnosis and the output of the algorithm [43]. The Food and Drug Administration (FDA) in the United States (U.S.) has also authorized an AI-based software, called Paige Prostate, to detect prostate biopsy diagnosis. The tool has reported contributing to a significant decrease in second opinion requests, and time for reporting, while maintaining highly accurate diagnostic standards [44, 45]. According to the review by McGenity et al., [41], applications in digital pathology exhibit high diagnostic accuracy, with average sensitivity and specificity surpassing 90% in numerous studies. In breast cancer pathology, AI has excelled in identifying invasive tumors and lymph node metastasis, with Paige breast lymph node, an AI-based tumor detection system reporting an overall efficiency gain of 55% when assisting pathologists in the detection of lymph node metastases [46]. AI is also playing a role in cancer staging, in which the AI model has been trained on hundreds, if not thousands, of curated images, allowing for cancer staging to be conducted quickly, resulting in appropriate and timely treatment.

Cytology (also known as cytopathology) is the study of cells from bodily tissue or fluids to diagnose diseases. It is often used to diagnose various cancers. Traditional cytology involves the microscopic examination of cell samples obtained through either intervention techniques such as fine-needle aspiration, or exfoliative methods such as manual tissue brushing or collecting tissues or fluids that the body naturally sheds. With the emergence of deep learning algorithms that can extract morphologic features from WSIs, there have been many studies detailing AI algorithms applied to cytology demonstrating successful cytomorphological analysis for diagnostic use and research discovery [47]. One example is the artificial intelligence cervical cancer screening (AICCS) system, an AI-based system for diagnosis of cervical cytology grades and cervical cancer which demonstrated remarkable accuracy, reporting AUC of 0.947, with high sensitivity (0.946) and specificity (0.890) in prospective assessment [48]. AI models using deep learning, such as DenseNet-121, have achieved high accuracy rates in classifying lung cancer cytology images, with accuracies of 94% for malignancy prediction and 90% for squamous cell carcinoma prediction at the patch level [49]. Similarly, in the diagnosis of pancreatic cancer, the "Mathematical Technology for Cytopathology (MTC)" algorithm has achieved accuracies of up to 74% in distinguishing between adenocarcinoma and benign tissues [50].

AI-powered digital pathology has revolutionized biomarker discovery and tumor analysis, enabling precise quantification critical for cancer diagnosis, prognosis, and therapy selection. For instance, AI can analyze immunohistochemistry (IHC)-stained slides to objectively quantify biomarkers like HER2 in breast cancer and PD-L1 in lung cancer [51, 52], providing reproducible results. Deep learning models also correlate biomarker patterns with patient outcomes, uncovering novel prognostic markers. Additionally, AI streamlines tumor grading and staging by analyzing nuclear morphology, a process which is crucial for assessing cancer severity and prognosis [53], and automate the detection and counting of mitotic figures in various cancers, such as breast cancer and uterine leiomyosarcoma [54, 55], reducing the subjectivity and time consumption associated with manual counting, offering a more consistent and reliable assessment.

AI further enhances cancer care by predicting treatment responses based on histopathological data. Models trained on whole-slide images (WSIs) can identify features associated with favorable or poor outcomes to chemotherapy and immunotherapy, facilitating personalized medicine by linking tissue morphology with genomic and molecular data. AI models have been developed to predict the response to neoadjuvant chemotherapy in HER2-positive breast cancer by analyzing histopathologic features from WSIs, using H&E and multiplex IHC images to assess the tumor immune microenvironment. They demonstrated superior performance compared to pathologist-derived features, achieving an AUC of 0.9005 in external validation [56]. Moreover, AI integrates multi-omics data, combining histological features with genomic alterations identified through next-generation sequencing (NGS) for comprehensive tumor profiling [57]. This holistic approach aids in discovering new therapeutic targets and enhances predictive modeling, advancing precision oncology.

AI-driven telepathology enables real-time analysis and decision support, allowing pathologists in remote areas to digitally analyze slides and ensure accurate diagnoses without requiring on-site experts. Through this process, telepathology fosters collaboration among global healthcare providers and researchers, enabling knowledge sharing and joint efforts to improve diagnostic accuracy and accessibility in underserved regions [58].

Liquid Biopsies and Biomarker Discovery

Liquid biopsy which can be used to identify factors such as cell-free DNA and circulating tumor DNA (ctDNA) are normally obtained from patients' blood. This approach is considered to be a non-invasive technique, and has been used in the diagnosis of some cancers [59, 60]. Liquid biopsy techniques focus on biomarker analysis, providing minimally invasive, safe, and highly sensitive alternatives to traditional tissue biopsies [61]. Along with the genomic information obtained during liquid biopsies, certain tumor biomarkers can be screened [62, 63]. AI is making headways in both the proteomic and genomic field of early biomarker detection. By combining both proteomic and genomic datasets from the same patient obtained from one non-invasive sampling period, these AI models can detect cancer earlier than is possible with traditional techniques and reduce workload, resulting in increased overall survival [64, 65].

AI applications involve detecting ctDNA, RNA, and cell-free nucleic acids from blood samples. These non-invasive diagnostics offer a safer and more convenient alternative to tissue biopsies than traditional diagnostic techniques. AI enhances biomarker identification by integrating large, complex datasets from genomics and proteomics. For example, the CancerSEEK test, which combines AI with ctDNA and protein biomarker analysis, detects eight cancer types with over 99% specificity and a sensitivity of 69–98% depending on the cancer type [66]. Similarly, Grail's Galleri test employs AI to analyze methylation patterns in cfDNA, enabling the detection of over 50 cancers, including hard-to-diagnose diseases like pancreatic and ovarian cancer [67].

AI-powered proteomic analysis complements genomic insights by identifying protein biomarkers associated with cancer progression. In one study, machine learning models analyzing plasma proteomes distinguished colorectal cancer patients from healthy individuals with over 90% accuracy [68]. AI also excels in monitoring tumor evolution and treatment response, to track changes in tumors over time and predict how they might respond to therapies. For instance, ctDNA analysis can detect minimal residual disease (MRD), predicting recurrence before imaging techniques in colorectal cancer (CRS) patients [69]. ctDNA analysis has produced high sensitivity and specificity in predicting cancer recurrence. Natera's AI-assisted ctDNA tracking achieved an overall sensitivity of 95% (95% CI: 92–99%) and a specificity of 91% (95% CI: 88–94%) in CRS patients [70]. In addition, ctDNA analysis has been found to be more effective than traditional biomarkers like carcinoembryonic antigen (CEA) in predicting recurrence [71, 72].

The integration of AI and liquid biopsies provides numerous advantages. Liquid biopsies minimize patient discomfort and allow frequent sampling to monitor disease progression. AI accelerates data processing, reduces clinician workload, and identifies subtle biomarkers that traditional methods might miss. Case studies such as Guardant360, which uses AI to analyze ctDNA for actionable mutations [73], and Freenome's multi-omics approach for detecting early-stage cancers [74], highlight

AI's transformative potential. These tests have demonstrated high concordance with tissue biopsies and support early intervention, improving patient outcomes.

The success of AI-enhanced liquid biopsies relies on interdisciplinary collaborations between researchers, clinicians, and technology companies. Partnerships like Grail, a leader in multi-cancer early detection (MCED) through liquid biopsy, and the Mayo Clinic, a collaboration focused on large-scale clinical studies to ensure the accuracy, reliability, and clinical utility of the Galleri test [75, 76], are crucial for scaling these technologies, ensuring robust dataset development, and integrating liquid biopsies into routine clinical workflows. AI applications in liquid biopsies are reshaping cancer research, enabling early detection, real-time monitoring, and personalized treatment, ultimately making them a cornerstone of precision oncology.

Omics Data Integration

The integration of multi-omics data—genomics, proteomics, metabolomics, transcriptomics, and epigenomics—has become a cornerstone of cancer research, offering a holistic understanding of tumor biology [77]. By leveraging artificial intelligence (AI) and machine learning (ML), researchers can analyze complex and large-scale datasets to uncover insights that traditional methods often miss. These advancements enhance cancer diagnostics, prognostics, and treatment strategies, paving the way for precision oncology.

AI-driven approaches enable the seamless integration of diverse omics datasets, combining genomic mutations, protein expression, metabolic profiles, and transcriptional changes to identify key molecular mechanisms driving cancer progression. For example, the Pan-Cancer Atlas applied integrative clustering to data from over 10,000 tumors, incorporating genomic, epigenomic, and proteomic information. This AI-driven analysis identified novel cancer subtypes linked to specific biological pathways, offering new therapeutic targets [78]. Similarly, the deep learning model DeepMO, a model using deep neural networks based on multi-omics data, integrates mRNA, DNA methylation, and copy number variation (CNV) data to classify breast cancer subtypes, achieving better results in terms of accuracy and area under the curve (AUC) [79].

Machine learning methods play a critical role in extracting insights from multi-omics data. Algorithms like Random Forests have been used to predict survival rates in glioblastoma by integrating transcriptomic and epigenomic data (Scientific Reports 2020). The integrative Glioblastoma Subtype (iGlioSub) classifier achieved a mean AUC of 95.9% in classifying glioblastoma molecular subtypes, paving the way for more effective subtype-specific treatment strategies [80]. Dimensionality reduction techniques, such as t-SNE and autoencoders simplify high-dimensional omics data while preserving essential biological information, improving interpretability and facilitating downstream analyses. Predictive modeling methods, including support vector machines (SVMs) and deep neural networks (DNNs), are commonly employed to classify cancer subtypes and forecast prognosis. For instance, an SVM-based model integrating metabolomic and proteomic data classified lung cancer subtypes with 95% accuracy.

AI-driven multi-omics integration has transformative applications in cancer research. AI has been used to identify novel biomarkers for early detection and treatment response. For example, a study integrating metabolomics and transcriptomics identified metabolites linked to immune checkpoint inhibitor response in melanoma patients (Cancer Cell 2021). In drug discovery and repurposing, platforms like DeepSyn combine genomic and proteomic data to predict synergistic drug combinations for colorectal cancer, significantly reducing experimental validation time (Nature Machine Intelligence 2021). Precision oncology also benefits greatly from AI; projects like The Cancer Genome Atlas (TCGA) use AI to stratify patients based on multi-omics profiles, enabling personalized treatment plans tailored to unique tumor characteristics.

AI's ability to integrate and analyze multi-omics data is revolutionizing cancer research by providing comprehensive insights into tumor biology, accelerating drug development, and advancing precision oncology. These advancements highlight the growing potential of AI as a transformative tool in the fight against cancer.

Clinical Trial Matching and Recruitment

AI is transforming the process of clinical trial matching and recruitment, addressing one of the most significant bottlenecks in cancer research. Traditionally, identifying eligible patients for clinical trials has been labor-intensive, relying on manual review of patient records and strict adherence to complex eligibility criteria. AI streamlines this process by analyzing large datasets, including electronic health records (EHRs), genomic data, and patient-reported information, to match patients with appropriate clinical trials in real time. For example, MatchMiner is an open-source AI precision medicine trial matching platform that matches patient genomic and clinical data with precision medicine trial eligibility data [81]. Based on the study of Kurnaz et al., [82], an AI-enabled multi-trial matching system increased cancer patients' matching rates to 1.82 times more trials and reduced matching time by 99.9%.

Machine learning algorithms can parse unstructured data in medical records to extract key eligibility factors, such as specific genetic mutations, tumor histology, or prior treatment history. For example, AI tools have been used to identify patients with rare genetic profiles, such as BRCA mutations, who are eligible for targeted therapies in cancer trials [83]. Trained BRCA-like classifiers effectively identify the majority of *BRCA-mutated* and methylated ovarian cancers, classifying a significant portion as *BRCA-like*. The *BRCA1-like* classifier achieved a 95.6% detection rate for *BRCA1* mutations and promoter hypermethylation [84]. Additionally, natural language processing (NLP) techniques can analyze clinical notes, and pathology reports to uncover relevant details that might be missed in traditional screenings. Using Natural Language Processing techniques, the AI system achieved 73.68%

precision, 77.78% accuracy, and 89.36% specificity in matching patients with phase 1 oncology clinical trials [85].

Platforms like IBM Watson and Mendel.ai for Clinical Trials leverage predictive analytics and personalized medicine recommendations to automate these processes, significantly reducing trial recruitment timelines and improving workflow efficiency. Implementing the Watson for Clinical Trial Matching (CTM) system in gastrointestinal oncology can significantly streamline patient screening for clinical trials. On average, CTM identified 7.66 clinical trials per patient, compared to 1.97 trials with manual screening. Additionally, CTM reduced screening time to 10.1 min per patient, compared to 30.5 min with the manual method [86]. Another recent development is the NIH-developed AI algorithm TrialGPT, which aims to accelerate the process of matching potential volunteers to relevant clinical trials. TrialGPT successfully identifies eligible participants and provides clear summaries explaining how each individual meets the criteria for study enrollment [87]. This tool has the potential to save clinicians time, streamline recruitment efforts, and speed up clinical research. TrialGPT accurately predicts patient eligibility for clinical trials for three cohorts of 183 synthetic patients with 87.3% accuracy and significantly reduces screening time by 42.6% [88].

AI also enhances patient recruitment by integrating real-world data from multiple sources, such as wearable devices, patient registries, and social media platforms. By doing so, AI can identify patients who may not be actively seeking trials but meet the eligibility criteria, expanding the recruitment pool [89]. For instance, AI-based recruitment tools have been used to locate underrepresented populations in oncology trials, ensuring more diverse participation and improving the generalizability of research findings. Patients who identify as non-English speaking were less likely to be enrolled in cancer clinical trials, and AI-based system, Clinical Trials Patient Matching (CTPM), was an effective tool to identify underrepresented populations [90]. Furthermore, AI applications in trial matching improve patient experience by personalizing recommendations. Patients can receive tailored suggestions for trials based on their medical history, preferences, and geographic location. This specificity not only improves recruitment efficiency but also enhances patient satisfaction and engagement. An open-source AI precision medicine trial matching platform called MatchMiner, developed by Dana-Farber Cancer Institute (DFCI), successfully matches patients with diverse genomic alterations and cancer types to precision medicine trials, with 87% of those matched going on trial [81].

By automating data extraction, improving matching accuracy, and increasing outreach, AI addresses critical challenges in clinical trial recruitment. These advancements accelerate the pace of cancer research, reduce trial costs, and improve the likelihood of successful outcomes by ensuring that trials are filled with the right patient populations in a timely manner.

AI in Cancer Treatment

Personalised Treatment Planning

AI is rapidly transforming the landscape of clinical oncology, offering innovative solutions to enhance cancer care across various touchpoints. From diagnosis to treatment planning and surgical interventions, AI-based systems are increasingly being developed with the objective of being integrated into clinical workflows to support oncologists in making more informed and personalized treatment planning [91, 92] (Fig. 6.1).

One of the prominent applications of AI in clinical oncology is the development of clinical decision support systems (CDSS). These AI-powered tools are designed to assist oncologists in navigating the complex landscape of cancer treatment options [93]. A prime example is IBM's Watson for Oncology (WFO) which has trained on vast amounts of medical data, including over 100 years of clinical cancer treatment information, to recommend appropriate chemotherapy regimens for specific cancer patients [94].

Other AI-based CDSS platforms have also emerged, each offering unique approaches to support clinical decision-making. For instance, xDECIDE provides personalized treatment recommendations by integrating clinical evidence, expert knowledge, and real-world outcomes [95]. Similarly, the Lung Cancer Assistant prototype uses probabilistic and guideline rule-based decision support to aid clinicians in lung cancer treatment planning [96].

Platforms such as CURATE.AI have shown promising results in recommending personalized chemotherapy doses, potentially reducing prescribed dosages by an average of 20% while maintaining efficacy [97]. Similarly, the National Institutes of Health (NIH), USA, have developed an AI tool called Logistic Regression-Based Immunotherapy-Response Score (LORIS) that uses routine clinical data, with six variables: patient's age, cancer type, history of systemic therapy, blood albumin

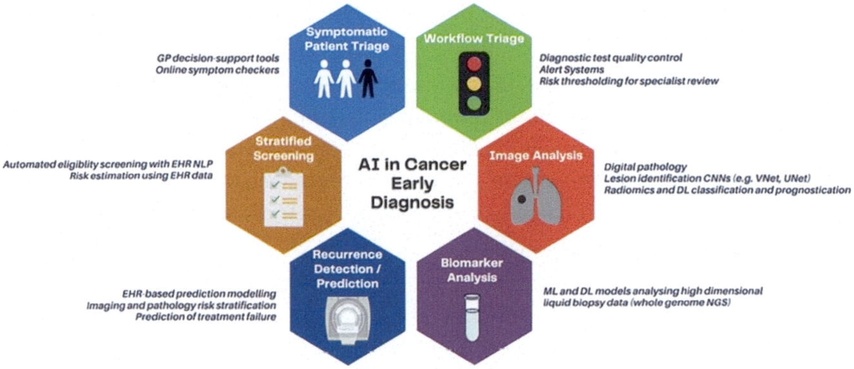

Fig. 6.1 AI applications in cancer treatment

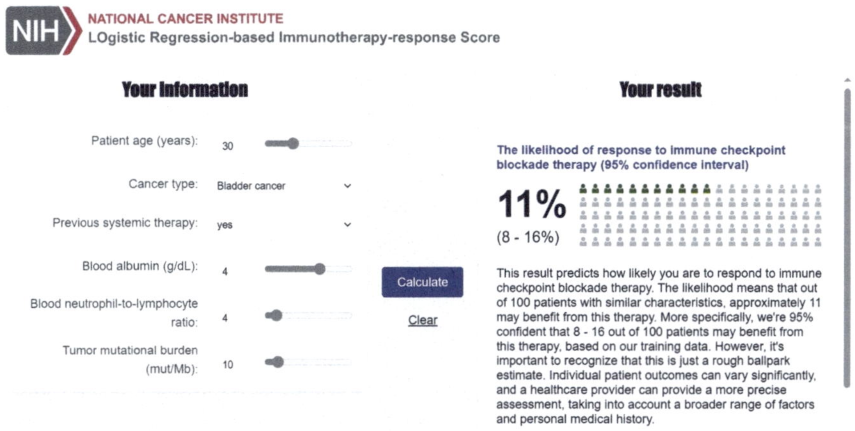

Fig. 6.2 LORIS tool developed by the National Institute of Health (NIH), USA. (Source: https://loris.ccr.cancer.gov/)

level, blood neutrophil-to-lymphocyte ratio, and tumor mutational burden, such as that from a simple blood test, to predict the likelihood of a patient responding to immune checkpoint inhibitors, a type of immunotherapy drug that helps immune cells kill cancer cells [98]. It is publicly available at https://loris.ccr.cancer.gov/ (Fig. 6.2).

AI platforms like Tempus and Foundation Medicine use genomic data to suggest targeted therapies or immunotherapies based on the patient's unique molecular profile. Tempus leverages AI and genomic data to analyze clinical and molecular data, enabling personalized treatment recommendations for cancer patients [99]. while the development of Foundation Medicine's genomic profiling test uses next generation sequencing to identify molecular alterations in cancer patients [100]. AI algorithms help oncologists predict potential side effects and optimize dosing strategies, enhancing both treatment efficacy and patient safety.

Radiotherapy Planning and Delivery

AI-powered contouring tools have significantly improved the precision of tumor delineation. Before conducting radiotherapy treatments, doctors manually need to outline organs on scans to protect healthy tissue from radiation. This is typically a time-consuming task and a potential candidate task which can be assisted by AI. AI-assisted clinical target volume (CTV) and organs at risk (OARs) delineation for postoperative radiotherapy significantly improves accuracy and efficiency compared to pure AI auto-segmentation or fully manual delineation by junior oncologists [101, 102]. One example is OSAIRIS, an open-source AI model for radiotherapy image segmentation. OSAIRIS reported a significant timesaving of 36% when used for prostate contouring and 67% for head and neck contouring, allowing the oncologists to plan radiotherapy 2.5 times faster [103]. This will ensure more patients can get treatment sooner and improve the likelihood of cure.

One of the most significant advancements in AI-assisted radiotherapy is the automation of radiotherapy planning, including tumor segmentation and dose distribution calculation. AI contributes to Magnetic Resonance-guided Radiotherapy (MRgRT) by safely and efficiently automating various manual operations, such as image segmentation, synthetic CT reconstruction, and automatic planning [104]. Traditionally, developing a sophisticated treatment plan has been a time-consuming process involving careful review of patient imaging data and multiple rounds of feedback within the medical team, which can span over days. However, AI algorithms which use deep learning technology can now generate optimal treatment plans within minutes or even seconds [105]. Automated radiotherapy treatment planning for head and neck radiotherapy using a probabilistic, atlas-based approach can generate dose distributions comparable to clinical doses, with fully automated plans generated in 12–13 min without user interaction [106]. This dramatic reduction in planning time allows patients to begin their radiation therapy sooner, potentially decreasing the odds of cancer spreading. Moreover, accurate treatment planning ensures that a patient receives only the required amount of radiation doses for specific locations identified as tumor, ensuring minimal damage to surrounding healthy tissues. This reduction in collateral damage can lead to fewer side effects for patients and potentially allow for more aggressive treatment of the tumor itself.

AI-powered tools like Varian's Ethos™ system provide real-time adaptive radiotherapy, adjusting treatment plans based on daily changes in tumor size or patient anatomy, enabling clinicians to better target treatment while significantly reducing the impact of radiation on healthy tissue [107]. Furthermore, predictive models are used to estimate patient response to radiotherapy, enabling oncologists to personalize treatment schedules and reduce adverse effects.

Drug Discovery and Development

AI is revolutionizing drug discovery and development in cancer research by significantly accelerating the process of identifying new therapies and repurposing existing drugs. Traditional drug discovery methods are time-consuming and costly, often taking over a decade and billions of dollars to bring a drug to market, and then therapeutic molecules may fail clinical trials and regulatory approval [108]. AI addresses these challenges by analyzing vast datasets of molecular, clinical, and omics data to identify promising drug targets, predict drug efficacy, and streamline development pipelines [109]. AI also streamlines the transition from discovery to testing by optimizing trial design and identifying suitable patient populations [108].

One of AI's key contributions is its ability to uncover novel drug targets by processing complex datasets, such as genomic and proteomic profiles of cancer cells. For instance, deep learning models can analyze molecular interactions and identify critical pathways driving cancer progression. Tools like Atomwise use AI (CNN) to predict the binding affinity between potential drug compounds and target proteins, accelerating the screening of millions of molecules for therapeutic potential [110]. Similarly, the AlphaFold[1] platform by DeepMind has revolutionized protein structure prediction, providing insights into how drugs interact with specific cancer-related proteins. By minimizing trial-and-error processes, AI reduces the overall cost of drug development.

AI also plays a vital role in predicting the efficacy and safety of drug candidates. Machine learning algorithms assess how a drug is likely to behave in different types of cancer by integrating data from preclinical studies, clinical trials, and patient records. For example, Drug Ranking Using Machine Learning (DRUML) ranks over 400 anti-cancer drugs by their efficacy across a wide range of pathologies using omics data [111]. A machine learning algorithm based on support vector machines (SVM) predicted individual cancer patient responses to chemotherapeutic drugs with >80% accuracy, potentially aiding in the identification of promising second-line treatments [112]. The Exscientia platform, a pioneer in precision medicine, uses generative AI models to optimize drug designs and identify candidates with higher probabilities of success in clinical trials. This approach has reduced the timeline for preclinical development from years to months in certain cases [113]. AI identifies synergistic drug combinations to enhance therapeutic efficacy while minimizing side effects. The platform DeepSynergy integrates genomic and proteomic data to predict synergistic effects of drug combinations for colorectal cancer treatment. Its application to the classification of drug combinations achieved a high predictive performance with an AUC of 0.90 [114]. This approach reduces the experimental workload and accelerates the clinical application of combination therapies.

Beyond discovering new drugs, AI has proven invaluable for drug repurposing, which involves finding new uses for existing drugs. By analyzing existing drug databases alongside cancer datasets, AI can identify drugs approved for other conditions that may also be effective against specific cancers. A notable example is the use of IBM Watson to analyze molecular pathways and suggest repurposing the diabetes drug metformin, a common anti-diabetic drug potentially used in anticancer therapy, for certain cancer types due to its impact on cellular metabolism [115]. Similarly, AI tools have identified cardiovascular drugs with potential anticancer properties by analyzing large-scale omics datasets [116]. AI combines clinical trial results with patient data to predict how repurposed drugs may perform in different cancer subtypes, tailoring recommendations to individual patients.

[1] https://deepmind.google/technologies/alphafold/

Surgical Oncology

In the realm of surgical oncology, AI is making significant strides in enhancing surgical precision and outcomes [117]. The da Vinci robotic surgical system, augmented with AI capabilities, has been successfully employed in thousands of minimally invasive procedures. AI technologies are also being leveraged to enhance intraoperative visualization, particularly in deep anatomical spaces [117]. Advanced image enhancement techniques powered by AI assist in optimizing the quality of intraoperative visuals through denoising, deblurring, and color correction of camera feeds [118].

AI is also contributing to surgical safety by identifying safe dissection planes and guiding intraoperative tasks to prevent cancer recurrence. Haptic feedback systems, driven by AI, are being developed to provide surgeons with tactile sensations during robot-assisted surgeries, helping them apply appropriate force during delicate procedures. Automation of specific surgical tasks, such as camera positioning, is another area where AI is making significant progress [117]. AI, such as Computer Vision (CV), can be trained to recognize surgical phases and actions with high accuracy, potentially enhancing intraoperative decision-making and guidance in colorectal cancer surgery [119]. Augmented Reality (AR) tools use AI to overlay 3D models of tumors onto the surgical field, guiding surgeons with visual cues for more precise excisions, particularly in complex surgeries such as breast, brain, and prostate cancer [120, 121].

AI is also being applied to surgical education and simulation. AI-powered systems are trained to provide personalized training experiences, analyzing a surgeon's performance and offering real-time feedback [117, 122]. AI systems like Biofourmis analyze postoperative data to detect early signs of complications, such as infections or blood clots. AI can effectively predict postoperative surgical site infections, with factors like comorbidity and minimally invasive surgery being protective against infection. In the study by Hopkins et al. [123], the positive predictive value (PPV), measuring the model's accuracy in predicting surgical site infections (SSI) when they were present, was 92.56% over all predictions, while the accuracy for predicted absence of SSI was 98.45%. Predictive models analyze patient data to estimate surgical risks, recovery times, and potential complications.

Remote Patient Monitoring and Teleoncology

Remote patient monitoring and teleoncology are emerging as attractive components in modern cancer care, leveraging AI-powered technologies to enhance patient outcomes and accessibility to specialized oncology services. These advancements are particularly significant in bridging healthcare disparities and improving access to specialised treatment, especially in underserved regions.

AI-powered platforms for remote monitoring of patients' symptoms, treatment adherence, and side effects have shown promising results in improving patient engagement and early detection of complications. Remote monitoring programs for cancer patients have been reported to improve symptom management as well as increased survival compared with usual care [124, 125].

Often patients living in remote or rural areas have reduced access to specialized care and, thus, have unacceptably high mortality and morbidity rates. Teleoncology, or the use of telemedicine to provide oncology services remotely by cancer specialists to geographically remote patients or primary care providers, can improve access to high-quality care and assist in alleviating the burden of some of the severe adverse events associated with cancer [126]. Teleoncology has proven particularly valuable in low-income nations and remote areas, allowing access to expert consultation and state-of-the-art technology which is otherwise unavailable [127].

Teleoncology solutions are leveraging AI to enable remote consultations and follow-ups, making cancer care more accessible. These tools have the potential to analyze patient data in real time, allowing oncologists to monitor patient progress and make informed decisions remotely while improving the efficiency and safety of telemedicine. The use of AI in teleoncology is anticipated to tackle the issue of avoidable medical errors and enhance workflow efficiencies, which are currently at a high rate in healthcare provision. The COVID-19 pandemic accelerated the adoption of teleoncology, protecting vulnerable cancer patients while ensuring continuity of care [127, 128]. Teleoncology also plays a crucial role in improving radiotherapy planning, monitoring chemotherapy side effects, and promoting clinical trial participation [126, 129]. Additionally, it significantly reduces healthcare costs by minimising travel expenses and lost work time for patients [126, 128].

Additional benefits of AI-powered remote patient monitoring and teleoncology include expanded collaborative opportunities at a global level and the enabling of access to a broad range of data from diverse participants across various regions and conditions. These tools facilitate remote palliative care by analyzing patient data to optimize comfort and symptom relief, ensuring better end-of-life care. AI also allows researchers to study long-term trends, such as how cancer therapies affect patients' quality of life over time, providing valuable insights for developing new treatments. Tools like Deep 6 AI use natural language processing to scan unstructured medical records and enhance clinical trial efficiency by integrating remote monitoring metrics with trial databases to identify eligible participants more effectively. Traditional recruitment efforts took 6 months to identify a dozen eligible patients for a trial, whereas Deep 6's software matched 80 potential participants within minutes. Moreover, AI-powered systems such as Apple HealthKit and Fitbit[2] collect and analyze data like heart rate, temperature, and activity levels in cancer patients, predicting potential issues in near-real time and enabling adaptive treatment approaches.

[2] https://apps.apple.com/us/app/fitbit-sync-to-health-app/id1637904679

Challenges and Future Directions

Challenges Associated with AI Implementation in Cancer Care

Data Privacy, Security, and Ethical Guidelines for AI in Cancer Care

AI models typically require large quantities of training data. In the absence of an appropriate quantity of training data, AI models tend to suffer from undesirable effects such as overfitting, reduced generalization, and lower model performance. However, in domains such as medicine, obtaining such large datasets can be constrained due to privacy concerns, regulatory restrictions, and ethical considerations [130, 131]. Since healthcare organizations manage large amounts of sensitive patient data, they are prime targets for cyberattacks, which can lead to identity theft, financial fraud, and compromised patient care [132]. Limited availability of data is also the biggest challenge for AI radiogenomics [19] (Fig. 6.3).

Key privacy challenges in AI-driven cancer care include ensuring the de-identification of patient data to prevent re-identification during AI model training and analysis, thereby safeguarding individual privacy. Consent management is another critical aspect, requiring explicit and informed consent from patients for the use of their data, particularly for secondary purposes such as research or algorithm refinement. Additionally, cross-border data sharing poses significant legal complexities, as many AI models rely on global datasets to enhance performance, but differing privacy regulations, such as the GDPR (General Data Protection Regulation) in Europe and HIPAA (Health Insurance Portability and Accountability Act) in the United States, make compliance a challenging yet essential requirement.

For instance, the medical domain deals with sensitive patient data which includes confidential information about a patient's medical history. Utilizing such sensitive data in healthcare applications, even those that do not apply AI, raises significant privacy concerns among the data owners. As a result, to ensure that the privacy and

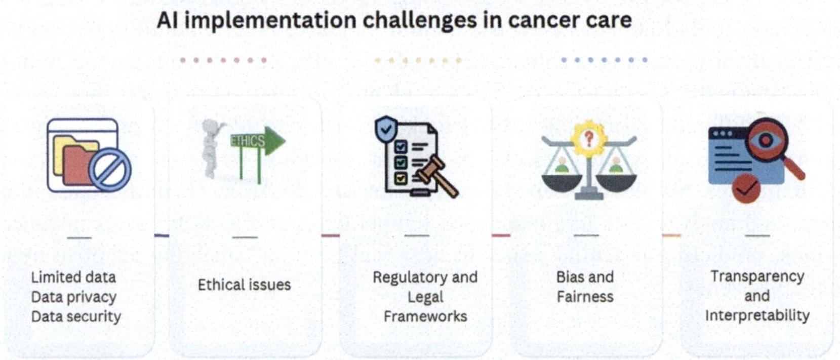

Fig. 6.3 AI implementation challenges in cancer care

security of patients' health information is protected, it is important to adhere to regulations such as the HIPAA, the GDPR and the Australian Privacy Act, which governs patient data access, storage, confidentiality, security and transmission [133]. Additionally, the establishment of robust data governance rules within individual institutions will also ensure clear standards are set for data anonymisation and patient consent management [134]. On the other hand, AI models in cancer care must align with medical ethics, particularly regarding patient autonomy, consent, and transparency. Oncologists should be able to explain to patients how AI works and obtain informed consent for its use in treatment decision-making. Consequently, ethical frameworks should address issues such as algorithmic fairness, transparency, and the potential impact on the patient-physician relationship. Explainable AI models, powered by patient data, enable personalized treatment recommendations and foster trust between medical practitioners and patients, propelling cancer care into the precision medicine era [135]. Ethical guidelines must also ensure that AI interventions respect the dignity, preferences, and choices of patients while prioritizing their safety and well-being. Patient autonomy must be preserved by ensuring that while AI provides recommendations, the final decisions rest with patients and healthcare providers, maintaining human oversight. Clear guidelines on data ownership are necessary to ensure that patients retain control over their personal health information. Additionally, ethical AI usage is paramount, avoiding practices that could harm patients, such as discriminatory insurance policies or exclusion from treatments based on predictive outcomes.

Regulatory and Legal Frameworks for AI-Driven Medical Devices and Software

AI-powered medical devices and software are generally subject to rigorous regulatory scrutiny before they can be used in clinical settings. For example, the FDA has frameworks to evaluate AI-driven tools to ensure that they are safe and effective for patient care. The FDA has cleared or approved more than 40 AI-based medical devices for clinical use [133, 136]. This process typically includes clinical trials, validation studies, and ongoing post-market surveillance. Similarly, the European Union (EU) has its own set of regulatory guidelines for medical devices, such as the Medical Device Regulation (MDR), which governs the production and distribution of medical devices in the EU. The EU MDR imposes stringent requirements on AI-based medical device software, requiring qualified medical physicist experts to ensure reliable and consistent product quality, safety, and performance [137]. In addition, AI software in the EU must undergo a conformity assessment procedure to be approved as a medical device, and common standards for clinical evaluation and transparency of evidence are needed [138]. These regulations aim to ensure the safety and effectiveness of AI tools while promoting innovation in patient care.

The regulation of AI in healthcare is complex, and varies by jurisdiction. While countries like the U.S. and EU have established frameworks for medical AI tools, others have yet to develop comprehensive regulatory standards. This disparity creates challenges for global adoption, particularly for companies wishing to bring AI innovations to multiple markets. Discrepancies in approval processes, data protection laws, and AI safety standards can create bottlenecks and inefficiencies in delivering AI-based solutions to clinical settings. A global regulatory convergence for AI in healthcare, similar to the voluntary AI code of conduct developed by the US-EU Trade and Technology Council, would be beneficial to all nations [139]. The harmonizing of these diverse regulatory environments is crucial for fostering international collaboration and ensuring equitable access to AI-driven cancer care solutions.

The use of AI in clinical decision-making raises complex liability issues. Therefore, healthcare providers must consider the potential legal ramifications if AI recommendations lead to adverse outcomes [133]. Clear guidelines on accountability and responsibility for AI-assisted decisions are necessary to protect both patients and healthcare professionals.

Bias and Fairness in AI Algorithms and Their Potential Impact on Patient Care

One of the main concerns of AI models is their vulnerability to model bias and discrimination. Generally model biases can occur from two sources: biases in training data (data bias) or biases in model design (algorithmic bias) [140–142]. However, in healthcare settings, additional biases can arise, such as the biases that originate from AI-clinician interactions and those that originate from AI-patient interactions [141, 142]. Biased AI models will make incorrect predictions which can result in inaccurate risk assessments or treatment recommendations for certain patient populations, particularly under-represented minorities. For instance, AI systems trained on data from predominantly urban or affluent populations may fail to address the unique needs of rural or underserved communities. As a result, such models will not be fair in providing their predictions in real-world settings. Similarly, AI models in orthodontics and craniofacial health can amplify racial biases when built on under-represented datasets, leading to poor performance for ethno-racial minorities [143].

Model biases can be detected and mitigated during the model development and training stages as well as during the usage of such models. Strategies for mitigating bias are multifaceted. One literature work suggests a set of recommendations, called "FAIR—Fairness of Artificial Intelligence Recommendations in healthcare" principles, which aim to ensure fair and equitable AI-driven healthcare solutions [142]. Following are the FAIR recommendations from Ueda et al., [142]:

1. Using diverse and representative data in AI development
2. Implementing independent audits and validation of AI algorithms
3. Education on AI biases for clinicians and patients
4. Strengthening data privacy and security measures
5. Establishing liability and accountability frameworks
6. Enhancing AI transparency and explainability

7. Collaboration between physicians, AI researchers, and developers
8. Policymaker and regulatory authority involvement
9. Patient and advocacy group participation in AI development and evaluation
10. Professional association support

Many datasets are currently available, including TCGA, HGP, and 1000 GP [144, 145], containing multi-omic data derived from a small subset of the human population, and particularly skewed [Segun Fatumo, Jinchuan Xing], although more work is being undertaken to diversify the samples collected for future multi-omic studies [Jinchuan Xing, All of Us (NIH)].

Importance of Transparency and Interpretability of AI Models for Building Trust and Accountability

Machine Learning models sometimes tend to be "black-box" models that do not explain their predictions in a sufficient manner that humans can understand [146]. This lack of transparency and accountability of machine learning models has had, and will have, severe consequences for its users, especially in high stake domains such as cancer care [146]. Without understanding the rationale behind AI-generated recommendations and predictions, clinicians will have no means to safely validate and integrate the AI outputs into clinical decision-making [146–148].

Deep learning models, particularly large-scale natural language processing models such as OpenAI's GPT (Generative Pretrained Transformer) and Meta AI's LLaMA models, demonstrate the way in which model performance improves with an increasing number of learnable parameters, with these models ranging from 7 to 175 billion parameters [149, 150]. However, as model complexity increases and performance improves, this enhancement often comes at the expense of reduced explainability and interpretability, presenting significant challenges in understanding and justifying model decisions. So how can we overcome this problem and enjoy the benefits of AI in cancer care?

One approach to addressing the trade-off between performance and interpretability is to use inherently human-interpretable machine learning models that are simple enough to be understood while still sufficiently sophisticated to capture the relationship between inputs and outputs, often referred to as white-box models [151, 152]. Examples of such models include traditional machine learning techniques, such as linear regression, support vector machines, and LASSO. Another approach involves applying explainable AI (XAI) techniques to trained models to gain insights into the learned relationships. These techniques include, among many others, inspecting learned features and their importance, analyzing feature interactions [153, 154], and using visual explanations such as saliency maps [155]. Additional methods for enhancing interpretability include generating heatmaps, prototypes, or even textual explanations [152]. Ultimately, the choice of approach depends on the trade-offs between model complexity, performance, and the need for transparency. Combining multiple XAI methods to generate clear reasoning of AI predictions can help in having clear communication between the clinician and patient, thereby building trust and safety in AI-assisted decision-making.

Regulatory frameworks for AI transparency are also emerging, with the EU's AI Act stating that high-risk AI systems must be designed to be transparent, so that those using them can understand as well as use them correctly while knowing the system's capabilities and limitations, and any potential risks (AI Act 2025). The FDA, Health Canada, and the United Kingdom's Medicines and Healthcare products Regulatory Agency (MHRA) have jointly identified guiding principles for transparency for machine learning-enabled medical devices (MLMDs), promoting safe, effective, and high-quality medical devices that use AI and ML [156]. Moreover, IBM's AI FactSheets 360 project[3] aims to foster trust in AI by increasing transparency and enabling governance by standardising AI system documentation.

By addressing the above critical aspects of data governance and ethics in AI based cancer care, the healthcare industry can harness the power of AI in cancer care while safeguarding patient rights and ensuring equitable, trustworthy, and effective implementation.

Future Directions and Opportunities

The role of AI in cancer care holds immense potential, with several key innovations poised to revolutionize the field. One of the most significant developments is the creation of platforms that can store, combine and manage data of multiple modalities, including medical imaging, genomics, pathology, and electronic health records from multiple sources. These comprehensive systems will not help manage medical data more securely and transparently amd also provide a holistic view of each patient's condition, enabling sharing of valuable information for research and treatment purposes.

The integration of multi-omics data for comprehensive patient profiling represents a significant opportunity in cancer care. By combining genomics, proteomics, metabolomics, and other -omics data, AI systems will be able to create more detailed and nuanced patient profiles. This holistic approach will enable more personalized treatment strategies and improve our understanding of cancer biology.

AI-powered CDSS are expected to play an increasingly important role in oncology. These systems will evolve to provide more sophisticated recommendations by analyzing vast amounts of clinical data, research findings, and patient-specific information. The integration of natural language processing and machine learning algorithms into electronic health records is anticipated to enhance the adoption of AI-driven CDSS into clinical workflows.

The democratization of AI tools holds the potential to widen access to advanced cancer care. As AI technologies become more user-friendly and accessible, they can

[3] https://aifs360.res.ibm.com/

be deployed in a variety of healthcare settings, including those with limited resources. This could help reduce disparities in cancer care by bringing advanced diagnostic and treatment planning capabilities to underserved areas.

As AI becomes increasingly integrated into cancer care, there is a growing focus on developing ethical AI and explainable models. Future research will prioritize the creation of AI systems that are not only accurate but also fair, transparent and interpretable, addressing current challenges related to the "black box" nature of some AI algorithms. This emphasis on explainability will be crucial in building trust among healthcare providers and patients, facilitating wider adoption of AI technologies in clinical practice.

The future of AI in cancer care will likely involve increased collaboration between clinicians, researchers, data scientists, and patients. This multidisciplinary approach will ensure that AI tools are clinically relevant, ethical, user-friendly, and aligned with patient needs. By addressing current challenges and capitalizing on these opportunities, AI has the potential to significantly improve cancer care outcomes, making treatments more effective, personalized, and accessible. As these advancements continue to unfold, they promise to reshape the landscape of cancer care, offering new hope and improved outcomes for patients worldwide.

References

1. WHO. (2025). *Cancer*. https://www.who.int/health-topics/cancer
2. NCI. (2021). *What Is Cancer?* (nciglobal,ncienterprise) [cgvArticle]. https://www.cancer.gov/about-cancer/understanding/what-is-cancer
3. Brown, J. S., Amend, S. R., Austin, R. H., Gatenby, R. A., Hammarlund, E. U., & Pienta, K. J. (2023). Updating the Definition of Cancer. *Molecular Cancer Research*, *21*(11), 1142–1147. https://doi.org/10.1158/1541-7786.MCR-23-0411
4. Hajdu, S. I. (2011). A note from history: Landmarks in history of cancer, part 1. *Cancer*, *117*(5), 1097–1102. https://doi.org/10.1002/cncr.25553
5. Bray, F., Laversanne, M., Sung, H., Ferlay, J., Siegel, R. L., Soerjomataram, I., & Jemal, A. (2024). Global cancer statistics 2022: GLOBOCAN estimates of incidence and mortality worldwide for 36 cancers in 185 countries. *CA: A Cancer Journal for Clinicians*, *74*(3), 229–263. https://doi.org/10.3322/caac.21834
6. Australian Bureau of Statistics (ABS) (2023). National Health Survey 2022, cat. no. 4364.0, ABS website, accessed 10 Feb 2025. https://www.abs.gov.au/statistics/health/health-conditions-and-risks/national-health-survey/2022
7. Bennett, H. S. (1956). The role of histology in medical education and biological thinking. *The Anatomical Record*, *125*(2), 327–354. https://doi.org/10.1002/ar.1091250210
8. Hussein, I., Raad, M., Safa, R., Jurjus, R., & Jurjus, A. (2015). Once Upon a Microscopic Slide: The Story of Histology. *Journal of Cytology & Histology*, *6*. https://doi.org/10.4172/2157-7099.1000377
9. Debela, D. T., Muzazu, S. G., Heraro, K. D., Ndalama, M. T., Mesele, B. W., Haile, D. C., Kitui, S. K., & Manyazewal, T. (2021). New approaches and procedures for cancer treatment: Current perspectives. *SAGE Open Medicine*, *9*, 20503121211034366. https://doi.org/10.1177/20503121211034366
10. NCI. (2023). *Tests and Procedures Used to Diagnose Cancer* (nciglobal,ncienterprise) [cgvArticle]. https://www.cancer.gov/about-cancer/diagnosis-staging/diagnosis

11. Neal, R. D., Tharmanathan, P., France, B., Din, N. U., Cotton, S., Fallon-Ferguson, J., Hamilton, W., Hendry, A., Hendry, M., Lewis, R., Macleod, U., Mitchell, E. D., Pickett, M., Rai, T., Shaw, K., Stuart, N., Tørring, M. L., Wilkinson, C., Williams, B., … Emery, J. (2015). Is increased time to diagnosis and treatment in symptomatic cancer associated with poorer outcomes? Systematic review. *British Journal of Cancer*, *112*(1), S92–S107. https://doi.org/10.1038/bjc.2015.48
12. Tørring, M. L., Frydenberg, M., Hansen, R. P., Olesen, F., & Vedsted, P. (2013). Evidence of increasing mortality with longer diagnostic intervals for five common cancers: A cohort study in primary care. *European Journal of Cancer*, *49*(9), 2187–2198. https://doi.org/10.1016/j.ejca.2013.01.025
13. Yun, Y. H., Kim, Y. A., Min, Y. H., Park, S., Won, Y. J., Kim, D. Y., Choi, I. J., Kim, Y. W., Park, S. J., Kim, J. H., Lee, D. H., Yoon, S. J., Jeong, S. Y., Noh, D. Y., & Heo, D. S. (2012). The influence of hospital volume and surgical treatment delay on long-term survival after cancer surgery. *Annals of Oncology*, *23*(10), 2731–2737. https://doi.org/10.1093/annonc/mds101
14. Jones, A. (2023). Pathology of Cancer: Causes, Pathophysiology, Diagnosis, Prevention and Treatment. *Journal of Medical & Surgical Pathology*, *8*(2), 1–2. https://doi.org/10.35248/2472-4971.23.08.267
15. Crosby, D., Bhatia, S., Brindle, K. M., Coussens, L. M., Dive, C., Emberton, M., Esener, S., Fitzgerald, R. C., Gambhir, S. S., Kuhn, P., Rebbeck, T. R., & Balasubramanian, S. (2022). Early detection of cancer. *Science*, *375*(6586), eaay9040. https://doi.org/10.1126/science.aay9040
16. Mamun, T. I., Younus, S., & Rahman, Md. H. (2024). Gastric cancer—Epidemiology, modifiable and non-modifiable risk factors, challenges and opportunities: An updated review. *Cancer Treatment and Research Communications*, *41*, 100845. https://doi.org/10.1016/j.ctarc.2024.100845
17. Boppana, V. R. (2020). *Ethical Implications of Big Data in Healthcare Decision Making* (SSRN Scholarly Paper 5005065). Social Science Research Network. https://doi.org/10.2139/ssrn.5005065
18. Mansour, R., Abdel-Razeq, H., Al-Hussaini, M., Shamieh, O., Al-Ibraheem, A., Al-Omari, A., & Mansour, A. H. (2024). Systemic Barriers to Optimal Cancer Care in Resource-Limited Countries: Jordanian Healthcare as an Example. *Cancers*, *16*(6), 1117. https://doi.org/10.3390/cancers16061117
19. Johnson, K. B., Wei, W., Weeraratne, D., Frisse, M. E., Misulis, K., Rhee, K., Zhao, J., & Snowdon, J. L. (2021). Precision Medicine, AI, and the Future of Personalized Health Care. *Clinical and Translational Science*, *14*(1), 86–93. https://doi.org/10.1111/cts.12884
20. Alowais, S. A., Alghamdi, S. S., Alsuhebany, N., Alqahtani, T., Alshaya, A. I., Almohareb, S. N., Aldairem, A., Alrashed, M., Bin Saleh, K., Badreldin, H. A., Al Yami, M. S., Al Harbi, S., & Albekairy, A. M. (2023). Revolutionizing healthcare: The role of artificial intelligence in clinical practice. *BMC Medical Education*, *23*, 689. https://doi.org/10.1186/s12909-023-04698-z
21. Olawade, D. B., David-Olawade, A. C., Wada, O. Z., Asaolu, A. J., Adereni, T., & Ling, J. (2024). Artificial intelligence in healthcare delivery: Prospects and pitfalls. *Journal of Medicine, Surgery, and Public Health*, *3*, 100108. https://doi.org/10.1016/j.glmedi.2024.100108
22. Vora, L. K., Gholap, A. D., Jetha, K., Thakur, R. R. S., Solanki, H. K., & Chavda, V. P. (2023). Artificial Intelligence in Pharmaceutical Technology and Drug Delivery Design. *Pharmaceutics*, *15*(7), 1916. https://doi.org/10.3390/pharmaceutics15071916
23. Karalis, V. D. (2024). The Integration of Artificial Intelligence into Clinical Practice. *Applied Biosciences*, *3*(1), Article 1. https://doi.org/10.3390/applbiosci3010002
24. Shao, D., Dai, Y., Li, N., Cao, X., Zhao, W., Cheng, L., Rong, Z., Huang, L., Wang, Y., & Zhao, J. (2022). Artificial intelligence in clinical research of cancers. *Briefings in Bioinformatics*, *23*(1), bbab523. https://doi.org/10.1093/bib/bbab523
25. El Mouddcn, M., Ahmcd, B. A., Amdaouch, I., Chaari, M. Z., Ruiz-Alzola, J., & Aghzout, O. (2024). High Directivity Improvements using the Theory of Characteristic Modes for

High-Resolution Imaging of Brain Tumors. *2024 International Conference on Computing, Internet of Things and Microwave Systems (ICCIMS)*, 1–5. https://doi.org/10.1109/ICCIMS61672.2024.10690765

26. Murugesan, G. K., McCrumb, D., Aboian, M., Verma, T., Soni, R., Memon, F., Farahani, K., Pei, L., Wagner, U., Fedorov, A. Y., Clunie, D., Moore, S., & Van Oss, J. (2024). AI-Generated Annotations Dataset for Diverse Cancer Radiology Collections in NCI Image Data Commons. *Scientific Data, 11*(1), 1165. https://doi.org/10.1038/s41597-024-03977-8
27. Nunna, B., Parihar, P., Wanjari, M., Shetty, N., & Bora, N. (2024). High-Resolution Imaging Insights into Shoulder Joint Pain: A Comprehensive Review of Ultrasound and Magnetic Resonance Imaging (MRI). *Cureus, 15*(11), e48974. https://doi.org/10.7759/cureus.48974
28. Viswanath, V., Chitalia, R., Pantel, A. R., Karp, J. S., & Mankoff, D. A. (2021). Analysis of Four-Dimensional Data for Total Body PET Imaging. *PET Clinics, 16*(1), 55–64. https://doi.org/10.1016/j.cpet.2020.09.009
29. Choma, A. (2023, September 4). AI in radiology and a reduction of interobserver variability in assessing patient response. *Graylight Imaging*. https://graylight-imaging.com/blog/ai-in-radiology-and-a-reduction-of-interobserver-variability-in-assessing-patient-response/
30. Frey, P., Mamilos, A., Minin, E., Banisch, R., Günther, S., Schmidt, C., Abele, N., Hartmann, A., Fasching, P. A., Rübner, M., Huebner, H., Lang, T., & Erber, R. (2023). AI-based HER2-low IHC scoring in breast cancer across multiple sites, clones, and scanners. *Journal of Clinical Oncology, 41*(16_suppl), 516–516. https://doi.org/10.1200/JCO.2023.41.16_suppl.516
31. Kwong, J. C. C., Khondker, A., Lajkosz, K., McDermott, M. B. A., Frigola, X. B., McCradden, M. D., Mamdani, M., Kulkarni, G. S., & Johnson, A. E. W. (2023). APPRAISE-AI Tool for Quantitative Evaluation of AI Studies for Clinical Decision Support. *JAMA Network Open, 6*(9), e2335377. https://doi.org/10.1001/jamanetworkopen.2023.35377
32. Tandon, Y. K., Bartholmai, B. J., & Koo, C. W. (2020). Putting artificial intelligence (AI) on the spot: Machine learning evaluation of pulmonary nodules. *Journal of Thoracic Disease, 12*(11). https://doi.org/10.21037/jtd-2019-cptn-03
33. Rahman, A., Gupta, M., Aarathi, S., T R, M., Vasanthan, V., Kumaran, S., & Guluwadi, S. (2024). Advanced AI-driven approach for enhanced brain tumor detection from MRI images utilizing EfficientNetB2 with equalization and homomorphic filtering. *BMC Medical Informatics and Decision Making, 24*. https://doi.org/10.1186/s12911-024-02519-x
34. Jackson, J. (2025). *AI improves mammography cancer detection rates in large cohort study*. Medical Xpress. https://medicalxpress.com/news/2025-01-ai-mammography-cancer-large-cohort.html
35. Mikhael, P. G., Wohlwend, J., Yala, A., Karstens, L., Xiang, J., Takigami, A. K., Bourgouin, P. P., Chan, P., Mrah, S., Amayri, W., Juan, Y.-H., Yang, C.-T., Wan, Y.-L., Lin, G., Sequist, L. V., Fintelmann, F. J., & Barzilay, R. (2023). Sybil: A Validated Deep Learning Model to Predict Future Lung Cancer Risk From a Single Low-Dose Chest Computed Tomography. *Journal of Clinical Oncology, 41*(12), 2191–2200. https://doi.org/10.1200/JCO.22.01345
36. Ehteshami Bejnordi, B., Veta, M., Johannes van Diest, P., van Ginneken, B., Karssemeijer, N., Litjens, G., van der Laak, J. A. W. M., & and the CAMELYON16 Consortium. (2017). Diagnostic Assessment of Deep Learning Algorithms for Detection of Lymph Node Metastases in Women With Breast Cancer. *JAMA, 318*(22), 2199–2210. https://doi.org/10.1001/jama.2017.14585
37. Liu, Y., Gadepalli, K., Norouzi, M., Dahl, G. E., Kohlberger, T., Boyko, A., Venugopalan, S., Timofeev, A., Nelson, P. Q., Corrado, G. S., Hipp, J. D., Peng, L., & Stumpe, M. C. (2017). *Detecting Cancer Metastases on Gigapixel Pathology Images* (arXiv:1703.02442). arXiv. https://doi.org/10.48550/arXiv.1703.02442
38. Annarumma, M., Withey, S. J., Bakewell, R. J., Pesce, E., Goh, V., & Montana, G. (2019). Automated Triaging of Adult Chest Radiographs with Deep Artificial Neural Networks. *Radiology, 291*(1), 196–202. https://doi.org/10.1148/radiol.2018180921
39. Shafi, S., & Parwani, A. V. (2023). Artificial intelligence in diagnostic pathology. *Diagnostic Pathology, 18*(1), 109. https://doi.org/10.1186/s13000-023-01375-z

40. Ibrahim, A., Gamble, P., Jaroensri, R., Abdelsamea, M. M., Mermel, C. H., Chen, P.-H. C., & Rakha, E. A. (2020). Artificial intelligence in digital breast pathology: Techniques and applications. *The Breast*, *49*, 267–273. https://doi.org/10.1016/j.breast.2019.12.007
41. McGenity, C., Clarke, E. L., Jennings, C., Matthews, G., Cartlidge, C., Freduah-Agyemang, H., Stocken, D. D., & Treanor, D. (2024). Artificial intelligence in digital pathology: A systematic review and meta-analysis of diagnostic test accuracy. *Npj Digital Medicine*, *7*(1), 1–19. https://doi.org/10.1038/s41746-024-01106-8
42. Zarella, M. D., Bowman, D., Aeffner, F., Farahani, N., Xthona, A., Absar, S. F., Parwani, A., Bui, M., & Hartman, D. J. (2018). A Practical Guide to Whole Slide Imaging: A White Paper From the Digital Pathology Association. *Archives of Pathology & Laboratory Medicine*, *143*(2), 222–234. https://doi.org/10.5858/arpa.2018-0343-RA
43. Pantanowitz, L., Quiroga-Garza, G. M., Bien, L., Heled, R., Laifenfeld, D., Linhart, C., Sandbank, J., Shach, A. A., Shalev, V., Vecsler, M., Michelow, P., Hazelhurst, S., & Dhir, R. (2020). An artificial intelligence algorithm for prostate cancer diagnosis in whole slide images of core needle biopsies: A blinded clinical validation and deployment study. *The Lancet Digital Health*, *2*(8), e407–e416. https://doi.org/10.1016/S2589-7500(20)30159-X
44. da Silva, L. M., Pereira, E. M., Salles, P. G., Godrich, R., Ceballos, R., Kunz, J. D., Casson, A., Viret, J., Chandarlapaty, S., Ferreira, C. G., Ferrari, B., Rothrock, B., Raciti, P., Reuter, V., Dogdas, B., DeMuth, G., Sue, J., Kanan, C., Grady, L., … Reis-Filho, J. S. (2021). Independent real-world application of a clinical-grade automated prostate cancer detection system. *The Journal of Pathology*, *254*(2), 147–158. https://doi.org/10.1002/path.5662
45. Eloy, C., Marques, A., Pinto, J., Pinheiro, J., Campelos, S., Curado, M., Vale, J., & Polónia, A. (2023). Artificial intelligence–assisted cancer diagnosis improves the efficiency of pathologists in prostatic biopsies. *Virchows Archiv*, *482*(3), 595–604. https://doi.org/10.1007/s00428-023-03518-5
46. Retamero, J. A., Gulturk, E., Bozkurt, A., Liu, S., Gorgan, M., Moral, L., Horton, M., Parke, A., Malfroid, K., Sue, J., Rothrock, B., Oakley, G., DeMuth, G., Millar, E., Fuchs, T. J., & Klimstra, D. S. (2024). Artificial Intelligence Helps Pathologists Increase Diagnostic Accuracy and Efficiency in the Detection of Breast Cancer Lymph Node Metastases. *The American Journal of Surgical Pathology*, *48*(7), 846. https://doi.org/10.1097/PAS.0000000000002248
47. Kim, D., Sundling, K. E., Virk, R., Thrall, M. J., Alperstein, S., Bui, M. M., Chen-Yost, H., Donnelly, A. D., Lin, O., Liu, X., Madrigal, E., Michelow, P., Schmitt, F. C., Vielh, P. R., Zakowski, M. F., Parwani, A. V., Jenkins, E., Siddiqui, M. T., Pantanowitz, L., & Li, Z. (2024a). Digital cytology part 2: Artificial intelligence in cytology: a concept paper with review and recommendations from the American Society of Cytopathology Digital Cytology Task Force. *Journal of the American Society of Cytopathology*, *13*(2), 97–110. https://doi.org/10.1016/j.jasc.2023.11.005
48. Wang, J., Yu, Y., Tan, Y., Wan, H., Zheng, N., He, Z., Mao, L., Ren, W., Chen, K., Lin, Z., He, G., Chen, Y., Chen, R., Xu, H., Liu, K., Yao, Q., Fu, S., Song, Y., Chen, Q., … Yao, H. (2024). Artificial intelligence enables precision diagnosis of cervical cytology grades and cervical cancer. *Nature Communications*, *15*(1), 4369. https://doi.org/10.1038/s41467-024-48705-3
49. Tanaka, R., Tsuboshita, Y., Okodo, M., Settsu, R., Hashimoto, K., Tachibana, K., Tanabe, K., Kishimoto, K., Fujiwara, M., & Shibahara, J. (2024). Artificial Intelligence Recognition Model Using Liquid-Based Cytology Images to Discriminate Malignancy and Histological Types of Non-Small-Cell Lung Cancer. *Pathobiology*, 52–62. https://doi.org/10.1159/000541148
50. Yamada, R., Nakane, K., Kadoya, N., Matsuda, C., Imai, H., Tsuboi, J., Hamada, Y., Tanaka, K., Tawara, I., & Nakagawa, H. (2022). Development of "Mathematical Technology for Cytopathology," an Image Analysis Algorithm for Pancreatic Cancer. *Diagnostics*, *12*(5), Article 5. https://doi.org/10.3390/diagnostics12051149
51. Brevet, M., Li, Z., & Parwani, A. (2024). Computational pathology in the identification of HER2-low breast cancer: Opportunities and challenges. *Journal of Pathology Informatics*, *15*, 100343. https://doi.org/10.1016/j.jpi.2023.100343

52. Yan, F., Da, Q., Yi, H., Deng, S., Zhu, L., Zhou, M., Liu, Y., Feng, M., Wang, J., Wang, X., Zhang, Y., Zhang, W., Zhang, X., Lin, J., Zhang, S., & Wang, C. (2024). Artificial intelligence-based assessment of PD-L1 expression in diffuse large B cell lymphoma. *Npj Precision Oncology*, *8*(1), 1–12. https://doi.org/10.1038/s41698-024-00577-y
53. Abel, J., Kirkup, C., Kos, F., Gerardin, Y., Srinivasan, S., Brosnan-Cashman, J., Leidal, K., Vasudevan, S., Rajan, D., Jain, S., Prakash, A., Padigela, H., Conway, J., Patel, N., Trotter, B., Yu, L., Taylor-Weiner, A., Krause, E. L., Bronnimann, M., … Wapinski, I. (2023). Abstract P4-09-08: AI-based quantitation of cancer cell and fibroblast nuclear morphology reflects transcriptomic heterogeneity and predicts survival in breast cancer. *Cancer Research*, *83*(5_Supplement), P4-09–08. https://doi.org/10.1158/1538-7445.SABCS22-P4-09-08
54. Balkenhol, M. C. A., Tellez, D., Vreuls, W., Clahsen, P. C., Pinckaers, H., Ciompi, F., Bult, P., & van der Laak, J. A. W. M. (2019). Deep learning assisted mitotic counting for breast cancer. *Laboratory Investigation*, *99*(11), 1596–1606. https://doi.org/10.1038/s41374-019-0275-0
55. Zehra, T., Anjum, S., Mahmood, T., Shams, M., Sultan, B. A., Ahmad, Z., Alsubaie, N., & Ahmed, S. (2022). A Novel Deep Learning-Based Mitosis Recognition Approach and Dataset for Uterine Leiomyosarcoma Histopathology. *Cancers*, *14*(15), Article 15. https://doi.org/10.3390/cancers14153785
56. Huang, Z., Parwani, A. V., Huang, K., & Li, Z. (2023). Abstract 5436: Developing artificial intelligence algorithms to predict response to neoadjuvant chemotherapy in HER2-positive breast cancer. *Cancer Research*, *83*(7_Supplement), 5436. https://doi.org/10.1158/1538-7445.AM2023-5436
57. Akhoundova, D., & Rubin, M. A. (2022). Clinical application of advanced multi-omics tumor profiling: Shaping precision oncology of the future. *Cancer Cell*, *40*(9), 920–938. https://doi.org/10.1016/j.ccell.2022.08.011
58. Ahuja, S., & Zaheer, S. (2025). Advancements in pathology: Digital transformation, precision medicine, and beyond. *Journal of Pathology Informatics*, *16*, 100408. https://doi.org/10.1016/j.jpi.2024.100408
59. Alix-Panabières, C., & Pantel, K. (2021). Liquid Biopsy: From Discovery to Clinical Application. *Cancer Discovery*, *11*(4), 858–873. https://doi.org/10.1158/2159-8290.CD-20-1311
60. Nikanjam, M., Kato, S., & Kurzrock, R. (2022). Liquid biopsy: Current technology and clinical applications. *Journal of Hematology & Oncology*, *15*(1), 131. https://doi.org/10.1186/s13045-022-01351-y
61. Darbandi, M. R., Darbandi, M., Darbandi, S., Bado, I., Hadizadeh, M., & Khorram Khorshid, H. R. (2024). Artificial intelligence breakthroughs in pioneering early diagnosis and precision treatment of breast cancer: A multimethod study. *European Journal of Cancer*, *209*, 114227. https://doi.org/10.1016/j.ejca.2024.114227
62. Hristova, V. A., & Chan, D. W. (2019). Cancer biomarker discovery and translation: Proteomics and beyond. *Expert Review of Proteomics*, *16*(2), 93–103. https://doi.org/10.1080/14789450.2019.1559062
63. Wu, L., & Qu, X. (2015). Cancer biomarker detection: Recent achievements and challenges. *Chemical Society Reviews*, *44*(10), 2963–2997. https://doi.org/10.1039/C4CS00370E
64. Bhinder, B., Gilvary, C., Madhukar, N. S., & Elemento, O. (2021). Artificial Intelligence in Cancer Research and Precision Medicine. *Cancer Discovery*, *11*(4), 900–915. https://doi.org/10.1158/2159-8290.CD-21-0090
65. Chen, Z.-H., Lin, L., Wu, C.-F., Li, C.-F., Xu, R.-H., & Sun, Y. (2021). Artificial intelligence for assisting cancer diagnosis and treatment in the era of precision medicine. *Cancer Communications*, *41*(11), 1100–1115. https://doi.org/10.1002/cac2.12215
66. Cohen, J. D., Li, L., Wang, Y., Thoburn, C., Afsari, B., Danilova, L., Douville, C., Javed, A. A., Wong, F., Mattox, A., Hruban, R. H., Wolfgang, C. L., Goggins, M. G., Dal Molin, M., Wang, T.-L., Roden, R., Klein, A. P., Ptak, J., Dobbyn, L., … Papadopoulos, N. (2018). Detection and localization of surgically resectable cancers with a multi-analyte blood test. *Science*, *359*(6378), 926–930. https://doi.org/10.1126/science.aar3247

67. Liu, M. C., Oxnard, G. R., Klein, E. A., Swanton, C., Seiden, M. V., Liu, M. C., Oxnard, G. R., Klein, E. A., Smith, D., Richards, D., Yeatman, T. J., Cohn, A. L., Lapham, R., Clement, J., Parker, A. S., Tummala, M. K., McIntyre, K., Sekeres, M. A., Bryce, A. H., … Berry, D. A. (2020). Sensitive and specific multi-cancer detection and localization using methylation signatures in cell-free DNA. *Annals of Oncology*, *31*(6), 745–759. https://doi.org/10.1016/j.annonc.2020.02.011
68. Gillette, M. A., Satpathy, S., Cao, S., Dhanasekaran, S. M., Vasaikar, S. V., Krug, K., Petralia, F., Li, Y., Liang, W.-W., Reva, B., Krek, A., Ji, J., Song, X., Liu, W., Hong, R., Yao, L., Blumenberg, L., Savage, S. R., Wendl, M. C., … Shi, Z. (2020). Proteogenomic Characterization Reveals Therapeutic Vulnerabilities in Lung Adenocarcinoma. *Cell*, *182*(1), 200-225.e35. https://doi.org/10.1016/j.cell.2020.06.013
69. Chan, H. T., Nagayama, S., Chin, Y. M., Hayashi, R., Kiyotani, K., Nakamura, Y., & Low, S.-K. (2019). The application of circulating tumor DNA analysis for detecting minimal residual disease and predicting recurrence in colorectal cancer patients. *Cancer Research*, *79*(13_Supplement), 1338. https://doi.org/10.1158/1538-7445.AM2019-1338
70. Natera.(2025).*NateratoPresentNewDataatthe2025ASCOGISymposium*.Natera.https://www.natera.com/company/news/natera-to-present-new-data-at-the-2025-asco-gi-symposium/
71. Kim, J.-S., Lee, Y. Y., Kim, M. Y., An, J., Shin, R., Park, J. H., Han, J., Choi, I. S., Heo, S. C., & Moon, Y. (2024b). Clinical validation of a novel circulating tumor DNA methylation assay for predicting recurrence of colorectal cancer in patients with curative-intent surgery by monitoring minimal residual disease. *Journal of Clinical Oncology*, *42*(16_suppl), 3620–3620. https://doi.org/10.1200/JCO.2024.42.16_suppl.3620
72. Nakamura, Y., Tsukada, Y., Matsuhashi, N., Murano, T., Shiozawa, M., Takahashi, Y., Oki, E., Goto, M., Kagawa, Y., Kanazawa, A., Ohta, T., Ouchi, A., Bando, H., Uchigata, H., Notake, C., Ikematsu, H., & Yoshino, T. (2024). Colorectal Cancer Recurrence Prediction Using a Tissue-Free Epigenomic Minimal Residual Disease Assay. *Clinical Cancer Research*, *30*(19), 4377–4387. https://doi.org/10.1158/1078-0432.CCR-24-1651
73. Gupta, R., Othman, T., Chen, C., Sandhu, J., Ouyang, C., & Fakih, M. (2019). Guardant360 Circulating Tumor DNA Assay Is Concordant with FoundationOne Next-Generation Sequencing in Detecting Actionable Driver Mutations in Anti-EGFR Naive Metastatic Colorectal Cancer. *The Oncologist*, *25*(3). https://doi.org/10.1634/theoncologist.2019-0441
74. Freenome. (2024). *Freenome | Outpacing cancer starts with early detection*. Freenome. https://www.freenome.com/
75. ADLM. (2017, June 1). *Grail Enlists Mayo Clinic Sutter Health to Develop Early Stage Cancer Tests*. https://myadlm.org/cln/articles/2017/june/grail-enlists-mayo-clinic-sutter-health-to-develop-early-stage-cancer-tests
76. Basharat, S., & Horton, J. (2022). *Emerging Multi-Cancer Early Detection Technologies: CADTH Horizon Scan*. Canadian Agency for Drugs and Technologies in Health. http://www.ncbi.nlm.nih.gov/books/NBK598992/
77. Hasin, Y., Seldin, M., & Lusis, A. (2017). Multi-omics approaches to disease. *Genome Biology*, *18*(1), 83. https://doi.org/10.1186/s13059-017-1215-1
78. Hoadley, K. A., Yau, C., Hinoue, T., Wolf, D. M., Lazar, A. J., Drill, E., Shen, R., Taylor, A. M., Cherniack, A. D., Thorsson, V., Akbani, R., Bowlby, R., Wong, C. K., Wiznerowicz, M., Sanchez-Vega, F., Robertson, A. G., Schneider, B. G., Lawrence, M. S., Noushmehr, H., … Laird, P. W. (2018). Cell-of-Origin Patterns Dominate the Molecular Classification of 10,000 Tumors from 33 Types of Cancer. *Cell*, *173*(2), 291-304.e6. https://doi.org/10.1016/j.cell.2018.03.022
79. Lin, Y., Zhang, W., Cao, H., Li, G., & Du, W. (2020). Classifying Breast Cancer Subtypes Using Deep Neural Networks Based on Multi-Omics Data. *Genes*, *11*(8), Article 8. https://doi.org/10.3390/genes11080888
80. Ensenyat-Mendez, M., Íñiguez-Muñoz, S., Sesé, B., & Marzese, D. M. (2021). iGlioSub: An integrative transcriptomic and epigenomic classifier for glioblastoma molecular subtypes. *BioData Mining*, *14*(1), 42. https://doi.org/10.1186/s13040-021-00273-8

81. Klein, H., Mazor, T., Galvin, M., Hansel, J., Mallaber, E., Trukhanov, P., Yu, J., Lindsay, J., Kehl, K., Hassett, M., & Cerami, E. (2023). MatchMiner: An open-source AI precision medicine trial matching platform. *Cancer Research, 83*(7_Supplement), 1067. https://doi.org/10.1158/1538-7445.AM2023-1067
82. Kurnaz, S., Loaiza-Bonilla, A., Carvallo Castañeda, D., Huner, O., Giritlioglu, D., & Precision Cancer Consortium. (2024). Effect of a novel artificial intelligence (AI)—enabled multi-trial matching system on patient matching using real-world data. *Journal of Clinical Oncology, 42*(16_suppl), e13501. https://doi.org/10.1200/JCO.2024.42.16_suppl.e13501
83. Nero, C., Boldrini, L., Lenkowicz, J., Giudice, M. T., Piermattei, A., Inzani, F., Pasciuto, T., Minucci, A., Fagotti, A., Zannoni, G., Valentini, V., & Scambia, G. (2022). Deep-Learning to Predict BRCA Mutation and Survival from Digital H&E Slides of Epithelial Ovarian Cancer. *International Journal of Molecular Sciences, 23*(19), Article 19. https://doi.org/10.3390/ijms231911326
84. Schouten, P. C., Richters, L., Vis, D. J., Kommoss, S., van Dijk, E., Ernst, C., Kluin, R. J. C., Marmé, F., Lips, E. H., Schmidt, S., Scheerman, E., Prieske, K., van Deurzen, C. H. M., Burges, A., Ewing-Graham, P. C., Dietrich, D., Jager, A., de Gregorio, N., Hauke, J., … Schmutzler, R. K. (2021). Ovarian Cancer–Specific BRCA-like Copy-Number Aberration Classifiers Detect Mutations Associated with Homologous Recombination Deficiency in the AGO-TR1 Trial. *Clinical Cancer Research, 27*(23), 6559–6569. https://doi.org/10.1158/1078-0432.CCR-21-1673
85. Ghosh, S., Abushukair, H. M., Ganesan, A., Pan, C., Naqash, A. R., & Lu, K. (2024). Harnessing explainable artificial intelligence for patient-to-clinical-trial matching: A proof-of-concept pilot study using phase I oncology trials. *PLOS ONE, 19*(10), e0311510. https://doi.org/10.1371/journal.pone.0311510
86. Jin, Z., Haddad, T., Hubbard, J., Hartgers, M. L., Leventakos, K., Cornwell, K., King, K., Franke, B. A., Pomerleau, K., Bibeau, V., Coverdill, S., Rammage, M., Helgeson, J., & Mahipal, A. (2019). A pilot study to implement an artificial intelligence (AI) system for gastrointestinal cancer clinical trial matching. *Annals of Oncology, 30*, v582. https://doi.org/10.1093/annonc/mdz257.029
87. NIH. (2024, November 18). *NIH-developed AI algorithm matches potential volunteers to clinical trials.* National Institutes of Health (NIH). https://www.nih.gov/news-events/news-releases/nih-developed-ai-algorithm-matches-potential-volunteers-clinical-trials
88. Jin, Q., Wang, Z., Floudas, C. S., Chen, F., Gong, C., Bracken-Clarke, D., Xue, E., Yang, Y., Sun, J., & Lu, Z. (2024). Matching patients to clinical trials with large language models. *Nature Communications, 15*(1), 9074. https://doi.org/10.1038/s41467-024-53081-z
89. George, R. D., Ellis, B. H., Sidey-Gibbons, C. J., & Swisher, C. (2023). Protecting against algorithmic bias of AI-based clinical decision making tools in oncology. *Cancer Research, 83*(7_Supplement), 1970. https://doi.org/10.1158/1538-7445.AM2023-1970
90. Corvese, L., Weiss, C., Huie, S., Zhou, B., Deng, Y., Gong, G., Kunz, P. L., & Fischbach, N. A. (2024). Using an AI trial screening tool to assess language as a barrier for enrollment of underrepresented minorities in cancer clinical trials. *Journal of Clinical Oncology, 42*(16_suppl), e13586–e13586. https://doi.org/10.1200/JCO.2024.42.16_suppl.e13586
91. Chen, P.-H. C. C., Jung, J.-J., Kim, Y., Lee, M., Sanchez-Bayona, R., Bröckelmann, P. J., Olson, R. A., Bernhardt, D., Goodman, C., Cecchini, M., Yan, M., Bahig, H., Lin, S., Cheng, J. Y., Giannikopoulos, P., Polkinghorn, W. R., Palma, D. A., & Lee, H.-B. (2024). AI-assisted clinical summary and treatment planning for cancer care: A comparative study of human vs. AI-based approaches. *Journal of Clinical Oncology, 42*(16_suppl), 1523–1523. https://doi.org/10.1200/JCO.2024.42.16_suppl.1523
92. Vandewinckele, L., Claessens, M., Dinkla, A., Brouwer, C., Crijns, W., Verellen, D., & van Elmpt, W. (2020). Overview of artificial intelligence-based applications in radiotherapy: Recommendations for implementation and quality assurance. *Radiotherapy and Oncology, 153*, 55–66. https://doi.org/10.1016/j.radonc.2020.09.008

93. Oehring, R., Ramasetti, N., Ng, S., Roller, R., Thomas, P., Winter, A., Maurer, M., Moosburner, S., Raschzok, N., Kamali, C., Pratschke, J., Benzing, C., & Krenzien, F. (2023). Use and accuracy of decision support systems using artificial intelligence for tumor diseases: A systematic review and meta-analysis. *Frontiers in Oncology*, *13*. https://doi.org/10.3389/fonc.2023.1224347
94. Jie, Z., Zhiying, Z., & Li, L. (2021). A meta-analysis of Watson for Oncology in clinical application. *Scientific Reports*, *11*(1), 5792. https://doi.org/10.1038/s41598-021-84973-5
95. Shapiro, M. A., Stuhlmiller, T. J., Wasserman, A., Kramer, G. A., Federowicz, B., Hoos, W., Kaufman, Z., Chuyka, D., Mahoney, W., Newton, M. E., Osking, Z., Wong, K. K., Kesari, S., & Shrager, J. (2024). AI-Augmented Clinical Decision Support in a Patient-Centric Precision Oncology Registry. *AI in Precision Oncology*, *1*(1), 58–68. https://doi.org/10.1089/aipo.2023.0001
96. Sesen, M. B., Peake, M. D., Banares-Alcantara, R., Tse, D., Kadir, T., Stanley, R., Gleeson, F., & Brady, M. (2014). Lung Cancer Assistant: A hybrid clinical decision support application for lung cancer care. *Journal of The Royal Society Interface*, *11*(98), 20140534. https://doi.org/10.1098/rsif.2014.0534
97. Blasiak, A., Truong, A., Tan, W. J., Lester, Kumar, K. S., Tan, S. B., Teo, C. B., Tan, B. K. J., Tadeo, X., Tan, H. L., Chee, C. E., Yong, W.-P., Ho, D., & Sundar, R. (2022). PRECISE CURATE.AI: A prospective feasibility trial to dynamically modulate personalized chemotherapy dose with artificial intelligence. *Journal of Clinical Oncology*, *40*(16_suppl), 1574–1574. https://doi.org/10.1200/JCO.2022.40.16_suppl.1574
98. Chang, T.-G., Cao, Y., Sfreddo, H. J., Dhruba, S. R., Lee, S.-H., Valero, C., Yoo, S.-K., Chowell, D., Morris, L. G. T., & Ruppin, E. (2024). LORIS robustly predicts patient outcomes with immune checkpoint blockade therapy using common clinical, pathologic and genomic features. *Nature Cancer*, *5*(8), 1158–1175. https://doi.org/10.1038/s43018-024-00772-7
99. TEMPUS. (2025). *Tempus | AI-enabled precision medicine*. Tempus. https://www.tempus.com/
100. Frampton, G. M., Fichtenholtz, A., Otto, G. A., Wang, K., Downing, S. R., He, J., Schnall-Levin, M., White, J., Sanford, E. M., An, P., Sun, J., Juhn, F., Brennan, K., Iwanik, K., Maillet, A., Buell, J., White, E., Zhao, M., Balasubramanian, S., … Yelensky, R. (2013). Development and validation of a clinical cancer genomic profiling test based on massively parallel DNA sequencing. *Nature Biotechnology*, *31*(11), 1023–1031. https://doi.org/10.1038/nbt.2696
101. Gungor, G., Michalet, M., Lombard, A., Roque, T., Atalar, B., Temur, B., Serbez, I., Azria, D., Vitry, L. de, Riou, O., Paragios, N., Ozyar, E., & Fenoglietto, P. (2021). Human-Level Precision Upper Abdominal OAR Contouring With Anatomically Preserving Deep Learning During Magnetic Resonance Imaging Guided Adaptive Radiotherapy (MRgRT). *International Journal of Radiation Oncology, Biology, Physics*, *111*(3), S44–S45. https://doi.org/10.1016/j.ijrobp.2021.07.122
102. Han, Z., Wang, Y., Wang, W., Zhang, T., Wang, J., Ma, X., Men, K., Shi, A., Gao, Y., & Bi, N. (2024). *Artificial Intelligence-Assisted Delineation for Postoperative Radiotherapy in Patients with Lung Cancer: A Prospective, Multi-Center, Cohort Study* (SSRN Scholarly Paper 4696974). Social Science Research Network. https://doi.org/10.2139/ssrn.4696974
103. Constantinou, A. D., Hoole, A., Wong, D. C., Sagoo, G. S., Alvarez-Valle, J., Takeda, K., Griffiths, T., Edwards, A., Robinson, A., Stubbington, L., Bolger, N., Rimmer, Y., Elumalai, T., Jayaprakash, K. T., Benson, R., Gleeson, I., Sen, R., Stockton, L., Wang, T., … Jena, R. (2025). OSAIRIS: Lessons Learned From the Hospital-Based Implementation and Evaluation of an Open-Source Deep-Learning Model for Radiotherapy Image Segmentation. *Clinical Oncology*, *37*, 103660. https://doi.org/10.1016/j.clon.2024.10.032
104. Cusumano, D., Boldrini, L., Dhont, J., Fiorino, C., Green, O., Güngör, G., Jornet, N., Klüter, S., Landry, G., Mattiucci, G. C., Placidi, L., Reynaert, N., Ruggieri, R., Tanadini-Lang, S., Thorwarth, D., Yadav, P., Yang, Y., Valentini, V., Verellen, D., & Indovina, L. (2021). Artificial Intelligence in magnetic Resonance guided Radiotherapy: Medical and physical consider-

ations on state of art and future perspectives. *Physica Medica*, *85*, 175–191. https://doi.org/10.1016/j.ejmp.2021.05.010

105. Kawamura, M., Kamomae, T., Yanagawa, M., Kamagata, K., Fujita, S., Ueda, D., Matsui, Y., Fushimi, Y., Fujioka, T., Nozaki, T., Yamada, A., Hirata, K., Ito, R., Fujima, N., Tatsugami, F., Nakaura, T., Tsuboyama, T., & Naganawa, S. (2024). Revolutionizing radiation therapy: The role of AI in clinical practice. *Journal of Radiation Research*, *65*(1), 1–9. https://doi.org/10.1093/jrr/rrad090
106. McIntosh, C., Welch, M., McNiven, A., Jaffray, D. A., & Purdie, T. G. (2017). Fully automated treatment planning for head and neck radiotherapy using a voxel-based dose prediction and dose mimicking method. *Physics in Medicine & Biology*, *62*(15), 5926. https://doi.org/10.1088/1361-6560/aa71f8
107. BC Cancer. (2023). *Cutting edge technology treats first patient in Kelowna*. http://www.bccancer.bc.ca/about/news-stories/stories/cutting-edge-technology-treats-first-patient-in-kelowna
108. Paul, D., Sanap, G., Shenoy, S., Kalyane, D., Kalia, K., & Tekade, R. K. (2021). Artificial intelligence in drug discovery and development. *Drug Discovery Today*, *26*(1), 80–93. https://doi.org/10.1016/j.drudis.2020.10.010
109. Pei, Z. (2024). Computer-aided drug discovery: From traditional simulation methods to language models and quantum computing. *Cell Reports Physical Science*, *5*(12), 102334. https://doi.org/10.1016/j.xcrp.2024.102334
110. Bess, A., Berglind, F., Mukhopadhyay, S., Brylinski, M., Griggs, N., Cho, T., Galliano, C., & Wasan, K. M. (2022). Artificial intelligence for the discovery of novel antimicrobial agents for emerging infectious diseases. *Drug Discovery Today*, *27*(4), 1099–1107. https://doi.org/10.1016/j.drudis.2021.10.022
111. Gerdes, H., Casado, P., Dokal, A., Hijazi, M., Akhtar, N., Osuntola, R., Rajeeve, V., Fitzgibbon, J., Travers, J., Britton, D., Khorsandi, S., & Cutillas, P. R. (2021). Drug ranking using machine learning systematically predicts the efficacy of anti-cancer drugs. *Nature Communications*, *12*(1), 1850. https://doi.org/10.1038/s41467-021-22170-8
112. Huang, C., Clayton, E. A., Matyunina, L. V., McDonald, L. D., Benigno, B. B., Vannberg, F., & McDonald, J. F. (2018). Machine learning predicts individual cancer patient responses to therapeutic drugs with high accuracy. *Scientific Reports*, *8*(1), 16444. https://doi.org/10.1038/s41598-018-34753-5
113. Exscientia. (2024). *Exscientia Launches AWS AI-powered Platform to Advance Drug Discovery*. https://investors.exscientia.ai/press-releases/press-release-details/2024/Exscientia-Launches-AWS-AI-powered-Platform-to-Advance-Drug-Discovery/default.aspx
114. Preuer, K., Lewis, R. P. I., Hochreiter, S., Bender, A., Bulusu, K. C., & Klambauer, G. (2018). DeepSynergy: Predicting anti-cancer drug synergy with Deep Learning. *Bioinformatics (Oxford, England)*, *34*(9), 1538–1546. https://doi.org/10.1093/bioinformatics/btx806
115. Halabitska, I., Petakh, P., Lushchak, O., Kamyshna, I., Oksenych, V., & Kamyshnyi, O. (2024). Metformin in Antiviral Therapy: Evidence and Perspectives. *Viruses*, *16*(12), 1938. https://doi.org/10.3390/v16121938
116. Joshi, I., Bhrdwaj, A., Khandelwal, R., Pande, A., Agarwal, A., Srija, C. D., Suresh, R. A., Mohan, M., Hazarika, L., Thakur, G., Hussain, T., Albogami, S., Nayarisseri, A., & Singh, S. K. (2023). Artificial intelligence, big data and machine learning approaches in genome-wide SNP-based prediction for precision medicine and drug discovery. In S. C. Basak & M. Vračko (Eds.), *Big Data Analytics in Chemoinformatics and Bioinformatics* (pp. 333–357). Elsevier. https://doi.org/10.1016/B978-0-323-85713-0.00021-9
117. Knudsen, J. E., Ghaffar, U., Ma, R., & Hung, A. J. (2024). Clinical applications of artificial intelligence in robotic surgery. *Journal of Robotic Surgery*, *18*(1), 102. https://doi.org/10.1007/s11701-024-01867-0
118. Ali, S., Jonmohamadi, Y., Fontanarosa, D., Crawford, R., & Pandey, A. K. (2023). One step surgical scene restoration for robot assisted minimally invasive surgery. *Scientific Reports*, *13*(1), 3127. https://doi.org/10.1038/s41598-022-26647-4

119. Quero, G., Mascagni, P., Kolbinger, F. R., Fiorillo, C., De Sio, D., Longo, F., Schena, C. A., Laterza, V., Rosa, F., Menghi, R., Papa, V., Tondolo, V., Cina, C., Distler, M., Weitz, J., Speidel, S., Padoy, N., & Alfieri, S. (2022). Artificial Intelligence in Colorectal Cancer Surgery: Present and Future Perspectives. *Cancers*, *14*(15), Article 15. https://doi.org/10.3390/cancers14153803
120. Gouveia, P. F., Costa, J., Morgado, P., Kates, R., Pinto, D., Mavioso, C., Anacleto, J., Martinho, M., Lopes, D. S., Ferreira, A. R., Vavourakis, V., Hadjicharalambous, M., Silva, M. A., Papanikolaou, N., Alves, C., Cardoso, F., & Cardoso, M. J. (2021). Breast cancer surgery with augmented reality. *The Breast*, *56*, 14–17. https://doi.org/10.1016/j.breast.2021.01.004
121. Tong, G., Xu, J., Pfister, M., Atoum, J., Prasad, K., Miller, A., Topf, M., & Wu, J. Y. (2024). Development of an augmented reality guidance system for head and neck cancer resection. *Healthcare Technology Letters*, *11*(2–3), 93–100. https://doi.org/10.1049/htl2.12062
122. Fazlollahi, A. M., Yilmaz, R., Winkler-Schwartz, A., Mirchi, N., Ledwos, N., Bakhaidar, M., Alsayegh, A., & Del Maestro, R. F. (2023). AI in Surgical Curriculum Design and Unintended Outcomes for Technical Competencies in Simulation Training. *JAMA Network Open*, *6*(9), e2334658. https://doi.org/10.1001/jamanetworkopen.2023.34658
123. Hopkins, B. S., Mazmudar, A., Driscoll, C., Svet, M., Goergen, J., Kelsten, M., Shlobin, N. A., Kesavabhotla, K., Smith, Z. A., & Dahdaleh, N. S. (2020). Using artificial intelligence (AI) to predict postoperative surgical site infection: A retrospective cohort of 4046 posterior spinal fusions. *Clinical Neurology and Neurosurgery*, *192*, 105718. https://doi.org/10.1016/j.clineuro.2020.105718
124. Basch, E., Deal, A. M., Dueck, A. C., Scher, H. I., Kris, M. G., Hudis, C., & Schrag, D. (2017). Overall Survival Results of a Trial Assessing Patient-Reported Outcomes for Symptom Monitoring During Routine Cancer Treatment. *JAMA*, *318*(2), 197–198. https://doi.org/10.1001/jama.2017.7156
125. Daly, B., Nicholas, K., Flynn, J., Silva, N., Panageas, K., Mao, J. J., Gazit, L., Gorenshteyn, D., Sokolowski, S., Newman, T., Perry, C., Wagner, I., Zervoudakis, A., Salvaggio, R., Holland, J., Chiu, Y. O., Kuperman, G. J., Simon, B. A., Reidy-Lagunes, D. L., & Perchick, W. (2022). Analysis of a Remote Monitoring Program for Symptoms Among Adults With Cancer Receiving Antineoplastic Therapy. *JAMA Network Open*, *5*(3), e221078. https://doi.org/10.1001/jamanetworkopen.2022.1078
126. Elder, A. J., Alazawi, H., Shafaq, F., Ayyad, A., & Hazin, R. (2023). Teleoncology: Novel Approaches for Improving Cancer Care in North America. *Cureus*, *15*(8), e43562. https://doi.org/10.7759/cureus.43562
127. Kumar, M., Rani, P., Joshi, B., Soni, R. K., Kumari, A., & Rohilla, K. K. (2022). Telemedicine as an unexpected catalyst during and beyond the COVID-19 Pandemic. *Nepal Journal of Epidemiology*, *12*(1), 1171–1174. https://doi.org/10.3126/nje.v12i1.42459
128. West, H. (Jack), Barzi, A., & Wong, D. (2022). Telemedicine in Cancer Care Beyond the COVID-19 Pandemic: Oncology 2.0? *Current Oncology Reports*, *24*(12), 1843–1850. https://doi.org/10.1007/s11912-022-01332-x
129. Kristensen, I., Lindh, J., Nilsson, P., Agrup, M., Bergström, P., Björk-Eriksson, T., Engellau, J., Hjelm-Skog, A.-L., Malmer, B., Martinsson, U., & Karlsson, M. (2009). Telemedicine as a tool for sharing competence in paediatric radiotherapy—Implementation and initial experiences from a Swedish project. *Acta Oncologica*, *48*(1), 146–152. https://doi.org/10.1080/02841860802409520
130. Carter, S. M., Rogers, W., Win, K. T., Frazer, H., Richards, B., & Houssami, N. (2020). The ethical, legal and social implications of using artificial intelligence systems in breast cancer care. *The Breast*, *49*, 25–32. https://doi.org/10.1016/j.breast.2019.10.001
131. Perera, C. R. D. (2024). *Deep Neural Networks for Limited Data Scenarios* [University of Melbourne]. https://findanexpert.unimelb.edu.au/scholarlywork/1935734-deep-neural-networks-for-limited-data-scenarios
132. Luong, K. (2024). *Challenges of AI Integration in Healthcare*. https://www.ominext.com/en/blog/challenges-of-ai-integration-in-healthcare

133. Gerke, S., Minssen, T., & Cohen, G. (2020). Chapter 12—Ethical and legal challenges of artificial intelligence-driven healthcare. In A. Bohr & K. Memarzadeh (Eds.), *Artificial Intelligence in Healthcare* (pp. 295–336). Academic Press. https://doi.org/10.1016/B978-0-12-818438-7.00012-5
134. Hantel, A., Clancy, D. D., Kehl, K. L., Marron, J. M., Van Allen, E. M., & Abel, G. A. (2022). A Process Framework for Ethically Deploying Artificial Intelligence in Oncology. *Journal of Clinical Oncology*, *40*(34), 3907–3911. https://doi.org/10.1200/JCO.22.01113
135. Lokare, R. R., Wadmare, J., Patil, S., Wadmare, G., & Patil, D. (2024). Transparent precision: Explainable AI empowered breast cancer recommendations for personalized treatment. *IAES International Journal of Artificial Intelligence*, *13*(3), 2694–2694.
136. Topol, E. J. (2019). High-performance medicine: The convergence of human and artificial intelligence. *Nature Medicine*, *25*(1), 44–56. https://doi.org/10.1038/s41591-018-0300-7
137. Beckers, R., Kwade, Z., & Zanca, F. (2021). The EU medical device regulation: Implications for artificial intelligence-based medical device software in medical physics. *Physica Medica*, *83*, 1–8. https://doi.org/10.1016/j.ejmp.2021.02.011
138. Fraser, A. G., Biasin, E., Bijnens, B., Bruining, N., Caiani, E. G., Cobbaert, K., Davies, R. H., Gilbert, S. H., Hovestadt, L., Kamenjasevic, E., Kwade, Z., McGauran, G., O'Connor, G., Vasey, B., & Rademakers, F. E. (2023). Artificial intelligence in medical device software and high-risk medical devices—a review of definitions, expert recommendations and regulatory initiatives. *Expert Review of Medical Devices*, *20*(6), 467–491. https://doi.org/10.1080/17434440.2023.2184685
139. Palaniappan, K., Lin, E. Y. T., & Vogel, S. (2024). Global Regulatory Frameworks for the Use of Artificial Intelligence (AI) in the Healthcare Services Sector. *Healthcare*, *12*(5), Article 5. https://doi.org/10.3390/healthcare12050562
140. Chen, R. J., Wang, J. J., Williamson, D. F. K., Chen, T. Y., Lipkova, J., Lu, M. Y., Sahai, S., & Mahmood, F. (2023). Algorithmic fairness in artificial intelligence for medicine and healthcare. *Nature Biomedical Engineering*, *7*(6), 719–742. https://doi.org/10.1038/s41551-023-01056-8
141. Rajkomar, A., Hardt, M., Howell, M. D., Corrado, G., & Chin, M. H. (2018). Ensuring Fairness in Machine Learning to Advance Health Equity. *Annals of Internal Medicine*, *169*(12), 866–872. https://doi.org/10.7326/M18-1990
142. Ueda, D., Kakinuma, T., Fujita, S., Kamagata, K., Fushimi, Y., Ito, R., Matsui, Y., Nozaki, T., Nakaura, T., Fujima, N., Tatsugami, F., Yanagawa, M., Hirata, K., Yamada, A., Tsuboyama, T., Kawamura, M., Fujioka, T., & Naganawa, S. (2024). Fairness of artificial intelligence in healthcare: Review and recommendations. *Japanese Journal of Radiology*, *42*(1), 3–15. https://doi.org/10.1007/s11604-023-01474-3
143. Allareddy, V., Oubaidin, M., Rampa, S., Venugopalan, S. R., Elnagar, M. H., Yadav, S., & Lee, M. K. (2023). Call for algorithmic fairness to mitigate amplification of racial biases in artificial intelligence models used in orthodontics and craniofacial health. *Orthodontics & Craniofacial Research*, *26*(S1), 124–130. https://doi.org/10.1111/ocr.12721
144. Olivier, P., Lana, G., Kumard, D., Sijia, H., & Zheng, J. (2021). *Multi-omic and survival datasets used for "DeepProg: An ensemble of deep-learning and machine-learning models for prognosis prediction using multi-omics data"* (Version v1) [Dataset]. https://doi.org/10.6084/m9.figshare.14832813.v1
145. Srikanth, M. S. (2017). *Analysis and Integration of Multi-Omics Datasets* [PhD Thesis, Centre for Bioinformatics, Pondicherry University]. http://dspace.pondiuni.edu.in/jspui/bitstream/123456789/2757/1/T6449.pdf
146. Rudin, C. (2019). Stop explaining black box machine learning models for high stakes decisions and use interpretable models instead. *Nature Machine Intelligence*, *1*(5), 206–215. https://doi.org/10.1038/s42256-019-0048-x
147. Colling, R., Pitman, H., Oien, K., Rajpoot, N., Macklin, P., Group, C.-P. A. in H. W., Snead, D., Sackville, T., & Verrill, C. (2019). Artificial intelligence in digital pathology: A roadmap

to routine use in clinical practice. *The Journal of Pathology*, *249*(2), 143–150. https://doi.org/10.1002/path.5310

148. MacDonald, S., Steven, K., & Trzaskowski, M. (2022). Interpretable AI in Healthcare: Enhancing Fairness, Safety, and Trust. In M. Raz, T. C. Nguyen, & E. Loh (Eds.), *Artificial Intelligence in Medicine: Applications, Limitations and Future Directions* (pp. 241–258). Springer Nature. https://doi.org/10.1007/978-981-19-1223-8_11
149. Brown, T., Mann, B., Ryder, N., Subbiah, M., Kaplan, J. D., Dhariwal, P., Neelakantan, A., Shyam, P., Sastry, G., Askell, A., Agarwal, S., Herbert-Voss, A., Krueger, G., Henighan, T., Child, R., Ramesh, A., Ziegler, D., Wu, J., Winter, C., … Amodei, D. (2020). Language Models are Few-Shot Learners. *Advances in Neural Information Processing Systems*, *33*, 1877–1901. https://proceedings.neurips.cc/paper/2020/hash/1457c0d6bfcb4967418bfb8ac142f64a-Abstract.html
150. Touvron, H., Lavril, T., Izacard, G., Martinet, X., Lachaux, M.-A., Lacroix, T., Rozière, B., Goyal, N., Hambro, E., Azhar, F., Rodriguez, A., Joulin, A., Grave, E., & Lample, G. (2023). *LLaMA: Open and Efficient Foundation Language Models* (arXiv:2302.13971). arXiv. https://doi.org/10.48550/arXiv.2302.13971
151. Murdoch, W. J., Singh, C., Kumbier, K., Abbasi-Asl, R., & Yu, B. (2019). Definitions, methods, and applications in interpretable machine learning. *Proceedings of the National Academy of Sciences*, *116*(44), 22071–22080. https://doi.org/10.1073/pnas.1900654116
152. Nauta, M., Trienes, J., Pathak, S., Nguyen, E., Peters, M., Schmitt, Y., Schlötterer, J., van Keulen, M., & Seifert, C. (2023). From Anecdotal Evidence to Quantitative Evaluation Methods: A Systematic Review on Evaluating Explainable AI. *ACM Comput. Surv.*, *55*(13s), 295:1-295:42. https://doi.org/10.1145/3583558
153. Lundberg, S. (2017). A unified approach to interpreting model predictions. *arXiv Preprint arXiv:1705.07874*.
154. Ribeiro, M. T., Singh, S., & Guestrin, C. (2016). "Why Should I Trust You?": Explaining the Predictions of Any Classifier. *Proceedings of the 22nd ACM SIGKDD International Conference on Knowledge Discovery and Data Mining*, 1135–1144. https://doi.org/10.1145/2939672.2939778
155. Zeiler, M. D., & Fergus, R. (2014). Visualizing and Understanding Convolutional Networks. In D. Fleet, T. Pajdla, B. Schiele, & T. Tuytelaars (Eds.), *Computer Vision—ECCV 2014* (pp. 818–833). Springer International Publishing. https://doi.org/10.1007/978-3-319-10590-1_53
156. Health, C. for D. and R. (2023). Good Machine Learning Practice for Medical Device Development: Guiding Principles. *FDA*. https://www.fda.gov/medical-devices/software-medical-device-samd/good-machine-learning-practice-medical-device-development-guiding-principles

Chapter 7
Artificial Intelligence for the Eye

Bhavna J. Antony and Iven M. Y. Mareels

Abstract In the last two decades, ophthalmology has seen rapid technological developments, particularly in medical imaging and AI for image interpretation. We discuss some of the innovations in imaging, including optical coherence tomography, and computer vision techniques such as convolutional neural networks, that have led to revolutionary advances in the detection of two vision threatening conditions: diabetic retinopathy and glaucoma. Throughout medical history the eye has been seen and used as a "window" into the body's internal state. Hippocrates, the father of Western medicine, identified a variety of eye characteristics associated with systemic conditions like hepatitis that causes yellowing of the sclera. In modern medicine, the eye continues to play a role in the management of systemic, cardiovascular and neurological conditions. We therefore also include recent advances in the analysis of retinal vasculature and optic nerve tissues, and the insights these analyses provide.

Introduction

The role of medical image analytics in precision medicine has been propelled by recent developments in deep learning and artificial intelligence (AI). Ophthalmology and optometry have experienced a surge of technological innovation over the last two decades. This situation may seem somewhat unexpected considering the relatively small scale of these specialties compared to disciplines such as radiology, neurology, and oncology, which rely even more heavily on medical imaging. The disparity can be attributed, in part, to a fundamental difference in image interpretation practices. Specialties, such as oncology and neurology, rely on radiologists to read, interpret, and generate reports regarding the imaging data, while

B. J. Antony (✉) · I. M. Y. Mareels
Institute of Innovation, Science and Sustainability, Federation University, Churchill, VIC, Australia
e-mail: b.antony@federation.edu.au

M. Chetty, J. Hallinan (eds.), *From Algorithms to Ailments*,
https://doi.org/10.1007/978-3-032-11023-7_7

ophthalmologists are typically tasked with interpreting their own images. This already arduous task became nearly impossible at the turn of the century, when optical coherence tomography (OCT) was able to create volumetric retinal scans almost instantaneously [1, 2]. The vast quantities of data so generated, can no longer be manually assessed. Thus, ophthalmologists, of necessity, sought automation earlier than other specialists. This is underscored by a recent study of clinicians reporting that ophthalmologists, compared to dermatologists, radiologists and radiation oncologists, are twice as likely to opt for AI tools to augment their workflows [3].

The scale of computer-aided analysis of ophthalmic images and their applications are too broad for discussion in a single chapter. Therefore, we limit ourselves to two conditions that make up the leading causes of blindness worldwide: diabetic retinopathy (DR) and glaucoma, and discuss the systems that have been proposed for their effective detection in ophthalmic images [4].

In 2019, diabetes was estimated to affect 463 million people worldwide. This number is expected to grow to 700 million by 2045 [5, 6]. Diabetic retinopathy, a key microvasculature complication of diabetes, affects 30–40% of diabetics, and its incidence is expected to grow at a similar rate [7, 8].

Glaucoma is less prevalent, but it is the leading cause of irreversible blindness worldwide, because presently its induced atrophies can only be slowed by treatment, not cured. In 2020, glaucoma affected approximately 76 million people worldwide. This number is expected to increase to 110 million by 2040 [9, 10]. Glaucoma is neurodegenerative and slowly developing, affecting the peripheral vision first. This change goes unnoticed by patients until significant portions of the visual field have been lost. About half of all patients experiencing glaucoma are unaware of their condition and therefore remain untreated [11–14].

In this chapter, we begin with the imaging modalities used in the diagnosis of these conditions (section "Imaging Modalities in Ophthalmology"), as well as the important biomarkers associated with them (sections "Detection and Grading of Diabetic Retinopathy" and "Proposed Disease Findings Observable on Level Dilated Ophthalmoscopy"). Early solutions to the detection of DR and glaucoma incorporated clinical knowledge, as they were designed to replicate a clinician's decision-making process, and are detailed in the section "Knowledge-Driven Analytics". More recently, AI-based computer vision approaches that utilize convolutional neural networks (CNN) were proposed for the detection of both conditions (section "Data Driven Analytics"). And finally, we discuss future directions, including AI models for prognostication, and the detection of other systemic conditions in the section "Extensions and Future Directions." The discussion of developments in medical image analytics would be incomplete without addressing computing resources, as computer vision as a whole, has seen symbiotic developments alongside improvements in processing units. As medical image analytics is fundamentally derived from computer vision, perhaps this is the best place to begin.

Developments in Computing Resources

In the early digital computing era (1960s–1980s), computer vision was more of a theoretical and experimental field than a practical technology. The fundamental challenges were rooted in the computational limitations of the time. Early computers possessed constrained processing capabilities, with a typical mainframe computer of the 1960s having much less computational power than a present-day smartphone. Memory was expensive and limited, measured in kilobytes rather than gigabytes. For context, early computers might have 464 kilobytes of RAM, compared to today's computers with gigabytes or terabytes. CPUs of this era were also fundamentally different. Clock speeds measured in megahertz, not gigahertz. A cutting edge CPU in 1975 operated at 12 MHz, compared to modern processors operating at 35 GHz. Memory bandwidth—the speed at which data could be transferred—was extremely limited, creating significant computational constraints.

Image processing is also particularly demanding, with each pixel manipulation requiring multiple computational steps, creating significant processing bottlenecks. As a result, pattern recognition was predominantly manual or semiautomated, with strictly defined feature extraction parameters. The process was more akin to computational assistance than autonomous machine learning. Early breakthrough research laid down critical theoretical foundations, such as computational models of visual processing, inspired by neurological understanding. These theoretical frameworks anticipated future technological capabilities, even if contemporary hardware could not implement them.

The field of CPU development saw significant improvements through the decades and is encapsulated in Moore's law: an empirical observation that the number of transistors per unit area in a chip doubles every 2 years (Fig. 7.1). This principle, expressed by and later named after Intel cofounder Gordon Moore, suggests that the number of transistors per area of an integrated circuit would double approximately every 2 years, leading to a corresponding exponential increase in computational power. This rapid enhancement in processing capabilities allowed computers to handle more complex tasks and run more sophisticated software applications.

Another major milestone was the introduction of multicore processors in the last 1990s. Unlike single core processors, which could only execute one instruction at a time, multicore processors featured multiple processing units (cores) on a single chip [15]. This innovation enabled parallel processing, in which multiple instructions could be executed simultaneously, significantly boosting overall performance and efficiency. Multicore processors became essential for handling demanding applications, such as video editing, gaming, and largescale data processing.

The 2000s and 2010s marked a transformative period in the field of computer vision, largely driven by advancements in Graphics Processing Units (GPUs). Initially designed to accelerate the rendering of images and graphics in video games and other visual applications, GPUs were soon recognized to possess remarkable capabilities for parallel computation [16]. Unlike traditional CPUs, which are optimized for sequential processing, GPUs are designed to handle thousands of

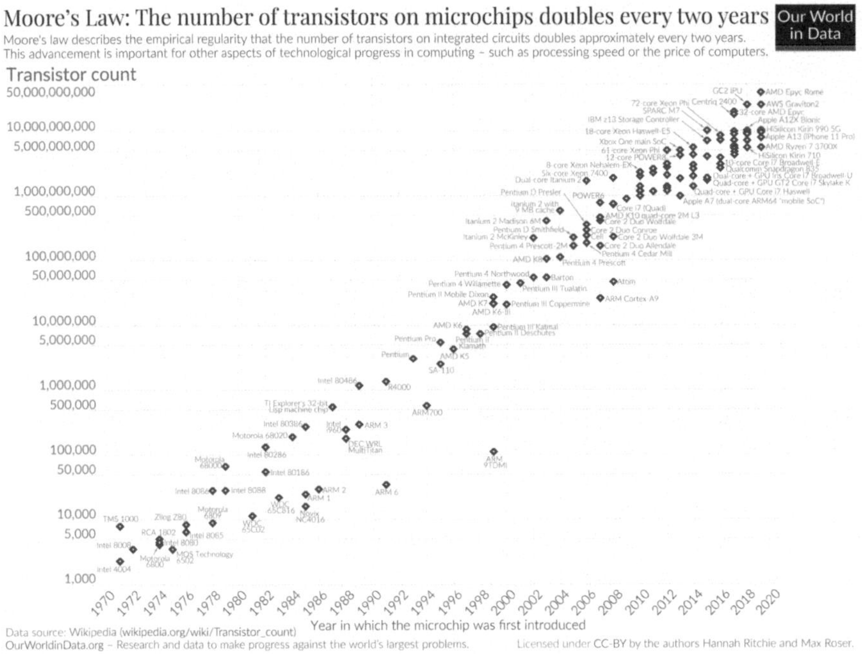

Fig. 7.1 Logplot of transistor counts for microprocessors and their introduction dates. Licensed under CCBY from authors Hannah Ritchie and Max Roser. (Reproduced from OurWorldinData.org)

operations simultaneously, making them ideal for tasks that require extensive parallel processing. One of the pivotal moments in this revolution was the introduction of NVIDIA's CUDA (Compute Unified Device Architecture) platform [17]. CUDA provided developers with the tools to harness the massive parallel processing power of GPUs for general purpose computing. This innovation enabled researchers and engineers to perform complex computations much faster than was previously possible with CPUs alone. The ability to execute many operations concurrently made GPUs particularly well suited for data intensive tasks, such as those found in scientific simulations, financial modeling, and computer vision. Convolutional neural networks (CNNs) (section "Data Driven Analytics") in particular, have greatly benefited from the computational power of GPUs. These neural networks are designed to process data with a gridlike topology, and thus are perfectly suited for the analysis of images.

The capabilities of CNNs became evident in 2012, when AlexNet, a deep CNN, won the ImageNet Large Scale Visual Recognition Challenge by a significant margin, demonstrating the potential of CNNs [18] in computer vision. This was one of the first examples of a CNN trained on GPUs, which drastically reduced the time required to train the network on large datasets. This architecture became the foundation of data-driven disease detection models that are so prevalent today.

Imaging Modalities in Ophthalmology

The story of analytics in ophthalmology would be incomplete without considering the development of imaging technology. The history of retinal imaging began in 1851 with a groundbreaking invention by Hermann von Helmholtz: the ophthalmoscope (or the mirror of the eye, as he called it) [19]. This revolutionary instrument allowed physicians to directly observe the interior of the eye, transforming medical understanding of ocular health. Prior to this invention, the internal structures of the eye were essentially a medical mystery, visible only during autopsy. Helmholtz's ophthalmoscope used a small mirror with a central hole, allowing light to be reflected into the eye and enabling direct visualization of the retina, optic disc, and blood vessels.

In the decades following Helmholtz's invention, medical professionals rapidly developed more sophisticated techniques for retinal examination. Physicians like Albrecht von Graefe in Germany and James Wardrop in Scotland refined ophthalmoscopic techniques, developing methods to examine the retina under various lighting conditions and from different angles [20, 21]. These early pioneers discovered that the retina could reveal critical information about systemic health, identifying signs of diabetes, hypertension, and other systemic diseases through changes in blood vessel appearance and retinal tissue. Julius Hirschberg described the natural history of DR and categorized DR into four types as early as 1880 using the ophthalmoscope [22, 23]. The transition to fundus photography began in the late nineteenth century, with the first successful retinal photographs produced in 1885 by Jackman and Webster [24]. It was not until the 1920s, that Noredson, in collaboration with Zeiss in Germany, was among the first to develop cameras capable of capturing detailed images of the retinal interior. These early photographic techniques were challenging, requiring precise alignment, extended exposure times, and significant patient cooperation. However, the general principles of these cameras form the basis of our modern cameras, and today a simple lens and smartphone will provide a rudimentary fundus image [25].

The next big breakthrough occurred in the 1990s, with the invention of optical coherence tomography (OCT) [26]. While similar to computed tomography, OCT uses a broadband light source instead of X rays, and generates images by comparing backscatter from tissue with a reference beam [2, 27]. The interference pattern generated depends on the time delay (or optical path length) between the reflections and the reference beam, thus resolving depth and generating a so-called Ascan. By repeating the process at incremental steps of a tissue sample, a 2dimensional (2D) image can be created (also called a B-Scan). The early time domain systems, were very slow, with a maximum speed of 400 Ascans per second [1, 2], but provided high resolution cross-sectional views with a resolution of approximately 10 μm.

The cross-sectional views proved invaluable in imaging macular pathologies such as edemas and detachments, and also enabled detailed measurements of clinically relevant structures that could be used to diagnose and manage a variety of conditions, such as glaucoma. Modern spectral domain (that utilize spectrometers) and swept source systems (that use a rapidly tunable light source) boast much faster speeds of acquisition in the MHz range, and are thus able to capture volumetric scans. These modern technologies can now capture microscopic changes in retinal structure, enabling early detection of disease, and provide quantitative measurements that were simply impossible with earlier imaging techniques.

From Helmholtz's simple mirror to today's sophisticated digital imaging systems, the history of retinal imaging is a remarkable journey of medical and technological miniaturization and innovation.

Detection and Grading of Diabetic Retinopathy

Diabetic retinopathy represents a serious microvascular complication of diabetes mellitus that affects the retina. The condition develops when chronic high blood sugar levels damage the small blood vessels in the retina, leading to vision problems and potentially blindness if left untreated. Several effective treatment options are available today, such as photocoagulation therapy for microaneurysms and intravitreal injections of inhibitors of vascular endothelial growth factor (VEGF), but their effectiveness rapidly decreases if treatments are left too late [28, 29]. Vision impairment and blindness are of course, devastating outcomes to patients, but they also have negative economic implications [30]. In 2006, vision impairment was estimated to cost the Australian healthcare system more than AUD 184 million in direct health-related costs, with an additional AUD 850 million paid out in benefits [31, 32]. As DR can occur in young individuals still part of the workforce, it also has broader, long lasting negative impacts on the community and its economy.

Replicating the expertise of a trained ophthalmologist in a computer program poses a significant technological challenge in itself, but to begin doing so, we needed a comprehensive, well-defined grading protocol approved by the clinical community. Efforts to do this began as early as 1908, and are reflected in the work of the researcher Arthur James Ballantyne. While the condition has long been associated with diabetes and descriptions of the retinal lesions associated with the condition improved in step with developments in the ophthalmoscope, his research gave us a fuller understanding of the progression of diabetic retinopathy [33]. He demonstrated that the retinal changes observed in diabetic patients were specifically related to their diabetes rather than being coincidental findings. He also noticed that the disease progresses through distinct stages, giving us the foundations for the grading systems used today.

Numerous clinical studies such as the Early Treatment Diabetic Retinopathy Study (ETDRS) [34], and The Wisconsin Epidemiologic Study of Diabetic Retinopathy [35] that began in the 1970s refined our understanding of the condition and established evidence-based treatment protocols. The DR grading protocols grew out of these studies and have seen a number of iterations beginning with Airlie house standard (and a modified version) [36], to the International Classification of Diabetic Retinopathy (ICDR) scale [37]. All of these standards established

Table 7.1 International Classification of Diabetic Retinopathy (ICDR) grading protocol

Proposed disease level	Findings observable on dilated ophthalmoscopy
No apparent retinopathy	No abnormalities
Mild NPDR	Microaneurysms only
Moderate NPDR	More than just microaneurysms but less than severe NPDR
Severe NPDR	Any of the following: more than 20 intraretinal haemorrhages in each of four quadrants; definite venous beading in two quadrants; prominent intraretinal microvascular abnormalities in one quadrant and no signs of proliferative retinopathy
PDR	One or more of the following: neovascularization, vitreous/preretinal haemorrhage

NPDR non-proliferative diabetic retinopathy; *PDR* proliferative diabetic retinopathy. Table modified from [37]

protocols for the detection and characterization of retinal lesions such as retinal hemorrhages, microaneurysms, cotton wool spots, and hard exudates. The biomarkers associated with DR at the various stages of the disease are summarized in Table 7.1. The gold standard imaging protocol recommended was the stereoscopic 7-field fundus imaging, which consisted of a mosaic constructed from seven 300 fundus photographs. This imaging protocol, however, requires significant patient cooperation and a well dilated pupil. The acquisition of 7-field images require a minimum of 16 images/flashes per eye and is therefore time consuming and uncomfortable for the patient. Further, the quality of the images varied by the skill of the photographer, and thus, is difficult to achieve consistently in demanding clinical settings. This led to the search for alternatives, ranging from ophthalmoscopic examinations of the retina [38], to the use of a limited number of fields [39]. While single fundus photographs were found to be poor substitutes for grading DR, they were found to be suitable for screening for the disease, such as determining whether to refer a patient for further ophthalmic evaluation [39, 40]. More recently, wide-field fundus imaging has proven to be effective for the clinical screening and grading of DR, showing comparative performance with the recommended 7-field imaging protocol [41, 42].

Proposed Disease Findings Observable on Level Dilated Ophthalmoscopy

No apparent retinopathy No abnormalities. Mild NPDR Microaneurysms only. Moderate NPDR More than just microaneurysms but less than severe NPDR. Severe NPDR Any of the following: more than 20 intraretinal hemorrhages in each of four quadrants; definite venous beading in two quadrants; prominent intraretinal microvascular abnormalities in one quadrant and no signs of proliferative retinopathy. PDR One or more of the following: neovascularization, vitreous/preretinal hemorrhage. NPDR: non-proliferative diabetic retinopathy; PDR: proliferative diabetic retinopathy. Table modified from [37].

The development of analytics for the detection of specific retinal lesions continued alongside this progression in grading standards, with approaches developed on the available and recommended imaging modalities. In the section "Diabetic Retinopathy and Fundus Photographs", we will discuss an approach proposed for detection of referable DR i.e., the detection of any DR-related abnormalities. The method assesses four fundus images, 2-field images of both eyes and assigns a label to the entire exam [43]. This system was the precursor to the one that was submitted to the FDA as a de novo application for approval as an autonomous DR referral system [44, 45]. The more recent deep learning-based approaches that detect referable DR and grade the disease without using any clinical a priori information is detailed in the section "DR in Fundus Photographs."

Biomarkers Associated with Glaucoma

The term "glaucoma" originated in ancient Greek medicine, where it was used to describe a bluish-green hue observed in affected eyes. The understanding of glaucoma as a pressure-related condition emerged much later, when in the mid nineteenth century, Mackenzie described the "hardness" of the eye as a biomarker of the disease [46]. This observation sparked increasing interest in the intraocular pressure (IOP), and elevated IOP outside the bounds of a normal range came to be considered a characteristic hallmark of glaucoma. The observation of normal pressure glaucoma (or normal-tension glaucoma (NTG)) [47] has since refined our understanding of glaucoma, and while the IOP remains a therapeutic target, it is not considered the defining characteristic of the condition. Today, glaucoma is understood to be a group of ocular disorders that may vary in presentation, with the common characteristic being the intraocular pressure-associated damage to the optic nerve, optic neuropathy [48–50]. All of the subtypes of glaucoma, if left untreated, will ultimately lead to blindness and glaucoma is currently the most common cause of irreversible blindness worldwide [51].

As early as the 1970s, the retinal nerve fiber layer (RNFL) was observed to atrophy in fundoscopy [48, 52]. Crucially, these early studies demonstrated that RNFL defects could be detected before visual field loss defects became apparent in glaucoma patients [53]. The 1990s marked a transformative period with the introduction of optical coherence tomography (OCT) [26, 54, 55]. The early time domain OCT (TDOCT) systems only acquired a small number of radial slices, but these images were sufficient to quantify the RNFL over time. The introduction of spectral domain OCT (SDOCT) scanners allowed for additional markers such as the ganglion cell layer (GCL) to be quantified more precisely, and currently the GCL is one of the key biomarkers used to detect and manage glaucoma. Visual function and its

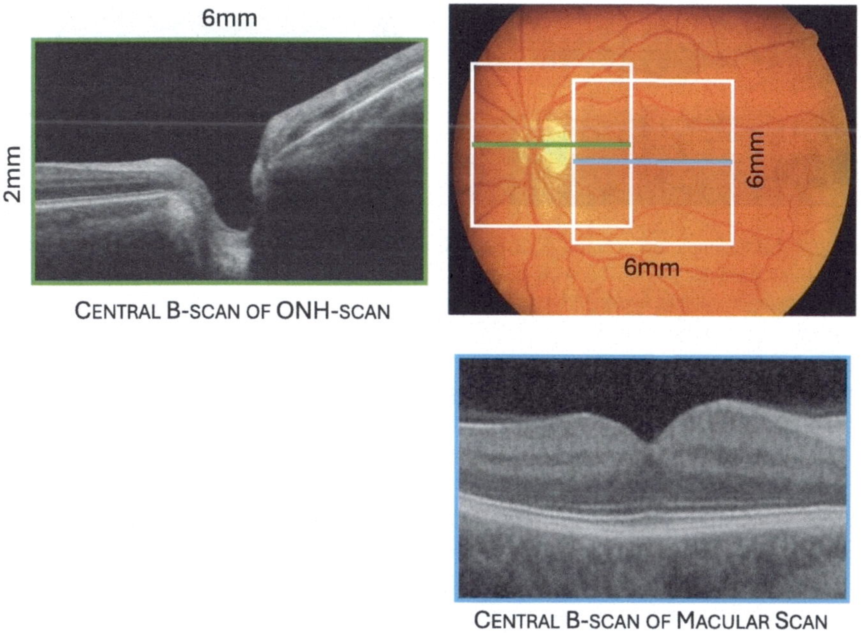

Fig. 7.2 Examples of OCT acquisition protocols centered on the fovea and the optic nerve head

deterioration that occurs in specific patterns is considered the gold standard test to assess glaucoma. However, OCT-based measurements have received increasing attention as RNFL and GCL atrophy has been shown to be highly correlated with visual field loss [56–59]. Moreover, OCT-based measurements show far less variability and inherent uncertainty as compared to visual field tests [60].

Figure 7.2 shows a fundus image, with examples of the central slices (B-Scans) of an ONH-centered and macular centered scan. The resolution, size and number of voxels in the volume varies considerably by scanner manufacturer and scan protocol. The scans are often 6 mm × 6 mm in size, but can vary, with some manufacturers supporting larger scan areas. While the depth of 2 mm is limited by the wavelength of the laser (850–1050 nm) used in SDOCT scanners, the voxel sizes in depth varies by scanner manufacturer, ranging from 1.95 to 3.95 μm. The number of frames or B-Scans can also vary from single to 200 B-Scans. Figure 7.3b shows the retinal layers that can be segmented in these scans. The RNFL and ganglion cell inner plexiform complex (GCIPC) are important for glaucoma management, while the photoreceptor bands are of importance in other conditions such as age-related macular degeneration (AMD) and retinitis pigmentosa (RP) [61]. The total retinal thickness, computed as the thickness from the inner limiting membrane (ILM) to the Bruch's membrane (BM) is also tracked, as atrophy or edema in the inner layers will be evident here. The equivalence between retinal structures and their appearance in OCT images remains an area of active research. The retina consists of stacks of cells, and the layers visualized in the OCT images are a result of varying optical

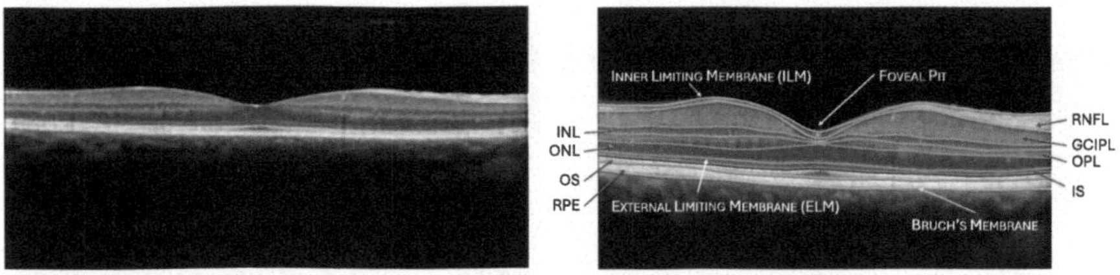

Fig. 7.3 (**a**) Example of a central macular B-Scan, (**b**) zoomed in showing the important retinal layers and surfaces: retinal nerve fiber layer (RNFL), ganglion cell inner plexiform complex (GCIPL), inner nuclear layer (INL), outer plexiform layer (OPL), myoid zone (MZ), outer segments (OS), retinal pigment epithelium (RPE)

properties. Histological studies certainly aided in identifying the specific structures, although the creation of slides can introduce significant distortions due to factors such as freezing and sectioning. This is especially true of the smaller structures, such as the photoreceptor bands. The nomenclature used here comes from the most recent study that combined electron microscopy, immunolocalizations, and histology [62].

There is a general consensus on the clinical utility of stratifying the severity of glaucoma into distinct grades. Such a grading system would not only provide a concise summary of a patient's condition but also serve as a quantifiable metric for monitoring disease progression and guiding therapeutic interventions. However, a lack of uniformity persists in the methodologies employed for this purpose. Although some researchers advocate the use of visual function assessments [63–65], citing their direct correlation with disease burden and patient quality of life, visual field tests are known for their inherent variability [60].

There is a growing interest in developing structure-based metrics, particularly those derived from Optical Coherence Tomography (OCT) scans [66]. Despite this interest, the numerous staging standards proposed present implementation challenges in clinical practice, often due to their subjective nature or excessive time requirements. Furthermore, the diverse modalities utilized in glaucoma diagnosis and management are not adequately represented in the existing staging frameworks. From a clinical standpoint, early detection remains paramount, as nearly half of the population of individuals suffering glaucoma is unaware of the condition [67]. We will therefore limit our discussion here to glaucoma detection methodologies using knowledge-driven approaches (section "Glaucoma and Optical Coherence Tomography") and deep learning networks (section "Glaucoma in OCT Volumes").

Knowledge-Driven Analytics

Prior to the introduction of neural networks, medical image analysis relied on the quantification in the images of biomarkers that can be associated with specific diseases. For instance, the automated diagnosis of DR in fundus images began with the detection of those pathologies specified in the ICDR grading protocol [37], namely, microaneurysms, cotton wool spots, and hemorrhages. The solutions proposed for the detection of these specific pathologies in the images utilized a two step approach beginning with the extraction of "image features" which were then classified using a machine learning approach. Feature extraction essentially transforms raw image data into a more compact and meaningful mathematical representation. This can be achieved by either convolving the images with predefined filters such as steerable Gaussian filters or Gabor filters [68], or by utilizing compressed representations such as principal component analysis (PCA) and wavelets [69]. For OCT scans, a variety of approaches were proposed for the segmentation and quantification of retinal layers, as the thicknesses of these layers are the crucial biomarkers.

The final disease detection methodology then utilizes the detected pathologies or quantified biomarkers to estimate the likelihood of the presence of a disease. The DR screening method detailed here [43, 44] utilized a machine learning based fusion of the identified lesions, while most glaucoma detection was achieved by comparing the measurements obtained to a normative baseline, deviations from which were used to identify disease [70]. This DR screening approach was the first to establish an automated methodology for referring patients to specialists. It also went on to be incorporated into the first FDA approved autonomous device for DR screening [45]. Similarly, the retinal segmentation approaches detailed in this section, continue to be utilized in many clinical studies and have not been superseded by deep learning methods.

Diabetic Retinopathy and Fundus Photographs

While the ICDR classification recommended the use of stereoscopic 7-field fundus photographs, Niemeijer et al. [43] showed that it was possible to build an accurate autonomous computer aided diagnosis (CAD) system using four fundus photographs; two for each eye, one centered on the macula and the second on the optic disc. This system (Fig. 7.4) consisted of a lesion detector and a final fusion step that combined the results of the lesions detected in the four fundus images as well as image quality metrics to provide a single soft label to indicate the likelihood that the patient should be referred to an ophthalmologist for further testing. This system was

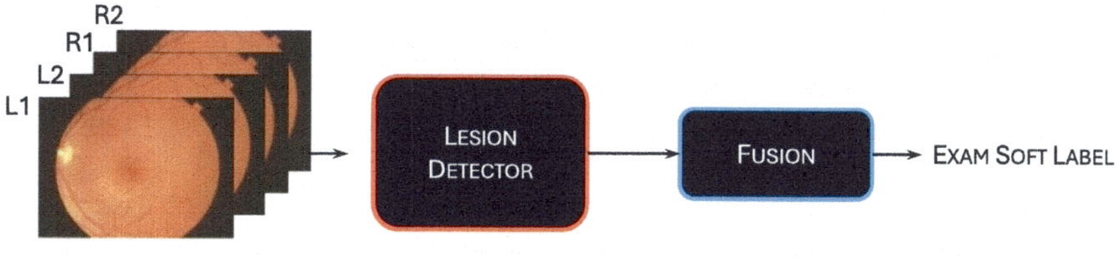

Fig. 7.4 Referable diabetic retinopathy detection system. (Modified from [43])

designed to screen patients and refer them to specialists rather than diagnose diseases.

Exam Classification via Label Fusion

The exam classification was obtained by fusing the lesion detection information from all four fundus images and their assessed image quality metrics. First, a posterior probability distribution normalization (PPDN)-based approach was used to fuse the information gathered regarding the lesions and the image quality of all the images, and then this soft label was incorporated into a supervised classification method—a k-Nearest Neighbor classifier—trained using descriptive features of the detected lesions. These descriptors were designed to capture the variety of lesions presentations possible, and included the posterior probabilities of lesions (maximum, sum, mean and standard deviation), as well as histograms of the lesion probabilities.

The image quality metrics generated by the lesion detector module where 1 represents the poorest quality, was combined into a single measure Q as follows: Q = min(max(Ql1, Ql2), max(Qr1, Qr2)), where Ql1, Ql2, Qr1, and Qr2 are the quality metrics for the two left and right eye images, respectively. This measure ensures that at least one good image per eye is available for the examination.

The PPDN fusion process aimed to fuse the information from the detected lesions (bright and red) as well as the image quality metric. First, the posterior probabilities for each lesion type is normalized, using the cumulative posterior probability distribution. The normalized posterior probabilities for all the lesions are then combined and represented by the maximum value Amax, thereby relying on the most confidently detected lesion. The final soft label for the exam is calculated as max(1 − Q, Amax). This incorporation of the image quality metric Q ensured that if the image quality is extremely low, the soft label assigned is dominated by the posterior probability associated with the detected lesions, and vice versa.

Preprocessing and Image Quality Estimation

The lesion detector consists of a preprocessing module and a feature extractor. The features were then used for image quality assessment, vessel detection, optic disc detection and finally red and bright lesion detection. The preprocessing module was designed to account for variations arising from using different fundus cameras, resulting in differing sizes of fields of view as well as borders around the fundus image. The sharp contrast difference between the fundus and the black border was especially important to remove as it could interfere with feature detection that follows the preprocessing steps.

A Gaussian filter bank at five different scales ($\sigma = 2i$, $i \in [0\ldots4]$) including derivatives up to the second order were computed. The final set of 31 features included these as well as the original image intensity per pixel. The image quality assessment was based on the assumption that all the important anatomical features will be visible in an image of good quality. Once the filter responses of an image were obtained, each pixel was compared to a set of five clusters generated using a set of good quality images [71], where the clusters were generated using a random set of fundus images.

Vessel Segmentation and Optic Disc Localization

The system also included the detection of major anatomical features, such as the vessels and the optic disc, as they share many similar features with the lesions. The vessels can mimic the red lesions and the optic disc appears quite bright in fundus images, and can therefore interfere with the bright lesion detection.

The same 31 features described earlier were used to train a k-NN classifier [72]. The dataset used to train this classifier came from a different dataset, DRIVE [73]. The optic disc segmentation relied on the brightness of the structure as well as the similarity in the vasculature structure and orientation across subjects. A k-NN regressor was used to identify the center of the optic disc using a feature-based template matching process. Image features were calculated within a circular region to create a feature vector v, and this was used to estimate the distance from the true center to the center of the template's current location [74]. The features computed within the template region consisted of pixel intensities and the direction and orientation of the blood vessels.

Red and Bright Lesion Segmentation

The lesion detection process aimed to identify microaneurysms and hemorrhages (collectively known as red lesions), and drusen, cottonwool spots, and exudates (collectively known as bright lesions). While drusen are not associated with diabetic retinopathy, they were still detected, as trying to differentiate them from the other bright lesions was extremely error prone. Moreover, drusen are a precursor to age-related macular degeneration (AMD) and therefore, it is best to refer these patients to specialists.

The red lesions were detected using two methods and then combined to include all potential candidates. The first method utilized a k-NN classifier trained using the 31 features detailed in the section "Preprocessing and Image Quality Estimation," while the second incorporated morphological features [75]. The red lesions were detected after the vessels were segmented and excluded from further analysis. These probability maps, containing the likelihood of each pixel belonging to a red lesion were then further analyzed to generate lesion candidates. This was achieved using a second k-NN classifier trained on an additional set of 69 features extracted from the fundus images describing the morphology of the lesion, textural properties, and color [76]. This classifier then assigned each lesion the likelihood of being a red lesion. The type of red lesion is not specified.

A similar process was followed for the detection of bright lesions, beginning with creating probability maps using a k-NN classifier trained on the 31 features described in the section "Preprocessing and Image Quality Estimation." Again, this step was only undertaken once the center of the optic disc had been identified, so that lesions close to the disc (within 60 pixels of the center) could be excluded from further analysis. The probability map was then locally clustered to separate the potential lesion candidates from the background. An additional set of 83 features were then computed, with the features capturing color, contrast, morphology, and location with respect to red lesions in the vicinity. Again, a k-NN classifier was used to assign each candidate a posterior probability of being a bright lesion [77].

Discussion

This approach was tested using 15,000 exams from patients with diabetes collected as part of the EyeCheck program [78]. Each exam was graded by an ophthalmologist into one of three categories: not suspect; suspect; and ungradable. Of these, only 394 exams were graded as suspect, while the remaining were not suspect, mimicking real-world screening scenarios in which the number of patients with diabetic retinopathy aligned with disease prevalence [6].

The big challenges identified by the authors included the correct detection of ungradable exams (the system failed to detect ungradable exams), hemorrhages connected to large blood vessels, and the presence of small exudates close to the fovea. Crucially, this system did not include a fovea detector, and the authors expected that inclusion of an additional fovea detector would likely improve their system overall. Despite these challenges, this system demonstrated that autonomous detection of referable DR was possible and could be done reliably [44, 79], and paved the way for the incorporation of autonomous diagnostic devices in healthcare [45].

Glaucoma and Optical Coherence Tomography

Evidence mounted that the thickness of the retinal nerve fiber layer (RNFL) and the combined ganglion cell inner plexiform layer (GCIPL) decreased as patients developed glaucoma, and was also found to correlate with the development of visual field defects [53, 56, 58, 59]. While the OCT scanners provided automated segmentation results, these measurements were found to vary in repeat scans as well as across the various scanners [80–82]. The reports were also limited to thicknesses averaged in predefined regions, and it was not possible to extract the entire retinal layer.

Numerous studies showed that machine learning classifiers trained using the RNFL and GCIPL thicknesses, averaged in predefined regions (typically the ETDRS grid [34]) can very accurately detect glaucoma [83, 84]. Other studies also incorporated visual field test parameters which further improved the classifier's stability [85]. However, as the diagnosis of glaucoma is tightly tied to the presence of visual field defects, the inclusion of these features probably explains the improved performance. These approaches were built using the measurements obtained from the scanners, which were known to be error prone. Thus, it appeared apparent that more reliable, reproducible measurements would lead to better diagnostic outcomes. The biomarker quantification in OCT analysis was necessarily more complicated, as the images are volumetric and the retinal layers, such as the RNFL, is a continuous structure present in every single frame of the volume. The proposed solutions for retinal layer segmentation ranged from 1D analysis to 2D and even 3D methods. The 1D methods analyzed individual columns (called Ascans) and sought to identify the boundaries between layers characterized by strong intensity changes in a smoothed intensity profile [86–96]. The 2D approaches incorporated active contours [97–99] as well as machine learning [100–103] to extract specific retinal structures from OCT images. In addition to these methods, two graph-theoretic approaches emerged that converted the segmentation problem into graph optimizations. One utilized the shortest path in 2D images [104–106], while the second utilized a 3D framework that supported the simultaneous segmentation of multiple surfaces [70, 107–112]. Their continued utilization in clinical studies is evidence of their accuracy and robustness and makes them appropriate for detailed discussion here.

Closed Set Formulation

The graph-theoretic approach [113] formulates the surface segmentation problem into the optimized identification of a closed set in a graph, in which a closed set is one where no edges leave the graph. The key novelty of this approach is in the construction of the graph with specific properties that then allow for the identification of minimum cost closed set, the envelope of which forms the segmented surface. Let us begin with a 2D image $I(x, y)$ with dimension $X \times Y$ where $x \in 1, \ldots X$ and $y \in 1, \ldots Y$, where X and Y represent the number of rows and columns in the image, respectively. The surface $S(y)$ is represented by a function, where $S(y) \in x$, and is therefore expected to intersect each column at a single location. The smoothness of the surface—the largest possible changes in the surface location between two adjacent columns—can also be enforced in this formulation. Let us represent this smoothness constraint by $\Delta = |x_p - x_q|$, where $S(y_p) = x_p$ and $S(y_p + 1) = x_q)$ are two adjacent pixels on the surface S.

A node-weighted graph $G(V, E)$ with nodes V and edges E is constructed such that each pixel in image $I(x, y)$ is represented by one and only one node $V(x, y)$ in the graph. The weights at the nodes are constructed as follows:

$$V(x,y) = ((x,y)\,\text{if}\; x = 0, (x,y) - (x-1,y) \tag{7.1}$$

where, $c(x, y)$ represents the cost function. The cost function can be constructed using a simple derivative $I'(x, y)$ or edge detector along the x-axis (negated, so that the surface of interest has the lowest possible cost). The cost function $c(x, y)$ input to the graph generator will in fact consist of the cumulative sum of the $I'(x, y)$. This ensures that when the node-weighted graph is generated as above, the final cost of the closed set will equal $\sum Y\ y = 1\ I'(S(y), y)$.

Two sets of edges, namely intracolumn and intercolumn edges are added to this graph as shown in Fig. 7.5. The intracolumn edges consist of directed edges connecting $V(x, y)$ to $V(x - 1, y)$, i.e., each node is connected to the vertex directly below it. The intercolumn edges enforce the smoothness constraints. Thus, a direct edge connecting $V(x_p, y_p)$ to $V(x_q, y_q)$ is added if if$(x_p - x_q) \leq \Delta$, where columns y_p and y_q are adjacent columns in the image. This graph can now be connected to terminal nodes s and t, and the minimum $s - t$ cut obtained using multiple polynomial-time algorithms [114–116], and the optimal surface is now represented by the envelope of a minimum cost closed set can extracted by identifying the minimum $s - t$ cut.

This formulation can be easily extended to 3D images where $I(x, y, z)$ has the dimension $X \times Y \times Z$ and $z \in 1\ldots, Z$; and the 3D image also contains multiple interacting sets of surfaces $S_n(x, y)$, where each surface is a function of an array of columns (x, y). Again, each surface is only allowed to intersect each column at one single location. In addition to the surface smoothness constraints, we now have an additional set of surface-interaction constraints that define the minimal and maximal allowed distances between two adjacent surfaces. For instance, a priori information regarding the surfaces of interest may inform us that surface i is known to occur above surface j, and $\delta_{ij}^{\min} \leq S_j(p) - S_i(p) \leq \delta_{ij}^{\max}$, as depicted in Fig. 7.5b.

The smoothness and surface-interaction constraints can be set globally for each surface [117], or be allowed to vary by location and be learned from a training set [107, 112]. Surface topology can also be influenced using additional edge weights that enforce shape penalties. These 'soft penalties' are in contrast to the previously defined smoothness and surface interaction constraints where the edge weights were

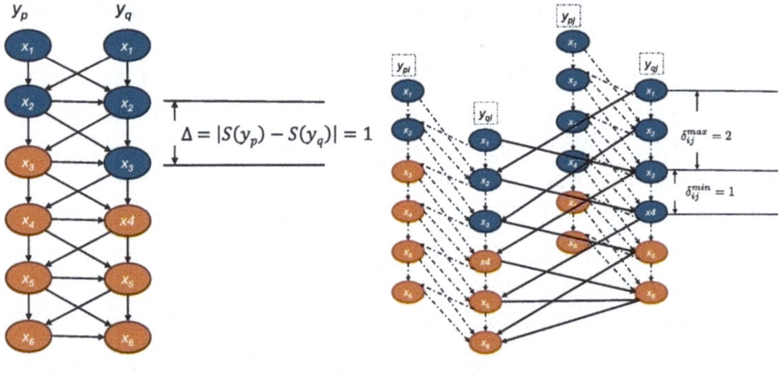

Fig. 7.5 Illustration of surface topology and surface interaction constraints enforced through hard connections in a graph. Here, nodes $S(y_p, \times 3)$ and $S(y_q, \times 4)$ represent the envelope of the closed set and the segmented surface in (**a**). (Modified from [107])

not rational numbers [118]; that is, they are 'hard constraints'. The shape penalties can also be extended beyond adjacent columns to enforce topological constraints with larger fields of view [109].

As the optimization is done with respect to the cost function, its careful design is a crucial step when using this approach. The cost can be defined in terms of on-surface as well as in-region costs. These two costs captured two different aspects of the retinal structures being segmented. The surfaces were characterized by intensity changes, while the retinal layers were of more or less similar intensity. The intensities in OCT scans do not have units and are normalized to either 8 bit or 16 bit grayscale intensities. Thus, there is a lot of variability seen in these images. These images are also characterized by significant speckle noise, making it difficult to identify hard thresholds for these different retinal layers. The earliest definition of the in region costs consisted of fuzzy membership functions defined to capture the three distinct bands seen in OCT retinal images [107]. The RNFL and the photoreceptor bands are 'bright', while the plexiform layers (inner and outer) are of medium 'gray' intensity and the nuclear layers (inner and outer) and the back ground have lower intensities and are 'dark'. Other formulations included the use of machine learning to further improve these in-region costs definitions [70, 112]. The on-surface costs could also be designed using machine learning, and the incorporation of this approach proved to be extremely advantageous [110, 112].

Antony et al. [112] utilized filter banks consisting of Haar features, Gaussian steerable features, Gabor filters [68], and additional intensity based features, which were then fed to a random forest classifier [119] to define the on-surface and in region costs. Lang et al. [110] utilized a much smaller set of features, which included the relative distance from the top and bottom of the retina as well as first and second order derivatives to define on-surface costs alone. Antony et al. also included learned smoothness constraints and surface-interaction constraints [70, 112] as well as shape priors [120]. It was found that the learned shape priors did not help the performance of the algorithm when using learned on-surface and in-region costs.

Shortest Path via Dynamic Programming

The shortest path approaches [104–106] also utilized graph-based representations. Unlike the closed set formulation, the surface segmentation problem was treated as a pathfinding one, involving looking for continuous paths from one side of the image to the other. This approach also required careful construction of the graph and a well-designed cost function.

In the approach proposed by Chiu et al. [104], an edge-weighted graph $G(V, E)$ was constructed such that each pixel in the image was represented by a node in the graph. The edges were added to allow a pathway from one side of the image to the other, and weighted to create path preferences. Careful setting of the edge weights was crucial, and was determined using the gradients of the image.

The shortest path algorithms require the specification of a root node and terminal nodes. To address this requirement, additional columns were added at each end of the image with edges along the vertical direction weighted with extremely small values. This allowed for the top left node to be set as the root node and the terminal node to be set as the node at the bottom right. The final surface segmentation was obtained by removing these two columns. Now any shortest path algorithm such as Dijkstra's algorithm could be used to find the shortest path.

As this algorithm can only find one path, the surfaces were segmented in a sequential manner, beginning with the outer surfaces and sequentially segmenting the inner surfaces one by one. At each step, the graph was created using a limited search space in the image, using expected retinal layer sizes. Thus, this approach was able to also incorporate expected layer distances.

Discussion

While both of these methods are graph based, there are two key differences. First, the closed set approach simultaneously segments multiple interacting surfaces in 3D, while assuring that the solution is at the global optimum with respect to the cost function. The shortest path approach ensures that each surface is optimal, but there is no way to enforce a global constraint on the set of surfaces. Second, the closed set formulation can explicitly incorporate a priori information such as surface topology and the interactions into the structure of the graph. The shortest path algorithm can enforce smoothness constraints in a similar way, but the only way to impose known retinal layer sizes was through the definition of limited regions of interest used when creating the graph for a specific retinal surface. This relies on the accurate segmentation of any previous surfaces and thus, errors can propagate through the process if the regions of interest are not created correctly.

While the closed set formulation may seem to be superior to the shortest path, in practice they were (and continue to be) utilized frequently for the segmentation of retinal surfaces in OCT images [121–126]. The closed set approach has proven to be excellent when segmenting dense OCT volumes with 40 200 B-Scans (frames) per volume as this allows for tight smoothness constraints to be applied in the slow scanning direction. This not only reduced the size of the graph, improving runtime performance, but also prevented the algorithm from latching onto spurious noise in the images. Similarly, the surface-interaction constraints proved to be a double-edged sword. Tight constraints helped improve the runtime performance as well as segmentation accuracy. However, if the structures of interest were affected by pathological changes the method fails often. Ultimately, the cost function is the most important aspect in this formulation, as the optimization is conducted with respect to it. Careful design, using machine learning, and even deep learning, has proven to be the best way to ensure accuracy as well as reasonable runtimes.

Data Driven Analytics

The ImageNet challenge, particularly the ImageNet Large Scale Visual Recognition Challenge (ILSVRC) [127, 128], was a pivotal event in the advancement of computer vision, especially in the field of deep learning. The challenge aimed to evaluate algorithms for object detection and image classification at a large scale and provided a benchmark dataset for researchers to compare the performance of their computer vision models. The ILSVRC used a subset of ImageNet, containing roughly 1.2 million training images belonging to 1000 different object categories. In 2012, AlexNet [18] achieved significantly lower error rates (>10% top1 and top5 accuracy) than previous methods, which relied on patch-based analysis [129]. The topn accuracy metric indicates the frequency with which the correct category occurs in the model's list of the top n most likely categories, ranked by their probability.

This marked a significant turning point in computer vision and immediately sparked interest in potential medical applications. However, these networks are prone to overfitting unless large datasets are available for training. The ILSVR utilized 1.2 million images. Transfer learning was proposed as a way to make the best of models trained on large natural scene datasets but reapplied in different applications. In transfer learning, a fully trained model is repurposed to new applications by retaining most of the weights and only adjusting a small number of layers in the network. Typically, the feature extraction backbone of a neural network, or the inner convolution layers, are frozen and only the last few layers, usually dense layers, are retrained using the medical images. This also allows for the number of classes identified to be adjusted to the new application. Occasionally, the entire network was also 'finetuned' over a small number of epochs to further improve the networks' performance on the medical data [130].

While this approach can be useful in some modalities, such as fundus photography where the images are in color, transfer learning was found to be less than ideal for grayscale modalities such as OCT. Volumetric images cannot be viewed as simple extensions of 3-channel color images. CNNs built for color images, and while capable of capturing detail in 2D, are not built to interpret structures that vary in 3D. In the following sections, we look at the deep learning approaches that successfully navigated these challenges and addressed DR detection and grading in fundus photographs (section "DR in Fundus Photographs"), and glaucoma detection in OCT volumetric scans (section "Glaucoma in OCT Volumes").

DR in Fundus Photographs

In 2015, Eye Picture Archive Communication System (EyePACS) introduced a challenge on the Kaggle website [131]. The dataset included nearly 90,000 fundus images with a DR grade associated with each image, ranging from 0 indicating normal to 4 as the most severe grade of DR. The images came from a variety of scanners, with varying resolution and image characteristics and were collected from a number of sites across the United States. The images were not quality controlled, with a number of initial studies indicating that nearly 20% of the images were in fact, ungradable [132].

Two primary methodologies emerged during the competition. The first approach involved explicit lesion detection using deep learning techniques, followed by subsequent DR grading. The second strategy employed large Convolutional Neural Networks (CNNs) for direct image grading. This paradigm shift represented a departure from earlier methods, which relied heavily on handcrafted feature engineering. The application of CNNs facilitated a data-driven feature learning process, wherein the internal representations of the convolutional filters remained implicit within the network architecture. In the subsequent sections, we discuss the work of Gulshan et al. [133], who put forward a retrained Inception model [134] that had been developed and tested on natural scene images; and Abràmoff et al. [135] where CNN based lesion detectors were used to identify lesions, but the grading followed the process detailed earlier [43].

Data Driven Grading

The model used was the Inception model [134], retrained using EyePACS as well as additional data obtained from three eye hospitals in India. In total, 128,175 images were used to train the model. The data was graded by 54 ophthalmologists or ophthalmology trainees, where the presence of DR severity was assessed as none, mild, moderate, severe or proliferative as per the ICDR protocol [37]. The images were also assigned a quality scale and assessed for the presence of diabetic macular edema. The model however, was trained to detect referable DR defined as moderate or worse DR, and the presence of macular edema.

The datasets used in the validation included the EyePACS dataset as well as MESSIDOR2 [44, 136]. This dataset, albeit smaller than the EyePACS dataset, was compiled and made available for retinal fundus image analysis in 2014. The images are macular centered images with one image acquired per eye. While the images are not graded, research groups have generated their own ground truths. The Inception model proved to be exceptional at the detection of referable DR, with an AUC > 0.99 on both datasets. The overall sensitivity and specificity of this model was >0.98 and >0.87, respectively, on both datasets, which was significantly higher than knowledge-driven approaches. The detection of macular edema was equally good on both datasets, with sensitivity and specificity at 0.90 and 0.98, respectively.

This approach demonstrated that lesion detection was not necessary for the detection of referable DR, and it was possible to train a large CNN using expert-generated labels alone. No additional information, feature engineering or expertise needed to be embedded in the system. The limitations encountered, ironically, came from the experts. The granular DR grades showed extremely high variability [137], stressing the need for better reference standards to be developed.

Recently, the focus has moved to the accurate identification of the grade of DR [138, 139], while others have also tried to emphasize the clinical need for explainability. For instance, Araujo et al. [140] proposed a CNN architecture to not only assess the grade of DR but also provide an explainability visualization map (section "Custom Architectures") and an estimate of model uncertainty. As the model provides a likelihood associated with each of the grades, it can be assumed that a confident model's output will resemble a Bernoulli distribution centered on the correct class; the likelihood scores of similar grades should be closer in value than likelihoods of further apart grades of DR. If this is found not to be the case, then the model output should be deemed of low certainty. All of these methods produced excellent performance, and the singular challenge that remains is the disparity among graders.

Lesion Detection Based Grading

One of the main drawbacks of CNNs is their opacity. It is very difficult, although not impossible, to identify the features that have been extracted. But understanding the relationship between the features and the output label, as well as any implicit feature engineering appears impossible to elucidate. The methods that incorporated explicit lesion detection into the grading process aimed to retain explainability of their models, by only replacing the lesion detectors with CNNs [135, 141, 142].

Abràmoff et al. [135] proposed to improve the previously described knowledge driven method [43, 44] through the use of CNN-based lesion detectors. AlexNet [18] formed the inspiration for the architecture used, while the final exam classification followed the process detailed in the section "Diabetic Retinopathy and Fundus Photographs." The dataset used to train the lesion detectors and the anatomical features vasculature and optic disc remained the same, while the testing was done on the MESSIDOR2 dataset. Since the MESSIDOR2 dataset only provides one fundus image per eye, the images were duplicated so that the rest of the system could remain the same. Other changes to the system included a fovea detector, which the authors had previously identified as a crucial missing component, and the fusion of the lesion probabilities was achieved using a random forest instead of a k-NN classifier.

The individual exams were graded into four categories: no DR, referable DR (ICDR levels ≥ 2, or macular edema), vision-threatening DR (ICDR level geq 3), and macular edema. All patients with macular edema fall into the second and third categories: referable DR and vision-threatening DR. This new model was found to detect referable DR with an AUC of 0.98, a significant improvement over the previously reported performance of 0.88. Moreover, vision-threatening DR was detected with a sensitivity of 100%, so no cases of vision-threatening DR were missed. The negative predictive value of the referable DR detection was also high at 0.99, indicating that patients could be confidently screened with this system.

Beyond the differences in the models, this approach also varied from many modern studies that assign an expert-derived grade based on a single image (e.g. [133])

rather than the recommended 7-field stereo fundus images. The grading on the MESSIDOR2 dataset was completed by three ophthalmologists using strict ICDR guidelines, and all differences in grades were adjudicated until consensus. Thus, the results in this study are far less affected by grader variability. Abràmoff et al. [135] also draws attention to the need to adhere to the grading protocols as strictly as possible. Failing to replicate the process as detailed in the grading protocol can lead to 'diagnostic drift' where the definitions slowly change as clinical standards become lax and our automated systems become more opaque. For instance, differentiating between a microaneurysm and a hemorrhage is important as one is a symptom of mild DR, while the other is indicative of moderate DR.

Glaucoma in OCT Volumes

The presentation of glaucoma in fundus imaging as well as OCT can be very subtle, unlike the often dramatic presentations of DR-related pathologies. Thus, CNN based approaches developed for the detection of glaucoma in OCT images have also been used to address the inherent opacity of these architectures.

One of the solutions proposed to help explain the outputs of the networks include class activation maps (CAM) [143]. CAMs essentially produce heatmaps indicating the regions of the image that the network has relied on most. Thus, they can be used to verify that the model is in fact learning important patterns in the images. The generations of CAMs requires the use of a global average pooling (GAP) layer (section "Custom Architectures") that averages the feature maps from the previous layer and connects it to the output dense layer. For instance, in a model with n convolutional layers, we can represent the features of the last layer by Fn and the weights that connect the GAP layer to the outputs by wn. The CAMs are computed for a specific class as a weighted average of the feature maps, i.e. $\sum c = 1 \;\; wc \;\; kFk$ will give us the CAM for class C. An extension of this, GradCAM [144], also incorporates the gradients with respect to the classification label. This allows for the method to be incorporated into any CNN architecture without the need to rely on specific layers such as the GAP.

Concept Activation Vectors (CAV) was another method proposed to improve in sights into the workings of neural networks [145]. This approach begins by defining specific concepts in the images and associating them with a specific class. For instance, it could include color (e.g., black vs. red) or in medical imaging it can be defined on the basis of a specific pathology. Passing examples and counterexamples of specific concepts through the network generates activations (i.e., CAVs) associated with the concept and its counterexamples. These can be drawn from any layers in the neural network but are typically drawn from the last convolutional layer. A linear model can now be trained to distinguish between the CAVs associated with a specific concept versus the counterexamples. This approach has been used successfully to understand the influence of specific concepts on the model's output and has helped greatly with interpretation of the results. We will see an example of its utility in the section "Transfer Learning."

Transfer Learning

One of the first examples of transfer learning for glaucoma detection in OCT images was proposed by Muhammad et al. [146], where AlexNet [18] was used as the CNN backbone, and the features extracted were used to train a Random Forest classifier [119]. The images analyzed consisted of thickness probability maps, which were generated using the scanner's onboard segmentation and rendered as color images. These images are not true thickness maps, as the colors are scaled to indicate the variations (regions of atrophy) with respect to a normative sample set. The method also incorporated RNFL and GCIPL thickness measurements as additional features. The authors reported that the inclusion of the RNFL thickness probability maps resulted in the best disease detection accuracy (92%). Thakoor et al. [147] also proposed a transfer learning approach utilizing an ensemble of CNN classifiers that boasted extremely good performance on the ImageNet Challenge, namely InceptionV3 [134], ResNet18 [148], VGG16 [149] and DenseNet121 [150]. Three dense layers were appended to the end of the pretrained networks and the entire model then finetuned using a small dataset consisting of 395 images. Transfer learning here was an excellent choice as the input images were thickness probability maps similar to those utilized above. The method boasted high accuracy rates (>90%) for individual CNNs as well as the ensembles, demonstrating that transfer learning on a small dataset was a viable option for disease detection.

The authors utilized CAVs to provide insight into the model output and verified the findings using by eye tracking data. The attention of experts was quantified through fixation counts and areas of interest while they studied OCT reports and graded the data as healthy or glaucomatous. This unique methodology revealed that the CAVs identified through the network coincided with the eye tracking data, with the RNFL probability maps showing the highest number of fixations.

Custom Architectures

The first CNN-based approach that analyzed raw OCT images was proposed by Maetschke et al. [151]. The architecture (see Fig. 7.6) was quite simple as the dataset was smaller than most used in deep learning applications, consisting of 1110 ONH centered OCT volumes. Unlike CNN architectures such as VGG16 [149], this model does not reduce the size of the input volume at each step. The size of the input volumes only reduced once and was achieved using a stride = 2 in the convolutional layer. The following layers use varying kernel sizes ($5 \times 5 \times 5$ in the second and $3 \times 3 \times 3$ in layers 35), but the stride is set to one, and the images are padded prior to the convolutions to retain the image size. Finally, the GAP layer averages the

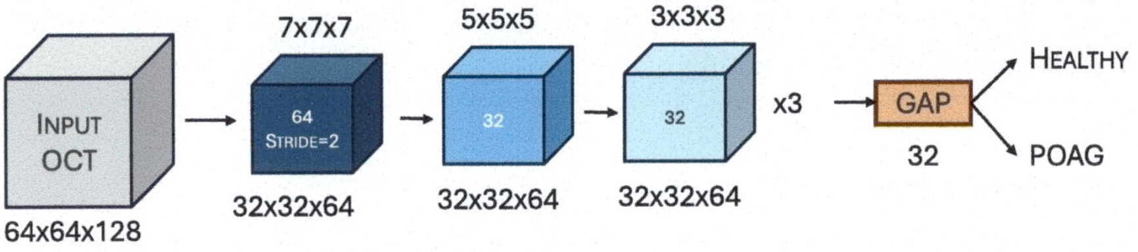

Fig. 7.6 Architecture of the 3D CNN used for glaucoma detection. (Modified from [151])

entire volumes resulting in a vector of size 32. This is then connected to a dense layer that provides the final classification of healthy or glaucoma.

Maetschke et al. did, however, have to down sample the images to meet the GPU memory constraints of the day. The images were down sampled from their original size of 200 × 200 × 1024 voxels to 64 × 64 × 128. Despite this loss of detail and a significant class imbalance between the number of healthy individuals and glaucoma patients, it was found that the CNN was very effective at detecting glaucoma (AUC > 0.90). The CNN required no preprocessing, such as denoising or contrast enhancement. This method was also found to improve over classical machine learning classifiers trained on segmented RNFL and GCIPL thicknesses. It was hypothesized that the segmentation process likely introduces noise that then propagates further into the disease detection module.

Maxpooling layers were avoided so that class activation maps (CAM) (see for example [143]) could be generated to visualize the regions of the volume to which the network paid attention. Using this technique, the authors verified that the model was in fact learning patterns in the images. The most commonly identified region of importance was the optic disc, with the anterior part of the lamina cribrosa also being identified in some instances. This is particularly interesting, as this structure, while known to be affected by glaucoma, is not completely visible in OCT images and is typically not quantified or analyzed. However, the network was able to pick up this pattern and deemed this area of the image important.

The down sampling of the volumes required in the above process is far from ideal, resulting in the loss of significant detail in the images. The human retina has a median size of 335 μm, while the depth image in OCT volumes is 2 mm. Thus, there are large portions of the image that are not really required. However, detecting the location of the retina in the volumes is akin to segmentation, which would not only degrade the runtime performance of the model but could also potentially introduce segmentation errors. George et al. [152] addressed this issue by introducing dynamic cropping, occluding unnecessary regions of the volume. The architecture, shown in Fig. 7.7, consists of three arms. One analyzes the original volume, while the second analyzes the volume with the unimportant section occluded, and the third analyzes a cropped volume consisting of only the regions identified as pertinent through an attention mechanism. The important regions were identified using gradCAM [144], and areas that were not deemed relevant were occluded. Note, the occlusion was done on the basis of B-Scans. The cropping in the third arm is done in the original image domain, retaining the 64 B-Scans with the most information

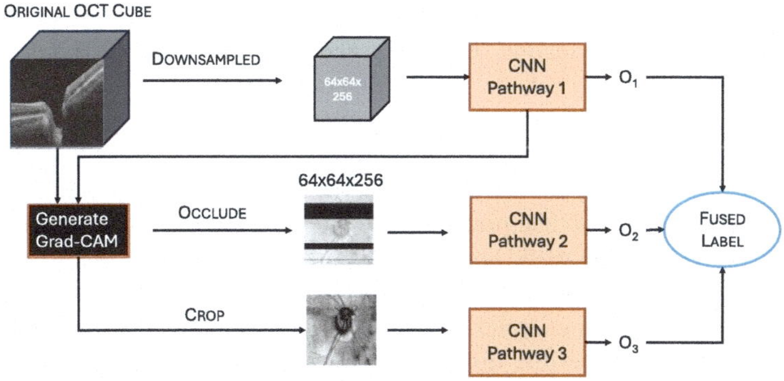

Fig. 7.7 Architecture of the attention guided framework for glaucoma detection. (Modified from [152])

and then resampling the remaining two axes to generate an image 64 × 64 × 256 in size. This enables potential weight sharing among the three arms. Each of the three arms generated an output classification, which was then fused to provide the final label.

An ablation study was used to identify the impact of the occluded and cropped volumes, as well as the impact of weight sharing among the networks. The authors found that weight sharing on arms 2 and 3 and utilizing the mean of the three outputs provided the best performance. This study proved that increasing the resolution of the input volumes was important, but not all areas of the volume are needed to provide an accurate diagnostic.

Overall, the glaucoma detection methods have not been validated using large datasets akin to DR, as data is not as easy to come by. Increasing data privacy and security concerns such as GDPR [153] are also a hindrance. While the necessity for these regulations is not in question, the technology to enable federated learning is not as mature [154]. Glaucoma does not have well established grading standards with defined gold standards of modalities or severity classification. Nevertheless, the clinical need for a robust screening tool remains, and as in DR, we will likely see the use of technological solutions in clinics soon.

Discussion

Deep learning networks revolutionized computer vision by introducing a paradigm shift in problem solving. Traditional approaches relied on explicitly mimicking expert behavior through handcrafted feature engineering. In contrast, the deep learning paradigm empowers data to autonomously reveal underlying patterns, at the price of requiring more data. Feature set definition, extraction, selection, and classification, previously distinct data processing stages, were unified within a single network capable of learning representations directly from raw data. It is also important to note that the choice to segment surfaces rather than layers (using the methods discussed in the section "Glaucoma and Optical Coherence Tomography") was not a biologically derived one, but one driven by the ease of annotating surfaces rather than layers. The semantic segmentation approaches, however, now segment retinal regions rather than surfaces.

This transformative approach yielded unprecedented performance on complex computer vision tasks that had previously defied resolution. However, this success comes at the cost of network opacity. The intricate decision making processes within these networks remain largely inscrutable. While individual learned features can be reconstructed, the complex interactions and combinatorial logic employed by the network are not readily discernible. This lack of transparency spurred the development of explainability techniques, such as Class Activation Maps (CAMs) [143] and Gradient weighted Class Activation Maps (GradCAM) [144], which provide insights into the image regions deemed salient by the network. Although these methods are not exhaustive, they serve as valuable tools for debugging during training and validating the network's focus on pertinent image features. Many traditional classifiers, including k-Nearest Neighbors, Support Vector Machines, and Random Forests, do not offer explicit definitions of decision boundaries. Consequently, the unease surrounding the opacity of deep learning networks may be amplified by their exceptional performance, reflecting a psychological response rather than an inherent methodological flaw.

In the domain of medical applications, explainability assumes paramount importance. This requirement is evident in approaches to Diabetic Retinopathy (DR) grading, where explicit lesion detection remains a fundamental component of many proposed methodologies. Likewise, in glaucoma assessment, considerable efforts are directed towards validating model outputs against expert clinical interpretations, exemplified by the integration of eye tracking data [147]. Similarly, the incorporation of CAM-generated insights, as proposed by George et al. [152] not only enhanced model performance but also provided crucial validation, confirming that the image regions identified by the network were indeed clinically relevant to the diagnostic task.

Extensions and Future Directions

Semantic Segmentation

The adoption of data-driven methodologies for disease detection in ophthalmic imaging offers several notable advantages. Primarily, it minimizes the requisite preprocessing of volumetric data and circumvents the need for explicit retinal layer segmentation. However, it is crucial to acknowledge that retinal layer integrity and the quantification of pathological features, such as intraretinal and subretinal fluid as sociated with age-related macular degeneration (AMD), constitute vital biomarkers for accurate diagnosis and disease monitoring. Semantic segmentation architectures have demonstrated exceptional efficacy in delineating specific anatomical structures within ophthalmic images. Notably, DenseNets [155, 156] and UNets have achieved remarkable success in retinal layer segmentation tasks [157]. The UNet architecture, in particular, has proven to be highly adaptable and effective across a diverse range of medical imaging applications. Nevertheless, the precise architectural configuration, including the number of down-sampling and up-sampling levels, as well as the filter count per convolutional layer, can exert a substantial influence on the final model's predictive accuracy. To address this challenge, the nnUNet framework was developed, which automates the optimization of network architecture based on the specific task requirements [158, 159]. Deep learning architectures have been effectively integrated within graph-theoretic frameworks (as described in the section "Closed Set Formulation"), wherein neural networks are employed to define the cost function [160]. This integration facilitates the incorporation of structural relationships within the data, enhancing the robustness and accuracy of disease detection.

Modeling Structure and Function

Deep learning has also shown significant promise in modeling the complex relationship between retinal structure and visual function, a crucial area of research in ophthalmology and neuroscience. While visual function tests are considered the gold standard for tracking progression in glaucoma, they are notoriously noisy, and are unreliable because they are difficult to execute and to administer [60, 161, 162]. These tests can be very long (may take as long as 40 min) and require patients to pay close attention for the entire duration of the test. The increasing interest in OCT based biomarkers came about due to the low reliability of visual function tests. As retinal structure is ultimately responsible for visual function, it is possible to model the relationship between the two. Retinal scans and derived thicknesses have shown very good reproducibility and thus estimates of visual function derived from the same ought to be very good. Bogunović et al. [163] proposed an approach that utilized segmented retinal thickness from a 9-field mosaic of OCT scans that spanned the entire field of a visual function test. Later, deep learning models would be proposed to estimate visual function from OCT volumes centered on the optic nerve head (ONH) and the macular alone [164, 165]. These efforts show that while the physiological function of each cell may remain unknown, the overall functioning of the tissue can be modeled effectively using deep learning methods.

Cardiovascular and Neurological Conditions

Oculomics [166], the comprehensive analysis of ocular structures and functions to derive systemic health insights, is rapidly gaining prominence in the management of cardiovascular and neurological conditions [167, 168]. The eye is often described as a window to the body as it is the only location in the body where neurological tissue—the ganglion cells, nerve fibers and the optic disc—as well as microvascular structures can be observed directly. Thus, the eye provides a noninvasive and very accessible avenue for observing microvascular and neural changes that reflect broader systemic pathologies.

The retina is particularly valuable in assessing cardiovascular risk. Retinal microvasculature, sharing similarities with cerebral and coronary vessels, is susceptible to damage from systemic conditions like hypertension, diabetes, and atherosclerosis [169–171]. Fundus photographs, and angiography enable detailed visualization of retinal vessel density, caliber, and tortuosity. These parameters serve as surrogate markers for microvascular dysfunction, which is a significant predictor of cardiovascular events such as stroke and myocardial infarction. Deep learning algorithms have enabled analysis of these images, quantifying subtle changes that may be missed by human observers. This allows for early identification of individuals at increased cardiovascular risk, facilitating timely interventions and preventive strategies [172].

Oculomics plays an increasingly vital role in the diagnosis and monitoring of neurological disorders. The retina, being an extension of the central nervous system, exhibits pathological changes in various neurodegenerative conditions. For instance, in Alzheimer's disease, retinal thinning and reduced retinal nerve fiber layer (RNFL) thickness have been observed [168]. OCT imaging allows for precise measurement of these structural changes, providing valuable insights into neuroaxonal degeneration. Similarly, in Parkinson's disease, alterations in retinal vascular density and RNFL thickness have been reported [173]. These ocular biomarkers can aid in the early detection and differentiation of neurodegenerative diseases, potentially complementing traditional neurological assessments. Retinal biomarkers have also been shown to be extremely useful in the management of patients with brain tumors, where these biomarkers have associated with survival outcomes [174] as well as cognitive decline [175].

The noninvasive nature of ocular imaging makes it particularly attractive for longitudinal monitoring and population-based screening. Unlike invasive procedures, retinal imaging can be performed quickly and comfortably, allowing for repeated assessments without significant patient discomfort or risk. This is especially important for chronic conditions that require long term monitoring, such as DR, glaucoma, and age-related macular degeneration, which are often comorbid with cardiovascular and neurological diseases.

This is a mere snapshot of ongoing research, and we anticipate significant advancements. The increasing resolution of ocular imaging, and the incredible insights that are gained into systemic conditions make it very likely that the next big strides in ophthalmic imaging will be made in management of cardiovascular and neuro logical conditions. In the future, even the diagnosis of metabolic disorders will come within reach through a new generation of biosensors enabling us to image metabolism in real time in the retina, and as the retina is perhaps the organ with the greatest metabolic demand in the body, it can reveal what metabolic disorders may lurk in the rest of the body.

Competing Interests The authors have no conflicts of interest to declare that are relevant to the content of this chapter.

References

1. T. C. Chen, B. Cense, M. C. Pierce, N. Nassif, B. H. Park, S. H. Yun, B. R. White, B. E. Bouma, G. J. Tearney, and J. F. De Boer, "Spectral domain optical coherence tomography: ultrahigh speed, ultrahigh resolution ophthalmic imaging," Archives of Ophthalmology, vol. 123, no. 12, pp. 1715–1720, 2005.
2. Z. Yaqoob, J. Wu, and C. Yang, "Spectral domain optical coherence tomography: a better octimaging strategy," Biotechniques, vol. 39, no. sup6, pp. S6–S13, 2005.
3. J. Scheetz, P. Rothschild, M. McGuinness, X. Hadoux, H. P. Soyer, M. Janda, J. J. Condon, L. Oakden-Rayner, L. J. Palmer, S. Keel, et al., "A survey of clinicians on the use of artificial intelligence in ophthalmology, dermatology, radiology and radiation oncology," Scientific Reports, vol. 11, no. 1, p. 5193, 2021.
4. V. Kavitha, M. M. Heralgi, and A. K. Gangrade, "Commentary: Understanding irreversible blindness the need of the hour; reversing it the need of the future!," Indian Journal of Ophthalmology, vol. 69, no. 10, pp. 2636–2637, 2021.
5. T. Y. Wong and T.E. Tan, "The diabetic retinopathy "pandemic" and evolving global strategies: the 2023 Friedenwald lecture," Investigative Ophthalmology & Visual Science, vol. 64, no. 15, pp. 47–47, 2023.
6. Z. L. Teo, Y.C. Tham, M. Yu, M. L. Chee, T. H. Rim, N. Cheung, M. M. Bikbov, Y. X. Wang, Y. Tang, Y. Lu, et al., "Global prevalence of diabetic retinopathy and projection of burden through 2045: Systematic review and metaanalysis," Ophthalmology, vol. 128, no. 11, pp. 1580–1591, 2021.
7. D. S. Fong, L. Aiello, T. W. Gardner, G. L. King, G. Blankenship, J. D. Cavallerano, F. L. Ferris III, R. Klein, and A. D. Association, "Retinopathy in diabetes," Diabetes Care, vol. 27, no. suppl 1, pp. s84–s87, 2004.
8. L. M. Aiello, "Perspectives on diabetic retinopathy," American Journal of Ophthalmology, vol. 136, no. 1, pp. 122–135, 2003.
9. K. Allison, D. Patel, and O. Alabi, "Epidemiology of glaucoma: the past, present, and predictions for the future," Cureus, vol. 12, no. 11, 2020.
10. Y.C. Tham, X. Li, T. Y. Wong, H. A. Quigley, T. Aung, and C.Y. Cheng, "Global prevalence of glaucoma and projections of glaucoma burden through 2040: a systematic review and metaanalysis," Ophthalmology, vol. 121, no. 11, pp. 2081–2090, 2014.
11. Y. Shaikh, F. Yu, and A. L. Coleman, "Burden of undetected and untreated glaucoma in the United States," American journal of Ophthalmology, vol. 158, no. 6, pp. 1121–1129, 2014.
12. R. Varma, M. Ying-Lai, B. A. Francis, B. B.T. Nguyen, J. Deneen, M. R. Wilson, S. P. Azen, L. A. L. E. S. Group, et al., "Prevalence of open angle glaucoma and ocular hypertension in Latinos: the Los Angeles Latino eye study," Ophthalmology, vol. 111, no. 8, pp. 1439–1448, 2004.

13. J. M. Tielsch, A. Sommer, J. Katz, R. M. Royall, H. A. Quigley, and J. Javitt, "Racial variations in the prevalence of primary open angle glaucoma: the Baltimore eye survey," JAMA, vol. 266, no. 3, pp. 369–374, 1991.
14. P. Mitchell, W. Smith, K. Attebo, and P. R. Healey, "Prevalence of open angle glaucoma in Australia: the Blue Mountains eye study," Ophthalmology, vol. 103, no. 10, pp. 1661–1669, 1996.
15. L. Chai, Q. Gao, and D. K. Panda, "Understanding the impact of multicore architecture in cluster computing: A case study with Intel dual core system," in Seventh IEEE International Symposium on Cluster Computing and the Grid (CCGrid'07), pp. 471–478, IEEE, 2007.
16. M. Lewis and J. Jacobson, "Game engines," Communications of the ACM, vol. 45, no. 1, p. 27, 2002.
17. R. S. Dehal, C. Munjal, A. A. Ansari, and A. S. Kushwaha, "GPU computing revolution: Cuda," in 2018 International Conference on Advances in Computing, Communication Control and Networking (ICACCCN), pp. 197–201, IEEE, 2018.
18. A. Krizhevsky, I. Sutskever, and G. E. Hinton, "Imagenet classification with deep convolutional neural networks," Advances in Neural Information Processing Systems, vol. 25, 2012.
19. A. Amireni, G. Bhasin, and L. Ganti, "History of the ophthalmoscope," Cureus, vol. 16, no. 8, p. e66387, 2024. Review 2024/09/09 Cureus. 2024 Aug 7;16(8):e66387. doi: 10.7759/cureus.66387. eCollection 2024 Aug.
20. C. R. Keeler, "The ophthalmoscope in the lifetime of Hermann von Helmholtz," Archives of Ophthalmology, vol. 120, no. 2, pp. 194–201, 2002.
21. W. McMullen, "The evolution of the ophthalmoscope," The British Journal of Ophthalmology, vol. 1, no. 10, p. 593, 1917.
22. W. Matuszewski, E. Bandurska-Stankiewicz, R. Modzelewski, U. Kaminska, and M. Stefanowicz-Rutkowska, "Diagnosis and treatment of diabetic retinopathy—historical overview," Clinical Diabetology, vol. 6, no. 5, pp. 182–188, 2017.
23. C. Fonseka, "The evolution in the treatment of diabetic retinopathy," Journal of the College of Ophthalmologists of Sri Lanka, vol. 26, no. 1, 2020.
24. R. B. Hildred, "A brief history on the development of ophthalmic retinal photography into digital imaging," Journal of Audiovisual Media in Medicine, vol. 13, no. 3, pp. 101–105, 1990.
25. U. Iqbal, "Smartphone fundus photography: a narrative review.," Int Journal of Retina and Vitreous, vol. 7, no. 44, 2021.
26. D. Huang, E. A. Swanson, C. P. Lin, J. S. Schuman, W. G. Stinson, W. Chang, M. R. Hee, T. Flotte, K. Gregory, C. A. Puliafito, et al., "Optical coherence tomography," Science, vol. 254, no. 5035, pp. 1178–1181, 1991.
27. J. S. Schuman, "Spectral domain optical coherence tomography for glaucoma (an AOS thesis)," Transactions of the American Ophthalmological Society, vol. 106, p. 426, 2008.
28. E. Y. Chew, F. L. Ferris III, K. G. Csaky, R. P. Murphy, E. Agron, D. J. Thompson, G. F. Reed, and A. P. Schachat, "The long term effects of laser photocoagulation treatment in patients with diabetic retinopathy: the early treatment diabetic retinopathy followup study," Ophthalmology, vol. 110, no. 9, pp. 1683–1689, 2003.
29. D. R. S. R. Group et al., "Photocoagulation treatment of proliferative diabetic retinopathy: Clinical application of diabetic retinopathy study (DRS) findings, DRS report number 8," Ophthalmology, vol. 88, no. 7, pp. 583–600, 1981.
30. K. D. Frick and A. Foster, "The magnitude and cost of global blindness: an increasing problem that can be alleviated," American Journal of Ophthalmology, vol. 135, no. 4, pp. 471–476, 2003.
31. H. Taylor, M. Pezzullo, and J. Keeffe, "The economic impact and cost of visual impairment in Australia," British Journal of Ophthalmology, vol. 90, no. 3, pp. 272–275, 2006.
32. A. P. Marques, J. Ramke, J. Cairns, T. Butt, J. H. Zhang, D. Muirhead, I. Jones, B. A. A. Tong, B. K. Swenor, H. Faal, et al., "Global economic productivity losses from vision impairment and blindness," eClinical Medicine, vol. 35, 2021.

33. A. Ballantyne, "Retinal changes associated with diabetes and with hypertension: A comparison and contrast," Archives of Ophthalmology, vol. 33, no. 2, pp. 97–105, 1945.
34. E. T. D. R. S. R. Group et al., "Early treatment diabetic retinopathy study report number 1; photocoagulation for diabetic macular edema," Arch Ophthalmol, vol. 103, pp. 1796–1806, 1985.
35. Klein R, Knudtson MD, Lee KE, Gangnon R, and Klein BE, "The Wisconsin epidemiologic study of diabetic retinopathy: Xxii the twenty five year progression of retinopathy in persons with type 1 diabetes," Ophthalmology, vol. 115, pp. 1859–68, 2008 Nov.
36. M. F. Goldberg and L. M. Jampol, "Knowledge of diabetic retinopathy before and 18 years after the Airlie house symposium on treatment of diabetic retinopathy," Ophthalmology, vol. 94, no. 7, pp. 741–746, 1987.
37. C. P. Wilkinson, F. L. Ferris III, R. E. Klein, P. P. Lee, C. D. Agardh, M. Davis, D. Dills, A. Kampik, R. Pararajasegaram, J. T. Verdaguer, et al., "Proposed international clinical diabetic retinopathy and diabetic macular edema disease severity scales," Ophthalmology, vol. 110, no. 9, pp. 1677–1682, 2003.
38. S. E. Moss, R. Klein, S. D. Kessler, and K. A. Richie, "Comparison between ophthalmoscopy and fundus photography in determining severity of diabetic retinopathy," Ophthalmology, vol. 92, no. 1, pp. 62–67, 1985.
39. S. Vujosevic, E. Benetti, F. Massignan, E. Pilotto, M. Varano, F. Cavarzeran, A. Avogaro, and E. Midena, "Screening for diabetic retinopathy: 1 and 3 nonmydriatic 45degree digital fundus photographs vs 7 standard early treatment diabetic retinopathy study fields," American Journal of Ophthalmology, vol. 148, no. 1, pp. 111–118, 2009.
40. G. A. Williams, I. U. Scott, J. A. Haller, A. M. Maguire, D. Marcus, and H. R. McDonald, "Single field fundus photography for diabetic retinopathy screening: a report by the American Academy of Ophthalmology," Ophthalmology, vol. 111, no. 5, pp. 1055–1062, 2004.
41. L. P. Aiello, I. Odia, A. R. Glassman, M. Melia, L. M. Jampol, N. M. Bressler, S. Kiss, P. S. Silva, C. C. Wykoff, J. K. Sun, et al., "Comparison of early treatment diabetic retinopathy study standard 7-field imaging with ultrawide-field imaging for determining severity of diabetic retinopathy," JAMA Ophthalmology, vol. 137, no. 1, pp. 65–73, 2019.
42. Y. Attiku, M. G. Nittala, S. B. Velaga, C. Ramachandra, S. Bhat, K. Solanki, C. Jayadev, N. Choudhry, S. M. A. Orr, S. Jiang, et al., "Comparison of diabetic retinopathy severity grading on ETDRS 7-field versus ultrawide-field assessment," Eye, vol. 37, no. 14, pp. 2946–2949, 2023.
43. M. Niemeijer, M. D. Abramoff, and B. Van Ginneken, "Information fusion for diabetic retinopathy CAD in digital color fundus photographs," IEEE Transactions on Medical Imaging, vol. 28, no. 5, pp. 775–785, 2009.
44. M. D. Abràmoff, J. C. Folk, D. P. Han, J. D. Walker, D. F. Williams, S. R. Russell, P. Massin, B. Cochener, P. Gain, L. Tang, et al., "Automated analysis of retinal images for detection of referable diabetic retinopathy," JAMA Ophthalmology, vol. 131, no. 3, pp. 351–357, 2013.
45. J. Carfagno, "Lumineticscore™ (formerly known as IDXDR), the first FDA approved AI system, is growing rapidly."
46. W. Mackenzie, "On glaucoma," Glasgow Medical Journal, vol. 3, no. 11, p. 254, 1830.
47. R. Ritch, M. B. Shields, and T. Krupin, The glaucomas: Glaucoma Therapy, vol. 3. Mosby, 1996.
48. L. E. Zimmerman, G. de Venecia, and D. I. Hamasaki, "Pathology of the optic nerve in experimental acute glaucoma," Investigative Ophthalmology & Visual Science, vol. 6, no. 2, pp. 109–125, 1967.
49. R. J. Casson, G. Chidlow, J. P. Wood, J. G. Crowston, and I. Goldberg, "Definition of glaucoma: Clinical and experimental concepts," Clinical & Experimental Ophthalmology, vol. 40, no. 4, pp. 341–349, 2012.
50. R. N. Weinreb, T. Aung, and F. A. Medeiros, "The pathophysiology and treatment of glaucoma: A review," JAMA, vol. 311, no. 18, pp. 1901–1911, 2014.

51. V. L. E. G. of the Global Burden of Disease Study et al., "Global estimates on the number of people blind or visually impaired by glaucoma: A metaanalysis from 2000 to 2020," Eye, vol. 38, no. 11, p. 2036, 2024.
52. W. F. Hoyt, L. Frisen, and N. M. Newman, "Fundoscopy of nerve fiber layer defects in glaucoma," Investigative Ophthalmology & Visual Science, vol. 12, no. 11, pp. 814–829, 1973.
53. H. A. Quigley, N. R. Miller, and T. George, "Clinical evaluation of nerve fiber layer atrophy as an indicator of glaucomatous optic nerve damage," Archives of Ophthalmology, vol. 98, no. 9, pp. 1564–1571, 1980.
54. E. Swanson, M. Hee, D. Huang, J. A. Izatt, J. G. Fujimoto, C. P. Lin, J. S. Schuman, and C. A. Puliafito, "Optical coherence tomography," in Conference on Lasers and ElectroOptics, p. CThB1, Optica Publishing Group, 1992.
55. J. S. Schuman, M. Hee, A. Arya, et al., "Optical coherence tomography," Curr Opin Ophthalmol, vol. 6, pp. 89–95, 1995.
56. J. S. Schuman, M. R. Hee, C. A. Puliafito, C. Wong, T. Pedut-Kloizman, C. P. Lin, E. Hertz mark, J. A. Izatt, E. A. Swanson, and J. G. Fujimoto, "Quantification of nerve fiber layer thickness in normal and glaucomatous eyes using optical coherence tomography: a pilot study," Archives of Ophthalmology, vol. 113, no. 5, pp. 586–596, 1995.
57. J. A. Izatt, M. R. Hee, D. Huang, J. G. Fujimoto, E. A. Swanson, C. P. Lin, J. S. Shuman, and C. A. Puliafito, "Ophthalmic diagnostics using optical coherence tomography," in Ophthalmic Technologies III, vol. 1877, pp. 136–144, SPIE, 1993.
58. C. Bowd, R. N. Weinreb, J. M. Williams, and L. M. Zangwill, "The retinal nerve fiber layer thickness in ocular hypertensive, normal, and glaucomatous eyes with optical coherence tomography," Archives of Ophthalmology, vol. 118, no. 1, pp. 22–26, 2000.
59. L. A. Kerrigan-Baumrind, H. A. Quigley, M. E. Pease, D. F. Kerrigan, and R. S. Mitchell, "Number of ganglion cells in glaucoma eyes compared with threshold visual field tests in the same persons," Investigative Ophthalmology & Visual Science, vol. 41, no. 3, pp. 741–748, 2000.
60. P. H. Artes, A. Iwase, Y. Ohno, Y. Kitazawa, and B. C. Chauhan, "Properties of perimetric threshold estimates from full threshold, SITA standard, and SITA fast strategies," Investigative Ophthalmology & Visual Science, vol. 43, no. 8, pp. 2654–2659, 2002.
61. S. P. Daiger, S. J. Bowne, and L. S. Sullivan, "Perspective on genes and mutations causing retinitis pigmentosa," Archives of Ophthalmology, vol. 125, no. 2, pp. 151–158, 2007.
62. L. Goerdt, T. A. Swain, D. Kar, G. McGwin, A. Berlin, M. E. Clark, C. Owsley, K. R. Sloan, and C. A. Curcio, "Band visibility in high resolution optical coherence tomography assessed with a custom review tool and updated, histology derived nomenclature," Translational Vision Science & Technology, vol. 13, no. 12, pp. 19–19, 2024.
63. R. P. Mills, D. L. Budenz, P. P. Lee, R. J. Noecker, J. G. Walt, L. R. Siegartel, S. J. Evans, and J. J. Doyle, "Categorizing the stage of glaucoma from prediagnosis to endstage disease," American Journal of Ophthalmology, vol. 141, no. 1, pp. 24–30, 2006.
64. M. Ng, P. A. Sample, J. P. Pascual, L. M. Zangwill, C. A. Girkin, J. M. Liebmann, R. N. Weinreb, and L. Racette, "Comparison of visual field severity classification systems for glaucoma," Journal of Glaucoma, vol. 21, no. 8, pp. 551–561, 2012.
65. P. Brusini and C. A. Johnson, "Staging functional damage in glaucoma: Review of different classification methods," Survey of Ophthalmology, vol. 52, no. 2, pp. 156–179, 2007.
66. J. D. Stein, A. P. Khawaja, and J. S. Weizer, "Glaucoma in adults—screening, diagnosis, and management: A review," JAMA, vol. 325, no. 2, pp. 164–174, 2021.
67. Z. Soh, M. Yu, B. K. Betzler, S. Majithia, S. Thakur, Y. C. Tham, T. Y. Wong, T. Aung, D. S. Friedman, and C.Y. Cheng, "The global extent of undetected glaucoma in adults: a systematic review and metaanalysis," Ophthalmology, vol. 128, no. 10, pp. 1393–1404, 2021.
68. S. E. Grigorescu, N. Petkov, and P. Kruizinga, "Comparison of texture features based on Gabor filters," IEEE Transactions on Image Processing, vol. 11, no. 10, pp. 1160–1167, 2002.

69. I. N. Figueiredo, S. Kumar, C. M. Oliveira, J. D. Ramos, and B. Engquist, "Automated lesion detectors in retinal fundus images," Computers in Biology and Medicine, vol. 66, pp. 47–65, 2015.
70. B. J. Antony, M. D. Abràmoff, K. Lee, P. Sonkova, P. Gupta, Y. Kwon, M. Niemeijer, Z. Hu, and M. K. Garvin, "Automated 3d segmentation of intraretinal layers from optic nerve head optical coherence tomography images," in Medical Imaging 2010: Biomedical Applications in Molecular, Structural, and Functional Imaging, vol. 7626, pp. 249–260, SPIE, 2010.
71. M. Niemeijer, M. D. Abràmoff, and B. van Ginneken, "Image structure clustering for image quality verification of color retina images in diabetic retinopathy screening," Medical Image Analysis, vol. 10, no. 6, pp. 888–898, 2006.
72. M. Niemeijer, J. Staal, B. Van Ginneken, M. Loog, and M. D. Abràmoff, "Comparative study of retinal vessel segmentation methods on a new publicly available database," in Medical Imaging 2004: Image Processing, vol. 5370, pp. 648–656, SPIE, 2004.
73. J. Staal, M. D. Abràmoff, M. Niemeijer, M. A. Viergever, and B. Van Ginneken, "Ridge based vessel segmentation in color images of the retina," IEEE transactions on Medical Imaging, vol. 23, no. 4, pp. 501–509, 2004.
74. M. D. Abràmoffand M. Niemeijer, "The automatic detection of the optic disc location in retinal images using optic disc location regression," in 2006 International Conference of the IEEE Engineering in Medicine and Biology Society, pp. 4432–4435, IEEE, 2006.
75. M. J. Cree, J. A. Olson, K. C. McHardy, P. F. Sharp, and J. V. Forrester, "A fully automated comparative microaneurysm digital detection system," Eye, vol. 11, no. 5, pp. 622–628, 1997.
76. M. Niemeijer, B. Van Ginneken, J. Staal, M. S. Suttorp-Schulten, and M. D. Abramoff, "Automatic detection of red lesions in digital color fundus photographs," IEEE Transactions on Medical Imaging, vol. 24, no. 5, pp. 584–592, 2005.
77. M. Niemeijer, B. van Ginneken, S. R. Russell, M. S. Suttorp-Schulten, and M. D. Abràmoff, "Automated detection and differentiation of drusen, exudates, and cottonwool spots in digital color fundus photographs for diabetic retinopathy diagnosis," Investigative Ophthalmology & Visual Science, vol. 48, no. 5, pp. 2260–2267, 2007.
78. M. D. Abràmoff and M. S. Suttorp-Schulten, "Web-based screening for diabetic retinopathy in a primary care population: The eyecheck project," Telemedicine Journal & eHealth, vol. 11, no. 6, pp. 668–674, 2005.
79. M. D. Abràmoff, J. M. Reinhardt, S. R. Russell, J. C. Folk, V. B. Mahajan, M. Niemeijer, and G. Quellec, "Automated early detection of diabetic retinopathy," Ophthalmology, vol. 117, no. 6, pp. 1147–1154, 2010.
80. L. Pierro, M. Gagliardi, L. Iuliano, A. Ambrosi, and F. Bandello, "Retinal nerve fiber layer thickness reproducibility using seven different OCT instruments," Investigative Ophthalmology & Visual Science, vol. 53, no. 9, pp. 5912–5920, 2012.
81. I. C. Han and G. J. Jaffe, "Comparison of spectral and time domain optical coherence tomography for retinal thickness measurements in healthy and diseased eyes," American Journal of Ophthalmology, vol. 147, no. 5, pp. 847–858, 2009.
82. U. E. Wolf-Schnurrbusch, L. Ceklic, C. K. Brinkmann, M. E. Iliev, M. Frey, S. P. Rothen Buehler, V. Enzmann, and S. Wolf, "Macular thickness measurements in healthy eyes using six different optical coherence tomography instruments," Investigative Ophthalmology & Visual Science, vol. 50, no. 7, pp. 3432–3437, 2009.
83. M.L. Huang and H.Y. Chen, "Development and comparison of automated classifiers for glaucoma diagnosis using stratus optical coherence tomography," Investigative Ophthalmology & Visual Science, vol. 46, no. 11, pp. 4121–4129, 2005.
84. J. S. Kim, H. Ishikawa, K. R. Sung, J. Xu, G. Wollstein, R. A. Bilonick, M. L. Gabriele, L. Kagemann, J. S. Duker, J. G. Fujimoto, et al., "Retinal nerve fibre layer thickness measurement reproducibility improved with spectral domain optical coherence tomography," British Journal of Ophthalmology, vol. 93, no. 8, pp. 1057–1063, 2009.
85. F. R. Silva, V. G. Vidotti, F. Cremasco, M. Dias, E. S. Gomi, and V. P. Costa, "Sensitivity and specificity of machine learning classifiers for glaucoma diagnosis using spectral domain

OCT and standard automated perimetry," Arquivos Brasileiros de Oftalmologia, vol. 76, pp. 170–174, 2013.
86. D. Koozekanani, K. Boyer, and C. Roberts, "Retinal thickness measurements from optical coherence tomography using a Markov boundary model," IEEE Transactions on Medical Imaging, vol. 20, no. 9, pp. 900–916, 2001.
87. D. Cabrera Fernandez, H. M. Salinas, and C. A. Puliafito, "Automated detection of retinal layer structures on optical coherence tomography images," Optics Express, vol. 13, no. 25, pp. 10200–10216, 2005.
88. M. Shahidi, Z. Wang, and R. Zelkha, "Quantitative thickness measurement of retinal layers imaged by optical coherence tomography," American Journal of Ophthalmology, vol. 139, no. 6, pp. 1056–1061, 2005.
89. H. Ishikawa, D. M. Stein, G. Wollstein, S. Beaton, J. G. Fujimoto, and J. S. Schuman, "Macular segmentation with optical coherence tomography," Investigative Ophthalmology & Visual Science, vol. 46, no. 6, pp. 2012–2017, 2005.
90. A. Chan, J. S. Duker, H. Ishikawa, T. H. Ko, J. S. Schuman, and J. G. Fujimoto, "Quantification of photoreceptor layer thickness in normal eyes using optical coherence tomography," Retina, vol. 26, no. 6, pp. 655–660, 2006.
91. M. Baroni, P. Fortunato, and A. La Torre, "Towards quantitative analysis of retinal features in optical coherence tomography," Medical Engineering & Physics, vol. 29, no. 4, pp. 432–441, 2007.
92. A. M. Bagci, M. Shahidi, R. Ansari, M. Blair, N. P. Blair, and R. Zelkha, "Thickness profiles of retinal layers by optical coherence tomography image segmentation," American Journal of Ophthalmology, vol. 146, no. 5, pp. 679–687, 2008.
93. T. Fabritius, S. Makita, M. Miura, R. Myllyla, and Y. Yasuno, "Automated segmentation of the macula by optical coherence tomography," Optics Express, vol. 17, no. 18, pp. 15659–15669, 2009.
94. O. Tan, G. Li, A. T.H. Lu, R. Varma, D. Huang, A. I. for Glaucoma Study Group, et al., "Mapping of macular substructures with optical coherence tomography for glaucoma diagnosis," Ophthalmology, vol. 115, no. 6, pp. 949–956, 2008.
95. O. Tan, V. Chopra, A. T.H. Lu, J. S. Schuman, H. Ishikawa, G. Wollstein, R. Varma, and D. Huang, "Detection of macular ganglion cell loss in glaucoma by Fourier domain optical coherence tomography," Ophthalmology, vol. 116, no. 12, pp. 2305–2314, 2009.
96. X. Zhang, S. Yousefi, L. An, and R. K. Wang, "Automated segmentation of intramacular layers in Fourier domain optical coherence tomography structural images from normal subjects," Journal of Biomedical Optics, vol. 17, no. 4, pp. 046011–046011, 2012.
97. M. Mujat, R. C. Chan, B. Cense, B. Hyle Park, C. Joo, T. Akkin, T. C. Chen, and J. F. De Boer, "Retinal nerve fiber layer thickness map determined from optical coherence tomography images," Optics Express, vol. 13, no. 23, pp. 9480–9491, 2005.
98. A. Mishra, A. Wong, K. Bizheva, and D. A. Clausi, "Intraretinal layer segmentation in optical coherence tomography images," Optics Express, vol. 17, no. 26, pp. 23719–23728, 2009.
99. A. Yazdanpanah, G. Hamarneh, B. R. Smith, and M. V. Sarunic, "Segmentation of intra retinal layers from optical coherence tomography images using an active contour approach," IEEE Transactions on Medical Imaging, vol. 30, no. 2, pp. 484–496, 2010.
100. R. J. Zawadzki, A. R. Fuller, D. F. Wiley, B. Hamann, S. S. Choi, and J. S. Werner, "Adaptation of a support vector machine algorithm for segmentation and visualization of retinal structures in volumetric optical coherence tomography data sets," Journal of Biomedical Op tics, vol. 12, no. 4, pp. 041206–041206, 2007.
101. K. Vermeer, J. Van der Schoot, H. Lemij, and J. De Boer, "Segmentation of retinal layers in volumetric OCT scans of normal and glaucomatous subjects," in Ophthalmic Technologies XXI, vol. 7885, pp. 267–271, SPIE, 2011.
102. F. Rossant, I. Ghorbel, I. Bloch, M. Paques, and S. Tick, "Automated segmentation of retinal layers in OCT imaging and derived ophthalmic measures," in 2009 IEEE International Symposium on Biomedical Imaging: From Nano to Macro, pp. 1370–1373, IEEE, 2009.

103. V. Kajic, B. Povazay, B. Hermann, B. Hofer, D. Marshall, P. L. Rosin, and W. Drexler, "Ro bust segmentation of intraretinal layers in the normal human fovea using a novel statistical model based on texture and shape analysis," Optics Express, vol. 18, no. 14, pp. 14730–14744, 2010.
104. S. J. Chiu, X. T. Li, P. Nicholas, C. A. Toth, J. A. Izatt, and S. Farsiu, "Automatic segmentation of seven retinal layers in SDOCT images congruent with expert manual segmentation," Optics Express, vol. 18, no. 18, pp. 19413–19428, 2010.
105. S. J. Chiu, J. A. Izatt, R. V. O'Connell, K. P. Winter, C. A. Toth, and S. Farsiu, "Validated automatic segmentation of AMD pathology including drusen and geographic atrophy in SDOCT images," Investigative Ophthalmology & Visual Science, vol. 53, no. 1, pp. 53–61, 2012.
106. Q. Yang, C. A. Reisman, Z. Wang, Y. Fukuma, M. Hangai, N. Yoshimura, A. Tomidokoro, M. Araie, A. S. Raza, D. C. Hood, et al., "Automated layer segmentation of macular OCT images using dual scale gradient information," Optics Express, vol. 18, no. 20, pp. 21293–21307, 2010.
107. M. K. Garvin, M. D. Abràmoff, X. Wu, S. R. Russell, T. L. Burns, and M. Sonka, "Automated 3d intraretinal layer segmentation of macular spectral-domain optical coherence tomography images," IEEE Transactions on Medical Imaging, vol. 28, no. 9, pp. 1436–1447, 2009.
108. K. Lee, M. Niemeijer, M. K. Garvin, Y. H. Kwon, M. Sonka, and M. D. Abràmoff, "Seg mentation of the optic disc in 3d OCT scans of the optic nerve head," IEEE Transactions on Medical Imaging, vol. 29, no. 1, pp. 159–168, 2009.
109. P. A. Dufour, L. Ceklic, H. Abdillahi, S. Schroder, S. De Dzanet, U. Wolf-Schnurrbusch, and J. Kowal, "Graph-based multi-surface segmentation of OCT data using trained hard and soft constraints," IEEE Transactions on Medical Imaging, vol. 32, no. 3, pp. 531–543, 2012. 1
110. A. Lang, A. Carass, M. Hauser, E. S. Sotirchos, P. A. Calabresi, H. S. Ying, and J. L. Prince, "Retinal layer segmentation of macular OCT images using boundary classification," Biomedical Optics Express, vol. 4, no. 7, pp. 1133–1152, 2013.
111. Q. Song, X. Wu, Y. Liu, M. Sonka, and M. Garvin, "Simultaneous searching of globally optimal interacting surfaces with shape priors," in 2010 IEEE Computer Society Conference on Computer Vision and Pattern Recognition, pp. 2879–2886, IEEE, 2010.
112. B. J. Antony, M. D. Abràmoff, M. M. Harper, W. Jeong, E. H. Sohn, Y. H. Kwon, R. Kardon, and M. K. Garvin, "A combined machine learning and graph-based framework for the segmentation of retinal surfaces in SDOCT volumes," Biomed. Opt. Express, vol. 4, pp. 2712–2728, Dec 2013.
113. K. Li, X. Wu, D. Z. Chen, and M. Sonka, "Optimal surface segmentation in volumetric images a graph theoretic approach," IEEE Transactions on Pattern Analysis and Machine Intelligence, vol. 28, no. 1, pp. 119–134, 2005.
114. A. V. Goldberg and S. Rao, "Beyond the flow decomposition barrier," Journal of the ACM (JACM), vol. 45, no. 5, pp. 783–797, 1998.
115. A. V. Goldberg and R. E. Tarjan, "A new approach to the maximum flow problem," Journal of the ACM (JACM), vol. 35, no. 4, pp. 921–940, 1988.
116. L. R. Ford Jr and D. R. Fulkerson, "Maximal flow through a network," Canadian Journal of Mathematics, vol. 8, pp. 399–404, 1956.
117. M. Haeker, M. D. Abràmoff, X. Wu, R. Kardon, and M. Sonka, "Use of varying constraints in optimal 3d graph search for segmentation of macular optical coherence tomography images," in International Conference on Medical Image Computing and Computer-Assisted Intervention, pp. 244–251, Springer Berlin Heidelberg Berlin, Heidelberg, 2007.
118. Q. Song, J. Bai, M. K. Garvin, M. Sonka, J. M. Buatti, and X. Wu, "Optimal multiple surface segmentation with shape and context priors," IEEE Transactions on Medical Imaging, vol. 32, no. 2, pp. 376–386, 2012.
119. L. Breiman, "Random forests," Machine Learning, vol. 45, pp. 5–32, 2001.
120. B. J. Antony, Q. Song, M. D. Abràmoff, E. Sohn, X. Wu, and M. K. Garvin, "Incorporation of learned shape priors into a graph theoretic approach with application to the 3d segmentation of intraretinal surfaces in SDOCT volumes of mice," in Medical Imaging 2014: Biomedical

Applications in Molecular, Structural, and Functional Imaging, vol. 9038, pp. 92–101, SPIE, 2014.
121. J. Y. Lee, S. J. Chiu, P. P. Srinivasan, J. A. Izatt, C. A. Toth, S. Farsiu, and G. J. Jaffe, "Fully automatic software for retinal thickness in eyes with diabetic macular edema from images acquired by cirrus and spectralis systems," Investigative Ophthalmology & Visual Science, vol. 54, no. 12, pp. 7595–7602, 2013.
122. N. Cassels, J. Wild, T. Margrain, L. Pearce, C. Blyth, S. Sivaprasad, V. Chong, and J. Acton, "Segmented SD-OCT imaging and microperimetry outcomes in age-related macular degeneration," Investigative Ophthalmology & Visual Science, vol. 57, no. 12, pp. 2656–2656, 2016.
123. J. Hedstrom, M. Nilsson, M. Engvall, and A. Venkataraman, "The ganglion cell complex thickness and visual function in Leber hereditary optic neuropathy," Acta Ophthalmologica, vol. 102, 2024.
124. F. A. Folgar, E. L. Yuan, M. B. Sevilla, S. J. Chiu, S. Farsiu, E. Y. Chew, C. A. Toth, A. R. E. D. Study, and S. Group, "Drusen volume and retinal pigment epithelium abnormal thinning volume predict 2year progression of age-related macular degeneration," Ophthalmology, vol. 123, no. 1, pp. 39–50, 2016.
125. G. Yiu, V. Manjunath, S. J. Chiu, S. Farsiu, and T. H. Mahmoud, "Effect of anti–vascular endothelial growth factor therapy on choroidal thickness in diabetic macular edema," American Journal of Ophthalmology, vol. 158, no. 4, pp. 745–751, 2014.
126. G. E. Nipp, S. S. Stinnett, S. J. Chiu, G.S. Ying, E. Daniel, M. G. Maguire, D. S. Grewal, and G. J. Jaffe, "Multimodal identification and quantification of subretinal fibrosis in eyes with neovascular AMD in CATT," Investigative Ophthalmology & Visual Science, vol. 64, no. 8, pp. 2384–2384, 2023.
127. J. Deng, A. Berg, S. Satheesh, H. Su, A. Khosla, and F. Li, "Imagenet large scale visual recognition challenge (ILSVRC)," LSVRC/index.php, 2010.
128. O. Russakovsky, J. Deng, H. Su, J. Krause, S. Satheesh, S. Ma, Z. Huang, A. Karpathy, A. Khosla, M. Bernstein, et al., "Imagenet large scale visual recognition challenge," International Journal of Computer Vision, vol. 115, pp. 211–252, 2015.
129. J. Sanchez and F. Perronnin, "High dimensional signature compression for largescale image classification," in CVPR 2011, pp. 1665–1672, IEEE, 2011.
130. H.C. Shin, H. R. Roth, M. Gao, L. Lu, Z. Xu, I. Nogues, J. Yao, D. Mollura, and R. M. Summers, "Deep convolutional neural networks for computer-aided detection: CNN architectures, dataset characteristics and transfer learning," IEEE Transactions on Medical Imaging, vol. 35, no. 5, pp. 1285–1298, 2016.
131. J. Cuadros and G. Bresnick, "Eyepacs: an adaptable telemedicine system for diabetic retinopathy screening," Journal of Diabetes Science and Technology, vol. 3, no. 3, pp. 509–516, 2009.
132. M. Voets, K. Møllersen, and L. A. Bongo, "Replication study: Development and validation of deep learning algorithm for detection of diabetic retinopathy in retinal fundus photographs," arXiv preprint arXiv:1803.04337, 2018.
133. V. Gulshan, L. Peng, M. Coram, M. C. Stumpe, D. Wu, A. Narayanaswamy, S. Venugopalan, K. Widner, T. Madams, J. Cuadros, et al., "Development and validation of a deep learning algorithm for detection of diabetic retinopathy in retinal fundus photographs," JAMA, vol. 316, no. 22, pp. 2402–2410, 2016.
134. C. Szegedy, V. Vanhoucke, S. Ioffe, J. Shlens, and Z. Wojna, "Rethinking the inception architecture for computer vision," in Proceedings of the IEEE Conference on Computer Vision and Pattern Recognition, pp. 2818–2826, 2016.
135. Abràmoff, M.D., Lou, Y., Erginay, A., Clarida, W., Amelon, R., Folk, J.C. and Niemeijer, M., 2016. Improved automated detection of diabetic retinopathy on a publicly available dataset through integration of deep learning. Investigative Ophthalmology & Visual Science, 57(13), pp. 5200–5206.
136. E. Decenciere, X. Zhang, G. Cazuguel, B. Lay, B. Cochener, C. Trone, P. Gain, J.R. OrdonezVarela, P. Massin, A. Erginay, et al., "Feedback on a publicly distributed image database: the Messidor database," Image Analysis & Stereology, pp. 231–234, 2014.

137. J. Krause, V. Gulshan, E. Rahimy, P. Karth, K. Widner, G. S. Corrado, L. Peng, and D. R. Webster, "Grader variability and the importance of reference standards for evaluating machine learning models for diabetic retinopathy," Ophthalmology, vol. 125, no. 8, pp. 1264–1272, 2018.
138. S. Wan, Y. Liang, and Y. Zhang, "Deep convolutional neural networks for diabetic retinopathy detection by image classification," Computers & Electrical Engineering, vol. 72, pp. 274–282, 2018.
139. H. Pratt, F. Coenen, D. M. Broadbent, S. P. Harding, and Y. Zheng, "Convolutional neural networks for diabetic retinopathy," Procedia Computer Science, vol. 90, pp. 200–205, 2016.
140. T. Araújo, G. Aresta, L. Mendonca, S. Penas, C. Maia, A. Carneiro, A. M. Mendonca, and A. Campilho, "Dr—graduate: Uncertainty aware deep learning based diabetic retinopathy grading in eye fundus images," Medical Image Analysis, vol. 63, p. 101715, 2020.
141. G. Quellec, K. Charriere, Y. Boudi, B. Cochener, and M. Lamard, "Deep image mining for diabetic retinopathy screening," Medical Image Analysis, vol. 39, pp. 178–193, 2017.
142. W. L. Alyoubi, M. F. Abulkhair, and W. M. Shalash, "Diabetic retinopathy fundus image classification and lesions localization system using deep learning," Sensors, vol. 21, no. 11, p. 3704, 2021.
143. B. Zhou, A. Khosla, A. Lapedriza, A. Oliva, and A. Torralba, "Learning deep features for discriminative localization," in Proceedings of the IEEE Conference on Computer Vision and Pattern Recognition, pp. 2921–2929, 2016.
144. R. R. Selvaraju, M. Cogswell, A. Das, R. Vedantam, D. Parikh, and D. Batra, "Gradcam: Visual explanations from deep networks via gradient-based localization," in Proceedings of the IEEE International Conference on Computer Vision, pp. 618–626, 2017.
145. B. Kim, M. Wattenberg, J. Gilmer, C. Cai, J. Wexler, F. Viegas, et al., "Interpretability be yond feature attribution: Quantitative testing with concept activation vectors (TCAV)," in International Conference on Machine Learning, pp. 2668–2677, PMLR, 2018.
146. H. Muhammad, T. J. Fuchs, N. De Cuir, C. G. De Moraes, D. M. Blumberg, J. M. Liebmann, R. Ritch, and D. C. Hood, "Hybrid deep learning on single widefield optical coherence tomography scans accurately classifies glaucoma suspects," Journal of Glaucoma, vol. 26, no. 12, pp. 1086–1094, 2017.
147. K. A. Thakoor, S. C. Koorathota, D. C. Hood, and P. Sajda, "Robust and interpretable convolutional neural networks to detect glaucoma in optical coherence tomography images," IEEE Transactions on Biomedical Engineering, vol. 68, no. 8, pp. 2456–2466, 2020.
148. K. He, X. Zhang, S. Ren, and J. Sun, "Deep residual learning for image recognition," in Proceedings of the IEEE Conference on Computer Vision and Pattern Recognition, pp. 770–778, 2016.
149. K. Simonyan and A. Zisserman, "Very deep convolutional networks for large scale image recognition," arXiv preprint arXiv:1409.1556, 2014.
150. G. Huang, Z. Liu, L. Van Der Maaten, and K. Q. Weinberger, "Densely connected convolutional networks," in Proceedings of the IEEE Conference on Computer Vision and Pattern Recognition, pp. 4700–4708, 2017.
151. S. Maetschke, B. Antony, H. Ishikawa, G. Wollstein, J. Schuman, and R. Garnavi, "A feature agnostic approach for glaucoma detection in oct volumes," PloS One, vol. 14, no. 7, p. e0219126, 2019.
152. Y. George, B. J. Antony, H. Ishikawa, G. Wollstein, J. S. Schuman, and R. Garnavi, "Attention-guided 3dcnn framework for glaucoma detection and structural-functional association using volumetric images," IEEE Journal of Biomedical and Health Informatics, vol. 24, no. 12, pp. 3421–3430, 2020.
153. R. N. Zaeem and K. S. Barber, "The effect of the GDPR on privacy policies: Recent progress and future promise," ACM Transactions on Management Information Systems (TMIS), vol. 12, no. 1, pp. 1–20, 2020.
154. H. Guan, P.T. Yap, A. Bozoki, and M. Liu, "Federated learning for medical image analysis: A survey," Pattern Recognition, p. 110424, 2024.

155. S. Jegou, M. Drozdzal, D. Vazquez, A. Romero, and Y. Bengio, "The one hundred layers tiramisu: Fully convolutional denseNets for semantic segmentation," in Proceedings of the IEEE Conference on Computer Vision and Pattern Recognition Workshops, pp. 11–19, 2017.
156. S. Sedai, B. Antony, D. Mahapatra, and R. Garnavi, "Joint segmentation and uncertainty visualization of retinal layers in optical coherence tomography images using Bayesian deep learning," in Computational Pathology and Ophthalmic Medical Image Analysis: First International Workshop, COMPAY 2018, and 5th International Workshop, OMIA 2018, Held in Conjunction with MICCAI 2018, Granada, Spain, September 1620, 2018, Proceedings 5, pp. 219–227, Springer, 2018.
157. O. Ronneberger, P. Fischer, and T. Brox, "Unet: Convolutional networks for biomedical image segmentation," in Medical image computing and computer-assisted intervention–MICCAI 2015: 18th International Conference, Munich, Germany, October 59, 2015, Proceedings, part III 18, pp. 234–241, Springer, 2015.
158. F. Isensee, P. F. Jaeger, S. A. Kohl, J. Petersen, and K. H. MaierHein, "nnU-Net: a self-configuring method for deep learning-based biomedical image segmentation," Nature Methods, vol. 18, no. 2, pp. 203–211, 2021.
159. Q. Cao, P. Söderberg, Z. Yu, K. Kisonaite, C. Wang, and J. Holm, "Automatic segmentation for early glaucoma detection using nnunet," in Ophthalmic Technologies XXXV, vol. 13300, pp. 77–86, SPIE, 2025.
160. Z. Chen, H. Zhang, E. F. Linton, B. A. Johnson, Y. J. Choi, M. J. Kupersmith, M. Sonka, M. K. Garvin, R. H. Kardon, and J.K. Wang, "Hybrid deep learning and optimal graph search method for optical coherence tomography layer segmentation in diseases affecting the optic nerve," Biomedical Optics Express, vol. 15, no. 6, pp. 3681–3698, 2024.
161. J. Flammer, S. M. Drance, F. Fankhauser, and L. Augustiny, "Differential light threshold in automated static perimetry: factors influencing short term fluctuation," Archives of Ophthalmology, vol. 102, no. 6, pp. 876–879, 1984.
162. J. Flammer, S. M. Drance, and M. Zulauf, "Differential light threshold: short and long term fluctuation in patients with glaucoma, normal controls, and patients with suspected glaucoma," Archives of Ophthalmology, vol. 102, no. 5, pp. 704–706, 1984.
163. Bogunović, H., Kwon, Y.H., Rashid, A., Lee, K., Critser, D.B., Garvin, M.K., Sonka, M. and Abramoff, M.D., 2015. Relationships of retinal structure and Humphrey 24-2 visual field thresholds in patients with glaucoma. Investigative Ophthalmology & Visual Science, 56(1), pp.259–271.
164. H.H. Yu, S. R. Maetschke, B. J. Antony, H. Ishikawa, G. Wollstein, J. S. Schuman, and R. Garnavi, "Estimating global visual field indices in glaucoma by combining macula and optic disc oct scans using 3dimensional convolutional neural networks," Ophthalmology Glaucoma, vol. 4, no. 1, pp. 102–112, 2021.
165. Z. Chen, H. Ishikawa, Y. Wang, G. Wollstein, and J. S. Schuman, "Deepl earning-based group pointwise spatial mapping of structure to function in glaucoma," Ophthalmology Science, vol. 4, no. 5, p. 100523, 2024.
166. S. K. Wagner, D. J. Fu, L. Faes, X. Liu, J. Huemer, H. Khalid, D. Ferraz, E. Korot, C. Kelly, K. Balaskas, A. K. Denniston, and P. A. Keane, "Insights into systemic disease through retinal imaging-based oculomics," Translational Vision Science and Technology, vol. 9, 2020.
167. M. Abdollahi, A. Jafarizadeh, A. Ghafouri-Asbagh, N. Sobhi, K. Pourmoghtader, S. Pedrammehr, H. Asadi, R.S. Tan, R. Alizadehsani, and U. R. Acharya, "Artificial intelligence in assessing cardiovascular diseases and risk factors via retinal fundus images: A review of the last decade," Wiley Interdisciplinary Reviews: Data Mining and Knowledge Discovery, vol. 14, no. 6, p. e1560, 2024.
168. C. Y. Cheung, V. Mok, P. J. Foster, E. Trucco, C. Chen, and T. Y. Wong, "Retinal imaging in Alzheimer's disease," Journal of Neurology, Neurosurgery & Psychiatry, vol. 92, no. 9, pp. 983–994, 2021.

169. W. Tan, X. Yao, T.T. Le, B. Tan, L. Schmetterer, and J. Chua, "The new era of retinal imaging in hypertensive patients," The Asia-Pacific Journal of Ophthalmology, vol. 11, no. 2, pp. 149–159, 2022.
170. C. Y.L. Cheung, M. K. Ikram, C. Sabanayagam, and T. Y. Wong, "Retinal microvasculature as a model to study the manifestations of hypertension," Hypertension, vol. 60, no. 5, pp. 1094–1103, 2012.
171. R. Del Pinto, G. Mule, M. Vadala, C. Carollo, S. Cottone, C. Agabiti Rosei, C. De Ciuceis, D. Rizzoni, C. Ferri, and M. L. Muiesan, "Arterial hypertension and the hidden disease of the eye: diagnostic tools and therapeutic strategies," Nutrients, vol. 14, no. 11, p. 2200, 2022.
172. A. Diaz-Pinto, N. Ravikumar, R. Attar, and et al., "Predicting myocardial infarction through retinal scans and minimal personal information," Nature Machine Intelligence, vol. 4, p. 55–61, 2022.
173. J.Y. Lee, A. Martin-Bastida, A. Murueta-Goyena, I. Gabilondo, N. Cuenca, P. Piccini, and B. Jeon, "Multimodal brain and retinal imaging of dopaminergic degeneration in Parkinson disease," Nature Reviews Neurology, vol. 18, no. 4, pp. 203–220, 2022.
174. R. Smith, R. Sapkota, B. Antony, J. Sun, O. Aboud, O. Bloch, M. Daly, R. Fragoso, G. Yiu, and Y. A. Liu, "A novel predictive model utilizing retinal microstructural features for estimating survival outcome in patients with glioblastoma," Research Square, pp. rs.3.rs-4420925, 2024.
175. A. Nisanova, A. Parajuli, B. Antony, O. Aboud, J. Sun, M. E. Daly, R. C. Fragoso, G. Yiu, and Y. A. Liu, "Retinal microstructural changes reflecting treatment-associated cognitive dysfunction in patients with lower-grade gliomas," Ophthalmology Science, vol. 4, no. 6, p. 100577, 2024.

Chapter 8
AI and Mental Health Research

Margaret Lech, Muhammad Shehram Shah Syed, and Zafi Sherhan Syed

Abstract This chapter delves into the role of artificial intelligence (AI) for the development of computer assisted mental health research, focusing specifically in the context of early Alzheimer's dementia diagnosis through speech analysis. It starts by discussing the recent intersection between AI and mental health, and stresses why early diagnosis is crucial in reducing the societal and economic burden of Alzheimer's disease. An overview of the clinical features of Alzheimer's-related language impairments based upon theories such as the Wernicke-Geschwind model and connectionist views is presented. It also outlines publicly available datasets like the Pitt and ADReSS corpora and their corresponding speaking tasks, used as benchmarks for the development of AI models.

This description is followed by a discussion on building an Alzheimer's dementia recognition pipeline. Important stages of the system are presented, including preprocessing of data and feature engineering. The various types of features used, such as, acoustic, textual, and disfluency-based elements, are also detailed in the chapter. Following this, the various challenges encountered by researchers are presented with a conclusion being provided at the end. The chapter serves as a starting point for researchers in the area of AI and mental health analysis to develop novel methodologies for AI based mental health disease diagnosis.

M. Lech (✉)
Royal Melbourne Institute of Technology (RMIT) University, Melbourne, VIC, Australia
e-mail: margaret.lech@rmit.edu.au

M. S. S. Syed · Z. S. Syed
Mehran University of Engineering and Technology (MUET), Jamshoro, Pakistan
e-mail: shehram.shah@faculty.muet.edu.pk; zafisherhan.shah@faculty.muet.edu.pk

M. Chetty, J. Hallinan (eds.), *From Algorithms to Ailments*,
https://doi.org/10.1007/978-3-032-11023-7_8

Introduction

The Intersection of AI and Mental Health

The intersection of artificial intelligence and mental health has ushered in a paradigm shift in research tending to the modalities of psychological and neurological evaluations. Mental health disorders have been increasing in prevalence globally and the demand for fast, dependable, and timely detection methods has become increasingly strained [1].

Mental health disorders range from mood disorders, anxiety as well as neurodegenerative diseases like Alzheimer and dementia [2]. Historically, mental health professionals have used clinical interviews, cognitive tests and self-reported questionnaires to screen for and diagnose these illnesses. Yet, the subjectivity of these methods and the challenges inherent in quantifying complex psychological states have prompted researchers to investigate the possibilities that AI-powered technologies could bring to mental health assessment [3].

While this is still an evolving field, the contribution of Artificial Intelligence (AI) has proven impressive for psychiatric assessment, leading to the creation of tools that can supplement or even supplant traditional forms of diagnosis [2, 3]. By analyzing diverse data inputs from behavioral data, physiological signals, and natural language, AI-powered systems are capable of detecting slight indicators of mental health conditions with high precision. However, one of the areas of AI application in mental health that has captured considerable interest is speech analysis for the early identification of Alzheimer disease.

The Urgency of Early Alzheimer's Dementia Detection

Alzheimer's Disease (AD) is a neurodegenerative illness that impacts millions of individuals around the globe. In 2020 the estimated total number of persons living with Alzheimer's and other dementias globally was 55 million, and it is projected to increase to 78 million in 2030 and 139 million in 2050 [4]. There is an enormous economic and social burden of Alzheimer's disease on health-care systems and caregivers which necessitates the crucial need for early detection and intervention.

Early diagnosis of Alzheimer's disease is important because early treatment, quality of life for patients, and support for caregivers depend on early identification. By recognizing the earliest signs of cognitive impairment, healthcare providers can initiate interventions at a time when they are most likely to be beneficial, manage symptoms more effectively, and allocate resources to provide adequate support for patients and their families.

Speech as a Non-invasive Biomarker

The scientific rationale for using speech as a diagnostic modality in Alzheimer's and other neurodegenerative diseases is the strong connection between cognition and language processing. There are brain changes—structural and functional—in people with Alzheimer's and these brain changes can, over time, be reflected in subtle but quantifiable changes in language used which is manifested in speech at the levels of vocabulary, syntax and fluency.

In the past 10 years, scientists have made great strides using speech analysis to discover Alzheimer's disease at an early stage. By employing natural language processing and machine learning methods, researchers have been able to identify speech biomarkers capable of differentiating between healthy individuals and those with cognitive decline. Speech as biomarkers has many unique advantages over traditional diagnostic methods such as their non-invasive nature, the ease of data collection, and remote application, allowing for early intervention and improving health care outcomes [5].

Fundamentals of Alzheimer's Dementia and Speech Analysis

How Alzheimer's Affects Cognitive Functions Related to Speech

Alzheimer's Dementia negatively impacts cognitive functions related to speech, such as language understanding and comprehension, verbal fluency and also the pragmatic aspects of communication. These impairments are caused by the damage to brain regions controlling language, memory and motor skills.

Language Comprehension in Alzheimer's Dementia

Initial symptoms of AD include having difficulties in processing complicated sentences or abstract ideas. Problems with understanding become more pronounced as the disease progresses. Patients may have difficulty following complex, multi-step verbal instructions or following conversation when it involves abstract or unfamiliar topics. Many of these deficits in comprehension can be accounted to damage to the posterior regions of the left hemisphere of the brain, specifically, Wernicke's area [6, 7].

Speech Production and Fluency

Speech production, that is, the ability to produce speech in a way that is coherent and interpretable, is another domain that is severely affected by AD. In the early stages, patients may start to catch themselves struggling to find words, marked by pauses, circumlocutions (talking around a word), or vague terms like "thing" or "stuff." This occurs as a result of poor access to the mental lexicon, the mental dictionary in which words and meanings are stored, due to the degeneration of neurons in language-related regions of the brain, such as Broca's area in the left frontal lobe [8, 9]. As the disease advances, the speech becomes more and more inarticulate, with more frequent pauses, repetitions and even nonsensical sound production. Such impairments in speech arise due to the loss of neurons in brain areas which are responsible for motor planning and speech execution, including the primary motor cortex that is responsible for muscle coordination in speech. Another condition that patients may sometimes develop is aphasia. Aphasia severely impairs speech, and can result in difficulty being able to choose the right words (anomic aphasia) or even an inability to utter anything coherent (global aphasia).

Pragmatics and Social Communication

Social rules governing language use, such as turn-taking in conversation, the use of appropriate tone and volume, and understanding non-literal language, such as metaphors or sarcasm, often also deteriorate due to Alzheimer's disease. Individuals may struggle to initiate or maintain conversations, demonstrate inappropriate or irrelevant responses, or fail to recognize social cues, leading to breakdowns in communication [10].

Apraxia of Speech and Dysarthria

In addition to the common language deficits observed in Alzheimer's disease, some individuals may also experience motor speech disorders such as apraxia of speech, and dysarthria conditions in which the brain has difficulty planning and coordinating the movements required for speech, leading to imprecise articulation and difficulty producing specific sounds [11].

Memory

Alzheimer's disease severely affects memory, particularly short-term and episodic memory. Patients may forget names, familiar phrases, or the topic of conversation, leading to frequent communication breakdowns. Long-term memory, while less affected in the early stages, becomes increasingly impaired as the disease progresses, resulting in a loss of autobiographical knowledge that can further hinder meaningful dialogue. The disruption of memory in Alzheimer's disease also affects the individual's ability to tell stories or recount events. As patients lose their ability to remember past experiences, they may struggle to form coherent narratives [12].

Neuropsychological Theories Linking Speech and Cognition

This interplay between speech and cognition has been a subject of interest, and various theories explaining this complexity have lent support to the field of neuropsychology. Neuropsychological models of language and cognition offer the foundational principles we need to understand how speech and cognition interact. Such theories of speech invariably reveal its dual nature, that is, as both a cognitive process and a social tool. Dysfunction of any of the cognitive systems serving language can result in severe speech deficiencies.

Traditional Wernicke-Geschwind Speech and Cognition Model

Classical models for speech and language generation propose that language abilities map to specific regions, like Broca's area for speaking and Wernicke's for understanding. The Wernicke-Geschwind Model is one of the earliest models that proposes interconnection between speech and cognition based on the various connected regions of the brain: Speech production involves Broca's area (in the frontal lobe), and Wernicke's area (located in the temporal lobe) is related to language comprehension. These two regions are connected by the Arcuate fasciculus, thereby closely associating comprehension with production. Damage to Broca's area usually leads to non-fluent aphasia, also called Broca's aphasia, in which production of speech is hindered but comprehension of sentences remains intact. In comparison, lesions in Wernicke's area are associated with Wernicke's aphasia or fluent aphasia, in which speech production is preserved, but comprehension is significantly diminished [13–15].

Connectionist Models of Speech and Cognition

Models which follow a connectionist approach propose that speech and cognition are connected via a network of neurons that cater to different features of language, such as phonology, AI and Mental Health Research 5 syntax, and semantics. This view of language suggests that language is not purely localized to one area of the brain but rather is distributed through a system of connected nodes, and information is processed in parallel in the various regions of the brain [16]. Such systems characterize speech output and recognition in terms of information propagation through this system of nodes. For example, retrieving a word depends on the activation of nodes in the semantic part of the network, and this then activates corresponding phonological nodes, triggering the generation of the output of speech. Disruption of these networks, as in the case of brain damage induced in Alzheimer's disease, produces specific language deficits [11].

In a connectionist system in which language processing is dynamic and flexible in nature, damage to one part of the network can affect the processing of other aspects of speech. This perspective stands in opposition to traditional models that localize language functions to specific regions of the brain. Working memory is a cognitive system that temporarily holds and processes the information needed for reasoning, problem-solving, and language comprehension. This perspective has led to the development of a prominent model, namely the working memory model [17], in which the working memory consist of three basic components: the central executive component that directs attentional skills and organizes cognitive processes; a phonological loop, which rehearses and stores phoneme elements of speech; and a visuospatial sketchpad, which is used to process visual and spatial information. It is well established that working memory deficits, as evidenced in frontotemporal dementia and related syndromes, can lead to impairments across both input and output forms of language, such as the capacity to understand and produce fluent speech, particularly under conditions in which an individual must remember multiple pieces of information at once [18].

The Interactive Activation Model of Sentence Processing

The interactive activation model of sentence processing proposes the integration of different cognitive functions which facilitate the production and understanding of language such as syntax, semantics, and phonology. The theory proposes that sentence comprehension and production are both interactive processes that depend on the simultaneous activation of multiple levels of language representations. These representations consist of syntactic structure (the rules that govern how sentences are formed), semantic meaning (the meaning of the words and sentences) and phonological representation (the sound of the words) [19].

The Cognitive Control Model of Speech Production

Speech production is also analyzed in terms of a cognitive control model which uses executive functions to modulate speech communication demands. These functions encompass choosing the right words, sustaining coherence, and modulating speech utterances according to the audience or context. Damage to executive function areas (like the prefrontal cortex) leads to disorganized and frequent word choice errors in speech along, with an inability to shift topics or adjust speech to different social contexts, as observed in frontal lobe damage or Alzheimer's disease [20].

Datasets and Tasks

Datasets

Progress in automated AD recognition relies on the availability of and access to well-curated datasets which allow the development of robust machine learning models for the detection of cognitive decline in different stages of the disease. Diversity in terms of speech samples from a large population, a variety of cognitive tasks, and multi-modalities can enable researchers to explore acoustic, linguistic, and behavioural markers of dementia. The inclusion of subjects with different diagnoses, from mild cognitive impairments to AD, which closely resembles real-life clinical conditions, enable the development of machine learning models that cater to real-life use-cases.

Another important point to note is that balanced demographic factors in datasets such as age, gender, and language help to alleviate bias in machine learning models while increasing generalizability across population groups [21, 22]. Datasets that capture speech and diagnoses in a longitudinal setting enable researchers to study changes in speech or behaviour over time and are not only essential for monitoring disease progression, but also determining how timely interventions may influence cognitive decline. As automated methods become critical to enable early diagnosis, diagnostic support, and continuous monitoring, datasets serve as the backbone of innovations that can enhance patient outcomes and aid in clinical decision-making.

A tabular summary of noteworthy datasets is provided in Table 8.1, brief details of which are provided in following sections.

Table 8.1 Speech datasets for dementia detection

Name	Ref.	Year	Speaking task(s)	Languages
Pitt Dataset	[23]	1994	PDT, SFT, PFT, SRT, SCT	English
CCC	[24]	2011	CRT	English
Dem@Care	[25]	2016	PDT	French and Greek
ADReSS	[21]	2020	PDT	English
ADReSSo	[22]	2021	PDT	English
ADReSS-M	[26]	2023	PDT	English and Greek
MDC	[27]	2024	CRT	English
TAUKADIAL	[28]	2024	PDT	English and Mandarin Chinese
PROCESS	[29]	2025	PDT, SFT, PFT	English

AI and Mental Health Research

Pitt Dataset

The Pitt corpus is a fundamental Natural Language Processing (NLP) corpus for dementia recognition. It has been widely used in studies focusing on the detection of dementia and the discovery of linguistic markers of cognitive impairment [23].

The corpus consists of speech and audio recordings, along with manually transcribed transcripts from subjects who were engaged in a variety of cognitive tasks designed to elicit language markers of cognitive decline. The corpus contains data for 104 healthy participants, 208 participants with a diagnosis of dementia, and 85 participants with an unknown diagnosis.

The Pitt corpus is entirely in English and features audio recordings of participants performing various language tasks, which include: Cookie Theft Picture Description: Here, participants are tasked with describing a picture depicting a detailed scene involving "Cookie Theft" from the Boston Diagnostic Aphasia Examination [30]. This task is commonly used in dementia research as it prompts connected speech and allows for the assessment of cognitive and linguistic abilities.

Verbal Fluency: Here, participants are asked to list as many words as they can that belong to a specific category, for example, animals or words starting with a particular letter. This task is meant to measure executive functioning and lexical retrieval.

Sentence Construction: In this task, participants receive words or prompts and are tasked to create meaningful sentences using these prompts. This task measures the syntactic and semantic processing abilities, which are key components of linguistic and cognitive functioning.

Story Recall: Here, participants are asked to listen to a short story and then retell it in their own words. This task evaluates memory retention and narrative structuring skills.

It is important to note that a recent study by Liu et al. [31] identified the presence of acoustic artifacts in the raw (unprocessed) audio recordings, which could introduce biases in machine learning models based on acoustic analysis. Therefore, it is recommended that the dataset be used whilst being mindful of this caveat. It should be mentioned that two popular datasets for AD research, the Alzheimer's Dementia Recognition through Spontaneous Speech (ADReSS) and Alzheimer's Dementia Recognition through Spontaneous Speech Only (ADReSSo) datasets, as described in subsequent sections, are derived from the Pitt corpus. The latter datasets were curated with the aim of creating balanced datasets for developing automated dementia recognition models that are more robust to population biases. The Pitt corpus is available through DementiaBank (https://dementia.talkbank.org).

Carolina Conversations Collection

The Carolina Conversations Collection (CCC) dataset consists of transcribed conversations about memories, daily life, and health, focusing on the health-related experiences of older adults aged 65 and above [24].

The dataset contains two cohorts of participants, the first of which is the 'Chronic Conditions Cohort' which contains more than 200 recorded conversations with adults who each had been diagnosed with at least one of 12 chronic medical conditions. For details of these medical conditions, the reader is referred to [24]. Members of this cohort were interviewed twice a year. The second cohort, called 'Cognitive Impairment Cohort', consists of more than 400 natural conversations from 125 individuals with an AD diagnosis. In both cohorts, participants were recorded at least biannually. This longitudinal nature of the corpus provides a solid groundwork for the extraction of cognitive decline via change in language patterns.

Unlike various other structured datasets, the dataset used here does not provide explicit diagnostic labels. Instead, it is created around the health conditions and cognition status of the participants in the conversations. This structure allows researchers to study communication patterns in the context of specific chronic illnesses and cognitive deficits. This data set is accessible at https://carolinaconversations.musc.edu/ccc/about.

Dem@Care Dataset

The Dem@Care project (Dementia Ambient Care) was an initiative for the creation of a platform-based system to offer personalized health services to dementia patients and medical professionals and caregivers. The Dem@Care dataset [25] takes a multi-modal approach to studying dementia by collecting data during controlled behavioral experiments at the Greek Alzheimer's Association and natural settings in the participants' homes. The dual nature of the data helped to shed light on dementia through structured cognition-neuropsychological tests and in-the-wild behavior. In addition to audio-visual data, the dataset contains physiological sensor data (for example, heart rate and skin conductance). This dataset provides the opportunity to develop truly multimodal models for dementia recognition. Further information about the project, including the dataset, is available at www.demcare.eu.

ADReSS Dataset

To overcome some of the limitations of the Pitt corpus, in particular the demographic imbalance, a new dataset, the Alzheimer's Dementia Recognition through Spontaneous Speech (ADReSS) dataset [21], was introduced as part of the ADReSS Challenge at the Interspeech 2020 conference. This dataset was created from a subset of the Pitt corpus in which participant groups were balanced across the training and testing partitions in terms of age, gender, and cognitive status; that is, AD and healthy controls (HC). This step was meant to ensure that results of analyses using this dataset are less likely to be affected by biased sampling of subgroups compared to the Pitt corpus. The ADReSS dataset consists of audio recordings and manually transcribed transcripts of structured conversations for the "Cookie Theft" speaking task. The dataset contains recordings from 156 subjects: 78 with AD diagnosis; and 78 from the HC cohort.

Since it is a subset of the Pitt corpus, all recordings are in the English language. The dataset is not only focused on binary classification (AD vs. HC) but also contains regression tasks predicting Mini-Mental State Examination (MMSE) [32] scores, providing each participant with a standard cognitive function metric.

ADReSSo Dataset

The Alzheimer's Dementia Recognition through Spontaneous Speech Only (ADReSSo) [22] dataset is also a subset of the Pitt corpus. It was released as part of the ADReSSo challenge at the Interspeech 2021 conference. The key aspect of this challenge was aimed at advancing dementia detection research from spontaneous language, as such manual transcripts were not provided, and participants of the challenge were encouraged to use Automated Speech Recognition (ASR) methods to transcribe speech from participants of the dataset. The ADReSSo dataset is based on structured interactions in a clinical setting, specifically the Cookie Theft picture description task. The dataset consists of 237 audio recordings, which includes 115 recordings from Healthy Controls and 122 recordings from the Alzheimer's Disease group. ADReSSo is like the ADReSS dataset in that it also contains an English-language dataset and includes cognitive status labels (Control or Probable AD) for each sample. It has MMSE scores which provide a standardized measure of cognitive function.

ADReSSo provides labels for both binary classification tasks, such as distinguishing healthy from AD participants, and regression tasks that aim to predict

MMSE scores. The ADReSSo dataset also contains a portion of the dataset that is labelled for cognitive decline.

ADReSS-M Dataset

The Alzheimer's Dementia Recognition through Spontaneous Speech-Multilingual (ADReSS-M) dataset [26] was introduced as part of the Signal Processing Grand Challenge at the 2023 IEEE International Conference on Acoustics, Speech, and Signal Processing (ICASSP). This dataset was a significant step towards such multilingual speech-based Alzheimer's detection and highlights the ever-increasing recognition of the importance of language diversity in dementia research.

The ADReSS-M dataset consists of 291 spontaneous speech recordings. Of these, 245 recordings form the training partition, which includes 237 in English and 8 in Greek, and 46 recordings were reserved for the testing partition, which are all in Greek. The data set is partitioned to three splits: One for English training, one for Greek samples and One for Greek testing.

The dataset provides binary classification labels for cognitive status in terms of healthy control or probable AD, whereas MMSE scores were used as indicator of cognitive status for the regression task.

The ADReSS-M dataset presented a new challenge for developing speech-based dementia detection systems, in which models were trained on one language but tested on another. The goal was to encourage the development of more inclusive and generalizable machine learning models that can function under diverse cultural contexts.

Multimodal Dementia Corpus

The Multi-modal Dementia Corpus (MDC) [27] is a longitudinal, multi-modal resource that captures the progression of dementia across different modalities of language production. This corpus differs from others in that it focuses on reminiscence material with recordings taking place in non-clinical settings rather than traditional clinical assessments, thus allowing for more naturalistic language use to be captured. The goal was to develop a dataset that can be used to investigate how language and communication change in real-world environments over time.

The corpus includes recordings of speech, with corresponding transcriptions, and written language data from pen and keyboard. The dataset consists of 22 participants (12 individuals with dementia and 10 healthy controls). This corpus serves as a valuable tool for the examination not just of verbal and linguistic changes in dementia but also writing actions at various stages of cognitive impairment. Through longitudinal tracking of subjects, the dataset enables studies examining the progression of dementias like Alzheimer's Disease, Frontotemporal Dementia and Mixed Dementia.

TAUKADIAL Dataset

The TAUKADIAL corpus [28] is a multilingual audio recording dataset of cognitive impairment in Mandarin Chinese and English, collected during a clinical setting picture description task. English speakers described three scenes (Cookie Theft, Cat Rescue, and Coming and Going) whereas Chinese speakers described culturally relevant Taiwanese images. It was presented during the TAUKADIAL Challenge at the Interspeech 2024 conference. The challenge comprised a classification and a regression task. The classification task involved developing models to differentiate between speech from healthy control individuals and those with Mild Cognitive Impairment (MCI) whereas the regression task aimed to predict cognitive test scores (i.e. MMSE) from spontaneous speech.

The TAUKADIAL dataset contains 507 speech recordings, of which 261 are in Mandarin Chinese and 246 in English. A key feature of this dataset, besides the multilingual aspects, is that the recordings have been matched for age and sex using propensity score analysis, so they are balanced and representative of the population for model training and evaluation. TAUKADIAL facilitates research on detection of cognitive impairment across different languages by incorporating multilingual speech data. The dataset is available in the DementiaBank respository.

PROCESS Dataset

The Prediction and Recognition of Cognitive Decline through Spontaneous Speech (PROCESS) dataset [29] was released as part of the Signal Processing Grand Challenge at the ICASSP 2025 conference. The goal was to facilitate research into the detection of cognitive decline, spanning from mild cognitive impairment to late-stage dementia, including Alzheimer's Disease. The dataset allows for a classification task to predict cognitive status in terms of healthy, MCI, or dementia and a regression task to estimate MMSE scores.

AI and Mental Health Research

Three prompts are used to elicit speech samples, intended to reflect real-world clinical assessments which include the semantic fluency task in which participants were asked to "name as many animals as you can in one minute", the phonemic fluency task where participants were asked to "name as many words that begin with 'P' in one minute", and the Cookie Theft picture description task, commonly used for evaluating memory, language comprehension, and executive function in dementia research. Further details about the dataset and methodologies will be available once proceedings of the ICASSP 2025 conference are published.

Speaking Tasks and Prompts

In Alzheimer's dementia research, speaking tasks are designed to assess the cognitive and language abilities of individuals, to screen them for dementia. Some common speaking tasks include structured tasks, such as picture description, fluency assessments, but spontaneous open-ended naturalistic conversations also exist in datasets.

The following sections provide a detailed overview of the key speaking tasks used in major dementia research datasets.

Picture Description Task

In the Picture Description Task (PDT), participants are asked to describe visual scenes in detail. Common prompts include describing the "Cookie Theft" image, "Cat Rescue" picture, or Norman Rockwell's "Coming and Going" scene. Chinese participants in the TAUKADIAL dataset describe culturally relevant images from Taiwanese culture. This task evaluates connected speech, narrative structure, memory, and language comprehension by analyzing how participants describe actions, objects, and relationships within the image. The PDT is most popular amongst speaking tasks for speech-based dementia assessment and is used in the Pitt, Dem@Care, ADReSS, ADReSSo, ADReSS-M, PROCESS, and TAUKADIAL datasets.

Semantic Fluency Task

In the Semantic Fluency Task (SFT), participants are asked to list (by speaking) as many items as possible within a specific category (for example, "animals") in a set time. This task is meant to assess lexical retrieval, category organization, and semantic memory, with the assumption that reduced fluency would indicate potential cognitive impairment. This type of speaking task was used in the Pitt and PROCESS datasets.

Phonemic Fluency Task

In the Phonemic Fluency Task (PFT), participants were asked to create words starting with a specified letter (for example, "P") within a set time. This task is meant to assess the executive functioning, working memory, and verbal fluency of participants. This speaking type of task is used in the Pitt and PROCESS datasets.

Story Recall Task

Here, participants are tasked to listen to a short story and then retell it in their own words. This task evaluates short-term memory, comprehension, and narrative recall, and aids in identifying issues with the retention and reproduction of information. The story recall task (SRT) type of speaking task was used in the Pitt and PROCESS datasets.

Sentence Construction Task

In this task, participants are provided with a collection of words or prompts and asked to create and complete sentences. This task assesses syntactic processing and language production so that individuals with cognitive decline may struggle with forming coherent and grammatically correct sentences. The sentence construction task (SCT) was used in the Pitt dataset.

Conversation and Reminiscence Task

In the Conversation and Reminiscence Task (CRT), participants are asked to discuss daily life, memories, or health topics in an open-ended speech setting. This type of task mirrors natural speech patterns and yields informative data about conversational flow and coherence, as well as emotional expression. The CCC and Multimodal Dementia Corpus used this type of speaking task.

Building the Alzheimer's Dementia Recognition Pipeline

An overview of the Alzheimer's Dementia Recognition Pipeline is shown in Fig. 8.1. It consists of multiple steps, including data preprocessing, feature computation, and feature engineering, which is then followed by model training, validation/evaluation

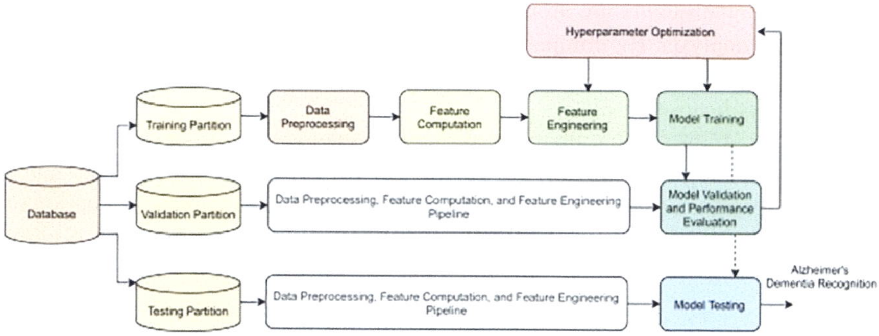

Fig. 8.1 Process flow diagram for AI based Alzheimer's dementia recognition

and testing. In this section, we discuss the data preprocessing and feature engineering aspects of the pipeline.

Data Preprocessing

Preprocessing is vital for ensuring that useful features can be extracted, which will determine a classifier model's classification success. If data is not pre-processed properly, models may learn unintended correlations because of signal and environmental noise. For example, in the Pitt Corpus, silent segments included background noise components that led to almost optimal AD detection accuracy [31]. To avoid such "Clever Hans" effects and to ensure that extracted features represent meaningful cognitive and linguistic markers rather than random acoustic artifacts, preprocessing and correctly identifying signal markers is critically important. The term "Clever Hans" [33] derives from the name of a horse that seemed to execute mentally advanced tasks such as arithmetic, only to reveal itself as responding to inadvertent signals from its trainer. This is a term used in machine learning, describing models that overfit on the spurious correlations in data, resulting in high test set performance, although learning was not performed for the pattern it was supposed to learn.

Recording Quality Assessment

The initial step of recording quality assessment is crucial to make sure that speech recordings are suitable for further processing and analysis. This step ensures that the recorded samples include speech which is clearly audible and has minimal noise and involves checks being performed manually as well as through an automated scheme. Manual assessment is performed as a sanity check to ensure that recordings that are of subpar quality are dropped, so that the whole dataset allows for a robust downstream analysis. By eliminating low-quality recordings, it is guaranteed that only high-quality recordings pass through to feature extraction, which is crucial for accurate classification results.

Background noise, microphone quality, and signal clarity are critical factors in the quality of recordings. Recording quality is typically evaluated in an automated manner, with indicators like signal-to-noise ratio (SNR) or perceptual evaluation of speech quality (PESQ) being calculated. While SNR measures the ratio of noise energy to speech energy, PESQ provides values calibrated against perceptual listening models.

It has been demonstrated in different studies that variations in sound recording conditions, such as room acoustics, background reverberations, and microphone inconsistencies, can lead to spectral distortions which may negatively impact feature extraction [34]. For instance, Ringeval et al. demonstrated how intonation contours were affected by changes in acoustic environments for speech-based assessments of developmental disorders [35].

Noise Removal and Filtering

Noise removal is crucial for isolating speech from environmental noise as it directly impacts the clarity of features like jitter, shimmer, and formant frequencies, which are important indicators of Alzheimer's-related changes [21]. Common approaches include spectral subtraction which removes steady background noise like hums and air conditioning by subtracting the estimated noise spectrum. Band-Pass filtering may also be used to retain only the frequency range relevant to speech (300 Hz to 3.4 kHz) to remove irrelevant components, however, one can argue that environmental noise may leave an imprint in the speech frequency band. In Alzheimer's detection tasks, improper noise removal can lead to models capturing background noise rather than meaningful speech patterns. For example, Liu et al. [31] demonstrated that background noise artifacts in the Pitt Corpus recordings significantly inflated AD classification accuracy when raw audio was used.

Segmentation

If there is the need to process the voice parts of the speech recordings only, then one can analyze them using utterance segmentation and segmentation based on voice activity detection (VAD). This preprocess splits continuous speech input into chunks of voiced speech to produce consistent temporal segments for analysis. VAD then separates speech from nonspeech, discarding non-essential silences and environmental sounds. Utterance segmentation splits a recorded speech into sentences or phrases to help with feature extraction, including speech rate and effort of articulation. Segmentation is critical for the capture of the temporal attributes of speech, such as pauses and speech rate, that are important indicators of Alzheimer's disease.

The need for well-performed segmentation is also emphasized by studies that indicate that even environmental noise, such as silence, if not properly excluded can carry signal signatures that bias any predictions made by the model [31]. Segmentation precisely delineates voiced from unvoiced sections, ensuring background noise and pauses do not confound aspects relating to speech rate and articulation patterns.

Standardization and Normalization

To ensure the comparability of features across speakers and sessions, normalization and standardization is used. When speech recordings are collected from multiple sources, it is crucial to standardize the sampling frequency to maintain consistency in data quality. Sampling at different rates may cause artifacts affecting the comparability of extracted features. In such situations, all audio recordings are resampled to a common sampling frequency, for example, of 16 kHz.

Amplitude normalization is equally important to reduce the effect of varying distance between speakers and the microphone. Variations in distance result in inconsistent volume levels which affect feature extraction, especially features related to the energy and amplitude. As shown by Eyben et al. [36], spectral energy features such as loudness and spectral flux tend to be very sensitive to amplitude inhomogeneity when normalization is not performed. Standardizing the loudness of recordings serves to mitigate the overfitting of models to differences between the loudness in sessions rather than meaningful components of cognition.

Feature Computation

The process of feature computation involves determining meaningful numerical representations from speech signals that can help distinguish between individuals with AD and healthy controls. These features are broadly categorized into audio-based and text-based modalities, both of which capture different aspects of cognitive decline.

Audio features aim to quantify acoustic biomarkers of AD, leveraging differences in speech production and vocal characteristics. Here, prosodic features, such as pitch variation and speech rhythm, provide insights into fluency and articulation deficits. Voice quality measures, including jitter, shimmer, and harmonic- to-noise ratio, capture changes in vocal stability. Spectral features, derived from frequency analysis, offer information on how speech energy is distributed across frequencies.

Additionally, temporal aspects like voice onset time (VOT) and speech rate—known to slow down in AD patients—serve as valuable indicators of cognitive decline.

Textual features also play a crucial role in dementia detection. Previous studies suggest that textual analysis can be even more effective than acoustic analysis for distinguishing between AD and healthy speech [37]. Linguistic deterioration manifests across multiple levels, leading to disruptions in syntax, semantics, lexical diversity, morphology, and narrative structure. For example, individuals with AD may produce short, fragmented sentences with reduced syntactic complexity, demonstrate reduced vocabulary richness, or struggle with maintaining coherent discourse. These characteristics are systematically captured through syntactic complexity metrics, word frequency analysis, morphological markers, and coherence scores. It should be noted that speech transcripts are required before textual features can be computed. While manual transcription has usually been used for this task, recent developments in AI have led to the development of robust approaches to automated speech recognition, as discussed below. A detailed description of audio and textual features is also provided below.

Feature Engineering

Once features are computed, they must be optimized before being used in ML models because the initial feature computing process often results in a high dimensional feature matrix, in which the number of features may exceed the number of training samples. This situation can lead to the "curse of dimensionality", making model training inefficient with potentially degraded performance. Feature engineering addresses this issue by refining the feature set to improve learning performance.

A widely used technique in this process is feature selection, in which only the most informative features are retained. Feature selection can be filter-based, wrapper-based, or embedded. Filter-based approaches use statistical metrics like mutual information or *t*-tests for selecting discriminative features. Wrapper-based approaches function by iteratively selecting features using model performance as a criterion, and in embedded approaches feature selection is integrated into model training, such as with LASSO regression. The main goal in feature selection is to eliminate redundant or irrelevant features while preserving those most relevant to dementia detection.

An alternate approach to optimizing the feature matrix can be achieved using dimensionality reduction techniques, such as Principal Components Analysis (PCA) which transform the original features into a lower-dimensional space while preserving as much variance as possible. Unlike feature selection, which directly removes features, PCA creates new features, the principal components, that are linear combinations of the original features, ranked by their contribution to total variance. While feature selection retains interpretability, PCA can reveal latent patterns in the data that may not be obvious from individual features.

Given the data-driven nature of AD classification and MMSE score prediction, it is essential to experiment with both feature selection and dimensionality reduction approaches, to determine the most effective strategy for a given dataset. We direct the reader to Guyon et al. [38] and Duboue [39] for comprehensive tutorials on feature selection and dimensionality reduction techniques for feature engineering.

Model Training, Validation, and Testing

Developing an ML model with an acceptable level of performance involves several crucial steps which extend beyond feature computation and engineering. A well-structured ML pipeline ensures that the model generalizes effectively to unseen data by systematically partitioning the dataset, optimizing hyperparameters, validating performance, and evaluating results on previously unseen benchmark data.

Data Partitioning into Training, Validation, and Testing Subsets

A typical ML pipeline requires the dataset to be divided into three subsets, each serving a distinct purpose in model development. As the names suggest, the training partition is where the ML algorithm learns from labeled data by mapping extracted features to cognitive status labels; for example, AD vs. healthy, or MMSE scores. This is the core learning phase where the model adjusts its internal parameters.

The validation partition consists of data previously unseen relative to the training set, but the labels are withheld during inference and provided afterwards for "validating" model performance using the current set of model parameters. This partition is used to assess model performance during the development process and helps to guide decisions on hyperparameter tuning to improve generalization and prevent overfitting the training partition. The validation set therefore plays a key role in optimizing parameters, although the types of parameters depend on the choice of ML algorithms. For example, the support vector machine classifier may only require optimization of the regularization parameter or at best the kernel function, whereas the random forest classifier has several parameters which may require optimization, such as the number of trees in the forest, the maximum depth of the tree, or the maximum number of features to consider. The optimization of learning rates, activation functions, and architecture choices are required for deep learning models.

Finally, the test partition serves as the ultimate performance benchmark. This subset remains untouched during the training and validation steps, to ensure an unbiased evaluation of the model's generalizability. Once hyperparameters have been optimized using the validation set, the final model is used to predict labels for the test partition and evaluate its performance. These performance results are used for comparative benchmarking in AD classification and cognitive score prediction.

Model Training and Hyperparameter Optimization

Training an ML model involves feeding the training data through an optimization algorithm that adjusts the model parameters to minimize the prediction error. Hyperparameter tuning is an integral part of training, as it controls aspects of model learning that cannot be directly optimized during training. A common approach to this end is to determine model performance over a grid of hyperparameters to find the set of hyperparameters that yield best performance.

Model Validation

Validation serves as an intermediate step to measure the model's generalization ability before final testing. A well-performing model should not only perform well on training data but should also maintain robust performance on unseen validation samples. Performance on the validation set determines whether further refinement is needed before moving to final testing. It also helps in guiding the change in hyperparameters of the training algorithm. For classification tasks, such as in the classification of AD vs. healthy samples, the performance of the ML model is typically measured using accuracy, precision, recall, and F1 score. For regression tasks, as used for MMSE score prediction, evaluation metrics include root mean squared error (RMSE) and mean absolute error (MAE), which assess the model's ability to accurately predict cognitive scores.

Model Testing

Once a model has been trained and validated, it undergoes final evaluation on the test partition, which contains unseen data meant to simulate real-world conditions. Unlike validation, where hyperparameters can still be adjusted, test partition predictions are made without any further modifications to the model. The performance metrics obtained on the test set provide the definitive measure of how well the model generalizes beyond its development environment.

Overview

Automatic Speech Recognition is a critical tool for analyzing speech data, especially useful in dementia research. ASR essentially transcribes spoken audio to written text, allowing for the extraction of linguistic features necessary for the detection and monitoring of cognitive decline. The general approach of ASR is to extract and process the acoustic features extracted from the speech signals and produce transcriptions using either end-to-end deep learning models or hybrid models that combine linguistic and acoustic approaches.

Recently introduced ASR technologies like wav2vec2 [40] and Whisper [41], which have delivered impressive transcription quality, even under challenging conditions. Despite the improvements, ASR systems still face huge challenges when dealing with pathological speech.

Challenges Specific to Transcribing Speech from Dementia Patients

Speech disfluencies, including hesitations, repetitions, and incomplete sentences, are prevalent in dementia individuals and present a unique challenge for an ASR system. These disfluencies, which are important diagnostic features of cognitive impairment, are often misrecognized or ignored by conventional ASR systems that are trained on fluent speech [42]. A study by Schultz et al. [43] has shown that ASR systems transcribe disordered speech less accurately than that of healthy controls due to lower intelligibility and increased background noise. Yet, in fact, this increase in the transcription errors is an important characteristic during the identification of disordered speech [44].

The reduced vocal intensity and inconsistent speech rates of dementia victims makes transcription even more difficult. People with dementia might talk at a lower volume, speak in whispers, or fluctuate between slow and fast-spoken sentences, requiring segmentation and transcription which makes the system prone to error. Transcripts generated by automatic speech recognition techniques can still serve a purpose. As shown in [44], they implicitly capture linguistic anomalies related to dementia and significantly contribute to the classification accuracy of cognitively healthy individuals and individuals with Alzheimer's disease. Patients with dementia also exhibit vastly different linguistic patterns to people with normal speech. Dementia patients speak in simplified phrases, with a mix of wrong words, or with unusual sentence structures that are not present in the data from which ASR models learn to recognize language. It was shown by [45], that features extracted from automatic transcription were able to achieve similar results as features extracted from manual transcription, pointing out that ASR might be a reliable tool to conduct linguistic analysis for dementia research.

Furthermore, acoustic variability—like the changes in tone, emotional swings during speech and distance from speaker to microphone—can also cause transcription accuracy to deteriorate. Ilias et al. [46] tackled this problem by unifying the acoustic and textual feature domains, showing that well-performing ASR systems can help dementia detection, as they can compensate for deviations in speech characteristics. Overall, ASR greatly assists in dementia research by leveraging its capabilities to transcribe speech quickly, and providing linguistic markers of cognitive decline. While ASR is challenged in understanding disordered speech, research suggests that even sub-optimal ASR outputs yield valuable information. Adaptive models, and the integration of features derived from causal structure enhance the impact of ASR in automating dementia recognition.

Tools and Software Options

Common commercial ASR systems like Google Cloud Speech-to-Text [47], IBM Watson Speech-to-Text [48], and Microsoft Azure AI Speech [49] have been used widely as off-the-shelf solutions that perform reasonably well on clean recordings of human speech. In recent years, open-source models such as Open AI's Whisper and Facebook AI's wav2vec2, as well as an open-source ASR toolkit, ESPnet [50], have been increasingly utilized for this task.

Feature Engineering from Speech

Feature engineering is a critical step in designing automated screening tools for Alzheimer's dementia using speech. Because the disease can disrupt both motor control and cognitive-linguistic abilities, subtle markers often appear in voice quality, word usage, and fluency. This observation motivates the extraction of three main types of features: acoustic (e.g., pitch, intensity), textual (e.g., lexical diversity, syntactic complexity), and disfluency-based (e.g., filled pauses, repeated words). Given the importance of feature computation, we provide more details in the following sections.

Speech Based Feature Computation

Acoustic Features

Speech-based assessment for Alzheimer's disease has gained significant attention in recent years due to its non-invasive nature and the wealth of information encoded in acoustic properties. This chapter explores various acoustic features, ranging from fundamental prosodic cues (e.g., pitch, rate) to advanced spectral and voice quality metrics, and discusses their potential in revealing early signs of cognitive decline.

A concise way to organize the broad range of acoustic features is to categorize them by their primary focus: prosodic, voice quality, spectral, temporal, energy based, or advanced. Table 8.2 provides examples of these features and highlights their relevance to Alzheimer's dementia. Each category pinpoints a different set of

Table 8.2 Categories of acoustic features for Alzheimer's dementia analysis

Feature category	Example	Features relevance to AD
Prosody	Pitch (mean, range, variability), intensity (mean and range), speaking rate, pause duration	Lower pitch variability and slower speech rate can reflect cognitive load. Frequent or long pauses may signal difficulty in word retrieval
Voice quality	Jitter, shimmer, harmonics- to-noise ratio (HNR), breathiness indices	Increased jitter and shimmer indicate irregular vocal fold control. A lower HNR may suggest a rough or breathy voice caused by motor deficits
Spectral	Formant frequencies (F1, F2, F3), mel-frequency cepstral coefficients (MFCCs), spectral centroid, spectral bandwidth	Shifts in formants or MFCC patterns can signify articulation issues. Changes in spectral shape may correlate with loss of fine motor control
Temporal/ segmental	Voice onset time (VOT), vowel/ consonant durations, inter-phoneme intervals, speech rate	Slower articulation, prolonged segments, and irregular timing often emerge as cognitive, and motor skills decline in Alzheimer's disease
Energy and signal-level features	Short-time energy, root mean square (RMS) energy, zero-crossing rate (ZCR)	Reduced energy or inconsistent amplitude can hint at weak breath support. Changes in ZCR patterns may reflect disordered articulation
Derived features	Trajectory-based analyses (pitch or formant slopes), composite scores from multiple features, machine learning-based embeddings	Complex patterns can detect subtle shifts in pitch, articulation, or voice quality that might not be clear in single-feature analysis

potential speech disruptions, from pitch changes and vocal instability to articulatory imprecision and slowed timing. A brief introduction of acoustic features is provided in the following sections:

Prosodic Features

Prosodic features focus on pitch, loudness, and timing in speech. They often reveal how Alzheimer's disease can slow down or disrupt normal speaking patterns [51]. For instance, a person may speak with a narrower pitch range, which indicates less variation in their fundamental frequency. They might also speak more quietly, with irregular changes in volume, and produce fewer changes in loudness across an utterance. In addition, patients with cognitive decline may pause frequently or produce long silences while searching for words. These disruptions mirror the effort needed to plan speech and retrieve linguistic information when memory and executive functions are compromised. Because prosody often reflects the speaker's overall cognitive and motor coordination, changes in pitch, volume, and pause patterns can serve as early indicators of Alzheimer's-related decline.

Voice Quality Features

Voice quality features measure how stable or clear a person's voice is. They quantify features such as how consistent the vibration of the vocal folds is, or how much noise is present in the signal. People with Alzheimer's disease might find it harder to control their vocal folds because of motor coordination problems or lack of cognitive monitoring. As a result, its pitch or amplitude may vary from one vocal cycle to the next, giving the voice a rough, breathy or shaky quality. When the variation is pronounced, it indicates less neuromuscular control and may indicate the progression of neurological symptoms. By analyzing the consistency of the voice or how much noise leaks into the signal, researchers can learn about a person's motor control and neurological health, both of which can be affected by dementia.

Spectral Features

Spectral features capture the way in which sound energy is distributed across the frequency bands in an audio signal. These features are highly correlated with the shape and motion of the vocal tract. In Alzheimer's disease, the precision of articulatory movements tends to falter, in part because the brain has difficulty coordinating the small movements of the tongue, lips and jaw. Formant frequencies, which are resonance frequencies within the vocal tract, might shift if articulation becomes unprecise. These shifts can also be captured with Mel-Frequency Cepstral Coefficients (MFCC), a common way to summarize the spectral shape that can help detect subtle changes in speech clarity. Because structural resonance patterns can provide clues about the way someone is shaping their vocal tract, spectral features give a glimpse into the breakdowns of fine motor control and cognitive processes that are part of speech production.

Temporal and Segmental Features

Temporal and segmental features refer to the spatiotemporal arrangement of speech sounds in terms of their timing and speech intervals. They analyze how fast a speaker moves from one sound to another, how long each vowel or consonant stays in the mouth, and how frequently voicing happens. In a person with Alzheimer's disease, the speed of speech may slow down, and speech may also become more irregular. Voice onset time—the interval between the release of a consonant and the onset of voicing—may increase if cognitive or motor control is compromised. The lengths of vowels and consonants may also vary. When these temporal rhythms are interrupted, it is typically indicative of its speaker's difficulty organizing and executing segments of speech. In turn, disorganized or slowed timing of speech can correlate with the severity of cognitive impairment.

Energy and Other Signal-Level Features

Energy and other signal level features are based on the raw amplitude of the voice and how it changes during speech. They aid in capturing changes in overall speaking effort, or breath support, which is thought to deteriorate in Alzheimer's disease. Patients may also have lower average energy which results in reduced vocal strength or uneven distribution of loudness (or low intensity). This can be seen by plotting short-time energy or RMS energy over small frames of speech. If the energy flags, or doesn't seem as stable as before, it might mean the speaker is having difficulty keeping consistent tone or controlling their breath. Another signal-level measure, the zero-crossing rate, can be used to show how frequently the speech waveform crosses the midpoint amplitude. A difference in the proportion of voiced to unvoiced sounds can further be discerned from changes in zero-crossing patterns. These differences reflect articulation problems due to dementia.

Advanced or Derived Features

Advanced or derived features combine several acoustic measures, or use machine learning to extract more profound structures in speech. They also can follow how pitch or spectral features vary across whole words or sentences, instead of just short stretches. Higher-order patterns can capture nuanced variations in speech organization that may not be detectable by individual features. Neural network models, for instance, may learn more abstract "embeddings" of speech that fuse prosody, voice quality, and spectral cues. Such representations can uncover early stages of Alzheimer's disease before more recognizable symptoms emerge. By integrating multiple speech dimensions into holistic scores or trajectories, they can help researchers and clinicians identify complex, interrelated impacts of dementia on speech.

Textual Features

Language is a highly sophisticated cognitive function that accesses memory, attention, and executive control. As Alzheimer's disease advances, it can hinder a person's ability to produce and organize language. By analyzing speech transcripts or written samples, researchers and clinicians can look for text-based features to reveal patterns that may indicate mild and even preclinical forms of cognitive decline.

Table 8.3 Categories of textual features for Alzheimer's dementia analysis

Feature category	Example	Features relevance to AD
Lexical	Type-token ratio, mean word frequency	Reduced vocabulary diversity or reliance on common words can indicate difficulty retrieving language
Morphological	Tense usage accuracy, plural markers, inflection errors	Grammatical errors in word endings or forms often point to declining cognitive and linguistic control
Syntactic	Mean length of utterance, subject-verb agreement	Simpler or error-prone sentences suggest an increasing struggle to manage grammatical rules
Semantic	Semantic diversity, semantic similarity	Repetitive or vague word choices reveal diminished ability to express a range of concepts
Pragmatic	Use of filler words, context-appropriate language	Breakdown in conversational norms or figurative language signals higher-level cognitive deficits
Discourse	Local coherence, global coherence	Disorganized or abrupt topic shifts reflect difficulties in linking ideas across extended passages
Narrative	Story grammar, event sequencing	Missing story elements or jumbled timelines highlight deficits in memory and event organization
Advanced features	Word embeddings	Computational analyses detect subtle patterns not evident in simpler linguistic measures

These features cover everything from simple measures of vocabulary (such as variety) to the more abstract aspects (like the logical flow of ideas). By examining a person's language production and contrasting it with typical norms, a researcher can identify small changes that may appear well before more visible symptoms emerge.

Table 8.3 provides a summary of these categories and describes the measures in a given category and how they may indicate language markers of dementia. The next sections provide brief details for each category.

Lexical Features

Lexical features refer to the vocabulary used in an utterance and include such factors as word choice and diversity. Some of these features reflect a diminished variety of language usage, which may indicate impairments in word-finding (limited access to the linguistic lexicon). For example, a type-token ratio—the ratio of unique words to total words—might decrease in people with dementia due to the use of repetitive or generic words. Mean word frequency (how common the chosen words are) could also go up, as speakers cluster around known, frequency-heavy words.

Morphological Features

Morphological features measure how well words are composed, including the proper use of tense and plural markers. In dementia, morphological error can reflect cognitive deterioration and speakers' inability to add or maintain appropriate inflections. For example, a patient might say "I walk yesterday" instead of "I walked yesterday," dropping the past-tense ending. Another example might be violation of plurality—"three cat" for "three cats"—which show failing grammatical processes.

Syntactic Features

Syntactic features characterize the construction of a sentence, for example, how complex or long an utterance is. In dementia, shorter or jumbled sentences suggest that the speaker's ability to handle linguistic rules has been reduced. Mean length of utterance, which measures how many words are in a sentence, usually goes down as patients speak in shorter, more direct phrases. Another item of interest is subject-verb agreement, errors (e.g., "He go" instead of "He goes") of which indicate trouble with grammatical planning.

Semantic Features

Semantic features describe what words mean and how concepts are communicated. They help flag dementia by revealing narrower, repetitive language use. For example, semantic diversity, which measures how many different topics or fields of words reappear, can mean difficulties coming up with fresh ideas when it is low. Another is semantic similarity between sentences: in dementia, excessive repetition or vague phrasing boosts similarity scores, an indication of less flexible thought.

Pragmatic Features

The pragmatic features assess the use of language in a particular context, such as conventions in conversation and clarity. They indicate dementia by exhibiting a lack of contextually appropriate verbal cue or an increase in inappropriate fillers. For example, a patient might have difficulty following shifts in topic, saying "um" or "you know" repeatedly. They might also be unable to use idioms or figurative forms of speech, therefore sounding more literal or blunt.

Discourse Features

Discourse level features assess how ideas interconnect multiple sentences. Keys to diagnosing dementia include noting whether a speaker changes topics abruptly while speaking, or whether their conversation consists of logical breakdowns. Local coherence can decline, with missing ties between successive sentences, and global coherence suffers if speakers lose their grip on the overall theme. Conversations may change from event to event haphazardly without proper transitions.

Narrative Features

Narrative features assess story-oriented structures, that is, with a clear beginning, middle, and end. They help identify dementia by marking incomplete or out-of-order storytelling. A person may leave out important parts of a narrative, leading to a disorganized order of events. Another behavior is repeating the same story point multiple times, a demonstration of short term memory problems that are detrimental to the narrative flow.

Advanced (Derived) Features

Basic metrics are sometimes mixed into advanced features using computational methods. They reflect patterns denoting dementia that are unobservable at the surface level. Word embeddings, for instance, positions words in high-dimensional space, uncovering unusual changes in used meaning. Topic modeling can follow a more limited range of themes or sudden derailments in topic focus. These sophisticated analyses detect subtle shifts in language associated with early cognitive decline.

Disfluency Features

Disfluency features focus on breaks and irregularities in speech that often signal underlying cognitive or motor planning difficulties. Table 8.4 lists the primary categories, provides specific examples, and explains how each might indicate a decline in linguistic function associated with Alzheimer's disease.

Table 8.4 Categories of disfluency features for Alzheimer's dementia analysis

Feature category	Example	Features relevance to AD
Filled pauses and filler words	"um", "uh", "er", frequent "you know" usage	Higher frequency and awkward placement of fillers suggest increased cognitive load or difficulty retrieving words
Silent pauses and hesitations	Unfilled breaks between words, extended silence before key terms	Longer or frequent pauses can signal problems in planning speech or recalling specific vocabulary
Repetitions	Repeated words or phrases ("I went… I went to the store.")	May reflect memory lapses or lexical retrieval issues, leading to unnecessary restatements
False starts and self-corrections	Abandoned utterances, mid-speech revisions ("I was going... wait... let me say...")	Indicate uncertainty or trouble maintaining a coherent plan for speech production
Prolongations (stretched words)	Extended vowels or consonants ("I w-a-a-a-s just thinking…")	Suggest motor or planning difficulty, often a tactic to buy time during word retrieval
Speech rate changes	Sudden slowing or speeding up of speech, uneven pacing	Can reflect varying degrees of cognitive load, with speakers adjusting pace when encountering linguistic challenges

Filled Pauses and Filler Words

Filled pauses are non-lexical vocalizations like "um," "uh," and "er." They are designed to capture instances when speakers require additional time to retrieve or plan their words, which can increase in Alzheimer's. For example, people with dementia might pepper conversations with multiple "um" sounds or position them uncomfortably in mid-sentence, showing that they are struggling cognitively to maintain fluent speech.

Silent Pauses and Hesitations

Silent pauses refers are unfilled breaks in speech. They allow quantification of the speaker's inability to maintain a stable stream of language, often mimicking word-finding or planning problems in dementia. For instance, patients might have longer pauses immediately preceding key nouns or verbs, or abruptly stop mid-sentence, both signs of heightened cognitive load.

Repetitions

Repetition is when one uses the same words or phrases repeatedly in a short time frame. Repetitions capture interruptions in fluent speech, as people with Alzheimer's may forget they have already used a word or have difficulty transitioning. Someone who has dementia might say "I went… I went to the market," which represents either a lexical retrieval problem or a failure of short-term memory.

False Starts and Self-Corrections

False starts are aborted utterances, and self-corrections refer to in-speech revisions. They offer a record of how often speakers lose sight of what they had been trying to say or notice mistakes they had made and try to correct themselves. A person with dementia might start a sentence ("I was going to—actually, wait… I think I should…") and then restart repeatedly, revealing trouble keeping a coherent plan for speech over time.

Prolongations (StretchedWords)

Prolongations measure stretched out production of sounds or syllables, such as lengthening of vowels ("I w-a-a-a-s there"). They do imply motor or planning difficulty, but they also tend to signal that the speaker is stalling for time to recall words or figure out how to structure a sentence. In dementia, these stretches may pop up more often, or at unexpected points in a sentence, highlighting increasing linguistic uncertainty.

Speech Rate Changes

Changes in speech rate measure how quickly or slowly words are spoken. They are relevant in dementia because speakers might slow down suddenly during challenging vocabulary or speed up in easier parts of the speech. Patients, also show uneven pace, speeding through common words and then pausing for too long on less familiar ones, which in turn reveals imbalanced cognitive load in conversation.

Challenges and Limitations

With an aging global population, the rates of neurodegenerative diseases such as Alzheimer's have quickly increased. Even with the progression in AI based systems for detecting such diseases, there are several challenges that are present in this task.

Data Quality and Quantity Challenges

One important limitation of applying AI for Alzheimer's analysis of speech is the limited amount of data, both in terms of quantity and quality [52]. Small dataset sizes (due to the difficulty of collecting them) and high variability in speech patterns for elderly and cognitively impaired patients are serious obstacles to overcome. To overcome these data challenges, researchers have proposed various methods including data augmentation, transfer learning, and synthetic data generation [53].

Data augmentation, the process of synthetically modifying existing speech samples to generate additional training examples, has been shown to increase model performance on some tasks. To alleviate this problem of limited domain-specific data, using transfer learning with models pre-trained on large, general speech datasets has also been proposed. Another focus is few-shot learning approaches that enable models to quickly adapt to new speakers with limited training data [53]. This finding underscores the potential for generative adversarial networks to synthesize realistic speech samples and augment poorly endowed real-world datasets. These developments remain limited in scope, encountering difficulties in obtaining good-quality speech samples for elderly and cognitively impaired individuals. Some of the logistical challenges encountered by researchers include obtaining informed consent, managing noise in the environment, and maintaining consistent recording setups.

Automatic Speech Recognition Limitations

Another important limitation of automatic speech recognition is its technical limitations, which serve as a barrier to effective Alzheimer's detection from speech beyond data scarcity. Current ASR systems fail to accurately process this type of speech, typified by slurred, incomplete, and repetitive speech output. Recognition accuracy tends to drop across the board for impaired speech processing, and [54] also point to particular hurdles with disfluencies, repetitions and background noise. Existing ASR technology is poorly suited to the speech patterns of Alzheimer's patients, and results in a high rate of errors. There have been several investigations aimed at improving automatic speech recognition (ASR) systems' performance for this speech, such as techniques for speaker adaptation, noise-robust feature extraction and language modeling in the Alzheimer's domain. Recent quantitative studies have shown how well the current ASR systems perform in parsing typical speech as opposed to Alzheimer's-related speech, highlighting the opportunity for further advances.

Ethical and Privacy Considerations

Extracting insights from speech data presents a host of ethical and privacy issues related to the collection and the application of this data for Alzheimer detection that will need to be properly handled. The nature of healthcare information is inherently sensitive; maintaining patient consent and data privacy is paramount. It is essential to observe regulatory requirements like Health Insurance Portability and Accountability Act (HIPAA) and General Data Protection Regulation (GDPR) with the right systems in place for secure data handling, anonymization, and long-term storage. Additionally, the ethical considerations behind the use of AI-based Alzheimer's diagnosis needs to be scrutinized. There is a possibility that biases in the underlying data or algorithms may result in false or unfair assessments with dire consequences to patients and their relatives. The ethical guidelines for the development and application of such AI systems should integrate ideas of transparency, accountability and patient empowerment. Recurrent engagement of researchers, clinicians, and ethicists will be needed to support the responsible, equitable use of these technologies. More research and further innovations in this area will be pivotal to solving those challenges and mining the full power of this non-invasive method for the early detection and monitoring of Alzheimer disease [55].

Conclusions

Detecting of Alzheimer's disease at an early stage from the analysis of speech using Artificial Intelligence is an innovative breakthrough in the fields of mental health and neurodegenerative research. The use of speech as a non-invasive biomarker is a potential practical, convenient and cheap solution compared to the traditional diagnostic methods where the patient often requires a costly or invasive procedure. AI's capability to detect slight shifts in speech patterns, including lexical diversity, fluency, and acoustic attributes, underscores its promise in the early identification of cognitive decline. This early detection not only improves the effectiveness of intervention but also greatly enhances the quality of life for the patients, and their caregivers. Furthermore, early diagnosis using such systems helps to take proper and timely therapeutic measures, better manage resources, and provide personalized help systems for the affected people. The continuous improvement on the data available, covering a diverse range of settings relating to subjects from different backgrounds when combined with advances in algorithms and methods for automated disease detection on the back of novel machine and deep learning frameworks will ensure that AI will play an ever increasing role in in the detection of mental health disorders. Research into improving data quality; developing robust algorithms for diverse populations; and navigating issues related to regulatory and ethical practices are expected to be of significant interest to researchers working at the intersection of AI, linguistics, and healthcare.

References

1. W. World Health Organization, "WHO Mental disorders Fact sheets," 2023. [Online]. Available: https://www.who.int/news-room/fact-sheets/detail/mental-disorders
2. F. Yang, T. Han, K. Deng, and Y. Han, "The application of artificial intelligence in the mental diseases," in Proceedings of the 2020 Conference on Artificial Intelligence and Healthcare, 2020, pp. 36–40.
3. F. Minerva and A. Giubilini, "Is AI the future of mental healthcare?" Springer Science + Business Media, vol. 42, no. 3, pp. 809–817, 05 2023. [Online]. Available: https://doi.org/10.1007/s11245-023-09932-3
4. W. H. Organization, "Dementia," 3 2023. [Online]. Available: https://www.who.int/news-room/fact-sheets/detail/dementia
5. B. Mohammad Abdallah Qasaimeh, A. Abdallah, and S. Ratte, "Detecting depression in alzheimer and mci using artificial neural networks (ANN)," in International Conference on Data Science, E-learning and Information Systems 2021, 2021, pp. 250–253.
6. M. Grossman, M. D'Esposito, E. Hughes, K. Onishi, N. Biassou, T. White-Devine, and K. M. Robinson, "Language comprehension profiles in Alzheimer's disease, multi-infarct dementia, and frontotemporal degeneration," Neurology, vol. 47, no. 1, pp. 183–189, 1996.
7. M.-M. Mesulam, Principles of behavioral and cognitive neurology. Oxford University Press, 2000.
8. H. H. Clark and T. Wasow, "Repeating words in spontaneous speech," Cognitive psychology, vol. 37, no. 3, pp. 201–242, 1998.
9. C. J. Mummery, K. Patterson, C. J. Price, J. Ashburner, R. S. Frackowiak, and J. R. Hodges, "A voxel-based morphometry study of semantic dementia: relationship between temporal lobe atrophy and semantic memory," Annals of neurology, vol. 47, no. 1, pp. 36–45, 2000.
10. H. Grice, "Logic and conversation," Syntax and semantics, vol. 3, 1975.
11. J. R. Duffy and Others, Motor speech disorders: Substrates, differential diagnosis, and management. Elsevier Health Sciences, 2013.
12. H. Jahn, "Memory loss in Alzheimer's disease," Dialogues in clinical neuroscience, vol. 15, no. 4, pp. 445–454, 2013.
13. N. Geschwind, "The Organization of Language and the Brain: Language disorders after brain damage help in elucidating the neural basis of verbal behavior." Science, vol. 170, no. 3961, pp. 940–944, 1970.
14. A. Baddeley, "The episodic buffer: a new component of working memory?" Trends in cognitive sciences, vol. 4, no. 11, pp. 417–423, 2000.
15. N. F. Dronkers, O. Plaisant, M. T. Iba-Zizen, and E. A. Cabanis, "Paul Broca's historic cases: high resolution MR imaging of the brains of Leborgne and Lelong," Brain, vol. 130, no. 5, pp. 1432–1441, 2007.
16. A. M. Collins and M. R. Quillian, "Retrieval time from semantic memory," Journal of verbal learning and verbal behavior, vol. 8, no. 2, pp. 240–247, 1969.
17. A. D. Baddeley and G. Hitch, "Working Memory," vol. 8, pp. 47–89, 1974. [Online]. Available: https://www.sciencedirect.com/science/article/pii/S0079742108604521

18. J. L. McClelland and J. L. Elman, "The trace model of speech perception," Cognitive psychology, vol. 18, no. 1, pp. 1–86, 1986.
19. J. L. McClelland, "An interactive activation model of context effects in letter perception: Part 2. The contextual enhancement effect and some tests and extensions of the model," Psychological Review, vol. 89, no. 1, pp. 60–94, 1982.
20. T. Ness, V. J. Langlois, A. E. Kim, and J. M. Novick, "The state of cognitive control in language processing," Perspectives on Psychological Science, p. 17456916231197122, 2023.
21. S. Luz, F. Haider, S. de la Fuente, D. Fromm, and B. MacWhinney, "Alzheimer's Dementia Recognition through Spontaneous Speech: The ADReSS Challenge," in INTERSPEECH, 2020, pp. 2172–2176.
22. ——, "Detecting cognitive decline using speech only: The ADReSSo Challenge," INTERSPEECH, pp. 3780–3784, 2021.
23. J. T. Becker, F. Boiler, O. L. Lopez, J. Saxton, and K. L. Mcgonigle, "The Natural History of Alzheimer's Disease: Description of Study Cohort and Accuracy of Diagnosis," Archives of Neurology, vol. 51, no. 6, pp. 585–594, 1994.
24. B. H. Davis and C. Pope, "Finding a balance: The Carolinas Conversation Collection," Corpus Linguistics and Linguistic Theory, vol. 7, no. 1, pp. 143–161, 2011.
25. A. Karakostas, A. Briassouli, K. Avgerinakis, I. Kompatsiaris, and M. Tsolaki, "The dem@ care experiments and datasets: a technical report," arXiv preprint arXiv:1701.01142, 2016.
26. S. Luz, F. Haider, D. Fromm, I. Lazarou, I. Kompatsiaris, and B. MacWhinney, "Multilingual alzheimer's dementia recognition through spontaneous speech: a signal processing grand challenge," in ICASSP 2023-2023 IEEE International Conference on Acoustics, Speech and Signal Processing (ICASSP). IEEE, 2023, pp. 1–2.
27. D. Gkoumas, B. Wang, A. Tsakalidis, M. Wolters, M. Purver, A. Zubiaga, and M. Liakata, "A longitudinal multi-modal dataset for dementia monitoring and diagnosis," Language Resources and Evaluation, pp. 1–20, 2024.
28. S. Luz, S. De La Fuente Garcia, F. Haider, D. Fromm, B. MacWhinney, A. Lanzi, Y.-N. Chang, C.-J. Chou, and Y.-C. Liu, "Connected Speech-Based Cognitive Assessment in Chinese and English," in Interspeech, 2024, pp. 947–951.
29. H. Christensen, S. Bell, D. Blackburn, B. Mirheidari, M. Pahar, F. Tao, D. Braun, H. ElGhazaly, C. Illingworth, R. O'Malley, F. Peters, S. Luz, and F. Haider, "Prediction and Recognition of Cognitive Decline through Spontaneous Speech Signal Processing Grand Challenge Proposal (PROCESS)," 2025. [Online]. Available: https://processchallenge.github.io
30. H. Goodglass, E. Kaplan, and B. Barresi, BDAE-3: Boston Diagnostic Aphasia Examination—Third Edition. Lippincott Williams & Wilkins Philadelphia, PA, 2001.
31. Y.-L. Liu, R. Feng, J.-H. Yuan, and Z.-H. Ling, "Clever Hans Effect Found in Automatic Detection of Alzheimer's Disease through Speech," Interspeech 2024, 2024.
32. I. Arevalo-Rodriguez, N. Smailagic, M. Roquei Figuls, A. Ciapponi, E. Sanchez-Perez, A. Giannakou, O. L. Pedraza, X. Bonfill Cosp, and S. Cullum, "Mini-Mental State Examination (MMSE) for the detection of Alzheimer's disease and other dementias in people with mild cognitive impairment (MCI)," Cochrane Database of Systematic Reviews, vol. 2015, no. 3, pp. 1–76, 2015.
33. O. Pfungst, Clever Hans:(the horse of Mr. Von Osten.) a contribution to experimental animal and human psychology. Holt, Rinehart and Winston, 1911.
34. D. Bone, T. Chaspari, K. Audhkhasi, J. Gibson, A. Tsiartas, M. Van Segbroeck, M. Li, S. Lee, and S. S. Narayanan, "Classifying Language-Related Developmental Disorders from Speech Cues: the Promise and the Potential Confounds," in INTERSPEECH, 2013, pp. 182–186.
35. F. Ringeval, J. Demouy, G. Szaszak, M. Chetouani, L. Robel, J. Xavier, D. Cohen, and M. Plaza, "Automatic intonation recognition for the prosodic assessment of language-impaired children," IEEE Transactions on Audio, Speech and Language Processing, vol. 19, no. 5, pp. 1328–1342, 2011.

36. F. Eyben, M. Wollmer, and B. Schuller, "OpenSMILE—The Munich versatile and fast open-source audio feature extractor," in ACM International Conference on Multimedia, 2010, pp. 1459–1462.
37. Z. S. Syed, M. S. S. Syed, M. Lech, and E. Pirogova, "Automated recognition of Alzheimer's Dementia using Bag-of-Deep-Features and Model Ensembling," IEEE Access, vol. 9, pp. 88 377–88 390, 2021.
38. I. Guyon and A. Elisseeff, "An introduction to variable and feature selection," Journal of Machine Learning Research, vol. 3, pp. 1157–1182, 2003.
39. P. Duboue, The art of feature engineering: essentials for machine learning. Cambridge University Press, 2020.
40. A. Baevski, H. Zhou, A. Mohamed, and M. Auli, "wav2vec 2.0: A framework for self-supervised learning of speech representations," in Advances in Neural Information Processing Systems, 2020, pp. 12 449—-12 460.
41. OpenAI, "Whisper: OpenAI's Speech Recognition Model," https://github.com/openai/whisper, 2022.
42. A. Meghanani, C. S. Anoop, and A. G. Ramakrishnan, "Recognition of Alzheimer's Dementia From the Transcriptions of Spontaneous Speech Using fastText and CNN Models," Frontiers in Computer Science, vol. 3, 2021.
43. B. G. Schultz, V. S. Tarigoppula, G. Noffs, S. Rojas, A. van der Walt, D. B. Grayden, and A. P. Vogel, "Automatic speech recognition in neurodegenerative disease," International Journal of Speech Technology, vol. 24, no. 3, pp. 771–779, 2021.
44. C. Li, W. Xu, T. Cohen, and S. Pakhomov, "Useful blunders: Can automated speech recognition errors improve downstream dementia classification?" Journal of Biomedical Informatics, vol. 150, 2024.
45. J. Weiner, M. Engelbart, and T. Schultz, "Manual and automatic transcriptions in dementia detection from speech," in INTERSPEECH, 2017, pp. 3117–3121.
46. L. Ilias and D. Askounis, "Multimodal Deep Learning Models for Detecting Dementia From Speech and Transcripts," Frontiers in Aging Neuroscience, vol. 14, 2022.
47. Google Cloud, "Google Cloud Speech-to-Text API," https://cloud.google.com/speech-to-text, 2025.
48. IBM, "IBM Watson Speech to Text API," https://www.ibm.com/cloud/watsonspeech-to-text, 2025.
49. Microsoft Azure, "Azure Cognitive Services: Speech API," https://azure.microsoft.com/en-us/products/cognitive-services/speech-to-text/, 2025.
50. S. Watanabe, T. Hori, S. Karita, T. Hayashi, J. Nishitoba, Y. Unno, N. E. Y. Soplin, J. Heymann, M. Wiesner, N. Chen, and Others, "ESPnet: End-to-End Speech Processing Toolkit," INTERSPEECH, pp. 2207–2211, 2018.
51. S. Saeedi, S. Hetjens, M. O. W. Grimm, and B. B. v. Latoszek, "Acoustic Speech Analysis in Alzheimer's Disease: A Systematic Review and Meta-Analysis," The Journal of Prevention of Alzheimer's Disease, vol. 11, no. 6, pp. 1789–1797, 2024.
52. C. Demiroglu, A. Besirli, Y. Ozkanca, and S. Celik, "Depression-level assessment from multilingual conversational speech data using acoustic and text features," EURASIP Journal on Audio, Speech, and Music Processing, vol. 2020, no. 1, p. 17, 2020.
53. K. Yang and E. A. Mohammed, "A review of artificial intelligence technologies for early prediction of alzheimer's disease," arXiv preprint arXiv:2101.01781, 2020.
54. S. Balne and A. Elumalai, "Machine learning and deep learning algorithms used to diagnosis of alzheimer's," Materials Today: Proceedings, vol. 47, pp. 5151–5156, 2021.
55. W. Holmes, K. Porayska-Pomsta, K. Holstein, E. Sutherland, T. Baker, S. B. Shum, O. C. Santos, M. T. Rodrigo, M. Cukurova, I. I. Bittencourt et al., "Ethics of ai in education: Towards a community-wide framework," International Journal of Artificial Intelligence in Education, pp. 1–23, 2022.

Epilogue

Madhu Chetty and Jennifer Hallinan

Artificial Intelligence (AI) has become a significant aspect of progress in health and healthcare, reshaping the foundations of medical science and practice. Across the eight chapters of this book, we present some basic theory plus AI applications in numerous subfields, from processing very large datasets to unraveling the complexities of biology. As we conclude this exploration, it is fitting to reflect on the significance of the first two chapters: the pillars that provide the framework for understanding the remarkable advancements covered in subsequent sections.

The opening chapter, devoted to presenting the evolution of computing from Data Science to Artificial Intelligence, establishes the foundation upon which the book's narrative is built. Data Science, with its tools and methodologies for managing and analyzing large datasets, laid the groundwork for AI to emerge as a powerful technological paradigm with which to address difficult problems in several domains, including healthcare. This chapter captures the progression from early statistical methods to sophisticated machine learning algorithms that can predict outcomes, identify patterns, and optimize decision-making with high accuracy. By following this trajectory, readers can gain insights into the way in which healthcare transitioned from data-driven strategies to AI-driven solutions. This progression underscores AI's capability to process vast amounts of information with unparalleled speed and accuracy, enabling breakthroughs in diagnostics, treatments, and patient care. It reveals how AI is transforming healthcare from reactive to proactive, empowering clinicians and researchers to anticipate and attempt to prevent diseases before they occur.

M. Chetty
Federation University, Churchill, VIC, Australia
e-mail: Madhu.chetty@federation.edu.au

J. Hallinan
BioThink, Brisbane, Redcliffe, QLD, Australia

M. Chetty, J. Hallinan (eds.), *From Algorithms to Ailments*,
https://doi.org/10.1007/978-3-032-11023-7

Following this foundational perspective, the second chapter shifts focus to molecular biology, delving into the realms of genomes and proteins. This chapter serves as a bridge between the computational prowess of AI and the intricate biological mechanisms that AI seeks to decode. Genomics, the study of an organism's complete set of genes, holds the key to understanding the genetic roots of diseases. Proteins, the molecules that carry out essential cellular functions, provide crucial insights into the way in which genes affect health and disease. By explaining these concepts, this chapter equips readers with the scientific context necessary to appreciate how AI can impact the well-established discipline of molecular biology. It highlights how AI-driven tools have accelerated genome sequencing, revealed genetic markers for diseases, and enabled the modeling of protein structures with astonishing accuracy. AI's ability to analyze genetic and protein data has paved the way for advancements in personalized medicine, in which treatments can be tailored to the unique genetic makeup of individual patients. This transformative approach represents a shift toward more targeted, effective, and personalized healthcare solutions.

As we draw the threads of this book together, the significance of these first two chapters resonates throughout its narrative. They establish a dual foundation: one rooted in the evolution of technology and the other in the intricacies of biological science. Together, they illustrate the synergy between AI and healthcare, showcasing the way in which computational intelligence enhances our understanding of human health. Throughout the chapters of this book, we have traversed the multifaceted landscapes of AI's applications, exploring the way in which its integration into health systems, diagnostics, treatments, and research has brought profound advancements. From patient care enhancements to breakthroughs in genetic disease research, AI has emerged as a tool of unparalleled power, bringing precision, and efficiency to areas that once demanded significant human effort and expertise.

One of the pivotal discussions in this book has been the impact of recent developments in Natural Language Understanding (NLU) and Large Language Models (LLMs): technologies at the heart of modern AI. These models have demonstrated remarkable abilities to process and interpret the intricate tapestry of human language. In healthcare, their applications range from analyzing clinical notes and medical records to offering conversational support for patients and professionals alike. When paired with genetic disease research, NLU and LLMs hold the promise of decoding complex genetic information, identifying novel markers for inherited conditions, and paving the way for personalized medicine tailored to genetic profiles. Their capabilities expand the boundaries of possibility, bringing insights and understanding to the complexities of human biology.

Central to this discussion on the application of AI in health and healthcare is the ability to understand and decipher the intricate mechanisms of life, thereby improving human well-being. The application of AI to the accurate modeling and inference of Gene Regulatory Networks (GRNs) is a challenging field within bioinformatics that epitomizes the marriage of computational ingenuity and biological processes. GRNs are a representation of the complex interplay of genes, proteins, and other molecules that regulate cellular functions. Decoding these networks is vital to understanding disease mechanisms, identifying potential therapeutic targets, and advancing precision medicine. AI and the subfield of evolutionary computation, with its unparalleled capacity to process vast amounts of data and discern hidden patterns, has emerged as a game-changer in unraveling these intricate networks. Techniques such as ensemble approaches (such as GRAMP) to harness the individual prowess of different modeling methods have enabled researchers to model GRNs with unprecedented accuracy, allowing for insights into conditions ranging from cancer to rare genetic disorders. These advancements are paving the way for developing tailored interventions that can address the unique genetic makeup of individual patients, bringing us closer to the promise of truly personalized healthcare. While the application of AI to health and healthcare is still in its early stages, it has boundless potential, much of which is yet to be realized. Accurate GRN modeling serves as a beacon for the way in which AI can tackle the most complex biological challenges.

As highlighted in this book, an important application of AI lies in its intersection with genomics and synthetic biology. These fields, rich with complexity and promise, exemplify the way in which AI is advancing our ability to manipulate and comprehend the building blocks of life, ushering in a new era of genetic engineering and biotechnological innovation. Genomics—the study of genomes and their functions—has long posed challenges due to the sheer scale and intricacy of genetic data. AI has emerged as a vital tool in tackling these challenges, enabling researchers to process vast datasets, uncover hidden patterns, and identify genetic variants associated with diseases. Machine learning algorithms, for example, have contributed to breakthroughs in understanding cancer genomes, rare genetic disorders, and hereditary diseases, helping to pave the way for targeted therapies and personalized healthcare. AI's ability to model and predict genetic outcomes has accelerated the journey from lab-based discoveries to clinical applications, benefiting countless lives. Synthetic biology—engineering biological systems to create new functionalities—has also gained momentum as a field in which AI is a critical ally. By optimizing experimental design, automating processes, and accurately predicting the behavior of synthetic biological components, AI has enabled scientists to create novel biotechnologies. From designing synthetic DNA to developing living therapies like engineered bacteria or gene-editing technologies, AI fuels innovation that holds the potential to address global health challenges. Together, genomics and synthetic biology embody the synergy between cutting-edge biology and computational intelligence, enabling breakthroughs that were once unimaginable. AI's role in genomics and synthetic biology offers glimpses into a world where healthcare is truly transformative, empowering humanity to solve some of its most pressing health challenges.

As this book has highlighted, AI is ushering in innovations that have profound implications, and is emerging as a transformative force in research in health, including cancer care. This intersection of technology and oncology represents one of the most promising frontiers in medicine, in which the union of human intelligence and machine learning is yielding outcomes that were once unattainable. AI has expedited the discovery of biomarkers, unraveling the genetic underpinnings of various cancers and identifying targets for novel therapies. The application of deep learning to genomic data is revealing insights into the way in which cancers develop and evolve, guiding the development of cutting-edge treatments such as immunotherapies and gene editing. AI-driven platforms are also transforming clinical trials, enhancing patient recruitment, and optimizing study designs to accelerate the evaluation of new treatments. These innovations not only bolster our understanding of cancer biology but also improve the speed and efficacy of bringing life-saving therapies to patients. AI-driven innovations in cancer care have revolutionized diagnostics by enabling earlier and more accurate detection of tumors. Advanced imaging algorithms, for instance, can identify subtle anomalies in medical scans that might be overlooked by human eyes, ensuring timely interventions that can save lives. AI is also paving the way for precision medicine, in which treatments are tailored to individual patients based on their genetic profiles, disease characteristics, and predicted response to therapies. Machine learning models are employed to predict the effectiveness of drugs and recommend personalized treatment plans, maximizing efficacy while minimizing side effects. These advancements will fundamentally change the way in which we approach cancer treatment, placing patient-centric care at the forefront. As we reflect on the progress outlined in this book, it is evident that AI's role in cancer care is just beginning to unfold.

While highlighting AI's transformative applications across various domains of medicine, we stop to explore one key topic having remarkable impact on ophthalmology: AI applied to diseases of the eye. This intersection of AI, image processing, and vision science is leading toward new paradigms in eye care, offering hope and solutions to millions worldwide. The eye is a window to overall health, capable of revealing not only ocular conditions like glaucoma, macular degeneration, and diabetic retinopathy, but also systemic diseases such as hypertension, diabetes, and even neurological disorders. AI-powered technologies have shown extraordinary promise in detecting, monitoring, and managing these conditions. Advanced machine learning algorithms are revolutionizing retinal imaging analysis, enabling the early detection of abnormalities that are often invisible to the human eye. Automated tools now assist clinicians in making accurate diagnoses faster than ever before, significantly improving outcomes for patients. Beyond diagnostics, AI is transforming therapeutic strategies in ophthalmology. Personalized treatment plans, informed by AI models analyzing patient-specific data, could be soon becoming a reality. Additionally, AI is optimizing surgical procedures for precision and efficiency, enhancing the quality of care. Virtual and augmented reality applications, powered by AI, are helping restore vision and assist individuals with visual impairments, opening up possibilities for improving the quality of life. It is important to make these technologies accessible globally, so their benefits extend to underserved communities and regions in which healthcare resources are scarce. However, the future of AI-driven ophthalmology is bright, and its journey has only begun.

Artificial Intelligence (AI) is also redefining mental health research, offering unprecedented insights into conditions that profoundly impact individuals and families worldwide. Amongst the various topics that are explored in this book, the application of AI in health and healthcare spans diverse areas, with one key topic highlighting its remarkable potential in advancing mental health research, particularly in understanding and addressing Alzheimer's disease. Alzheimer's disease, a progressive neurodegenerative disorder, presents profound challenges for patients and caregivers. Its complexity, combined with the need for early detection and intervention, has driven researchers to harness the power of AI. Machine learning models, for example, have been transforming the detection of Alzheimer's by analyzing subtle changes in brain imaging, speech patterns, and biomarkers. These tools are enabling earlier and more accurate diagnoses, providing the opportunity to intervene before the onset of significant cognitive decline. AI's ability to analyze large-scale data from patient populations offers new perspectives on risk factors, disease progression, and potential therapeutic targets. In Alzheimer's research, AI is enhancing drug development by identifying promising candidates and accelerating clinical trials. Deep learning algorithms are sifting through vast molecular datasets to uncover patterns that would be nearly impossible for humans to detect. AI is also revolutionizing personalized care for Alzheimer's patients, from creating tailored therapies based on individual genetic profiles to deploying technologies like wearable devices and virtual assistants to support daily living and monitor cognitive function. These innovations not only advance scientific understanding but also provide tangible benefits to those affected by the disease. The fight against Alzheimer's is a global effort, requiring collaboration between researchers, technologists, clinicians, and caregivers to ensure that AI-driven solutions are accessible to all.

From the commentary above, it is clear that Artificial Intelligence has emerged as a transformative force in healthcare, offering unparalleled opportunities to revolutionize the way in which we prevent, diagnose, and treat diseases. However, its rapid development also brings significant disadvantages and concerns that must be addressed thoughtfully. This epilogue must reflect not only on the promises but also the pitfalls of AI in health and healthcare, urging balanced and ethical approaches as we embrace this powerful technology. Among the foremost concerns surrounding AI is the issue of data privacy and security. The vast amounts of sensitive health data required to train AI systems pose risks of breaches and unauthorized access. Patients' privacy must be safeguarded to maintain trust and uphold ethical standards in healthcare. Moreover, the biases inherent in AI models present a troubling challenge, particularly in ensuring equitable access and treatment for diverse populations. If training data does not represent varied demographics, AI systems may perpetuate inequalities, leading to inaccurate predictions or disparities in care. Ethical concerns also extend to accountability and transparency. When AI systems make decisions, it can be difficult to understand or challenge the rationale behind their conclusions. The disadvantages are not limited to technical and ethical issues; there are also socioeconomic concerns. The implementation of AI in healthcare may widen the gap between developed and developing regions if access to AI-powered tools remains uneven. The costs associated with deploying and maintaining AI systems may disproportionately affect healthcare institutions with limited resources, creating barriers to equitable adoption. Furthermore, the increasing reliance on AI in clinical settings raises questions about the diminishing role of human intuition and empathy, which remain essential in providing compassionate care.

Despite these challenges, the applications of AI in healthcare have profound impacts. AI has revolutionized medical imaging, enabling faster and more accurate diagnoses for conditions such as cancer, cardiovascular disease, and neurological disorders. Predictive analytics powered by AI allow for the early detection of health risks, paving the way for preventive measures that save lives and reduce costs. In genomics, AI accelerates the discovery of genetic markers, advancing personalized medicine tailored to individual patients. Additionally, AI enhances drug development by optimizing molecular screening processes and predicting therapeutic efficacy, bringing innovative treatments to the market more efficiently. Even in mental health, AI-powered tools provide accessible support to patients, offering resources such as virtual therapy and the early detection of mental health disorders.

As we conclude this book, the need to approach AI in healthcare with both optimism and caution is clear. While its advantages are undeniable, addressing the disadvantages and concerns requires collaborative efforts among various stakeholders: technologists, clinicians, ethicists, policymakers, and patients. Responsible integration of AI into healthcare systems must prioritize fairness, transparency, and compassion, ensuring that its benefits are accessible to all.

This epilogue is a call to embrace the transformative power of AI while remaining vigilant to its challenges. The journey toward AI-driven healthcare is one of innovation and hope, guided by the principles of equity and ethics. Together, we can harness AI's potential to create a future in which healthcare is smarter, more inclusive, and profoundly impactful, transforming lives in ways previously unimaginable. The possibilities are vast, and the responsibility to shape them lies with us.

Index

M. Chetty, J. Hallinan (eds.), *From Algorithms to Ailments*,
https://doi.org/10.1007/978-3-032-11023-7

The manufacturer's authorised representative in the EU is Springer Nature Customer Service Centre GmbH, Europaplatz 3, 69115 Heidelberg, Germany. If you have any concerns regarding our products, please contact ProductSafety@springernature.com

Printed and bound by CPI Group (UK) Ltd, Croydon, CR0 4YY
07/10/2026
02229357-0001